Understanding Cardiomyopathy

Understanding Cardiomyopathy

Editor: Sasha Luther

FOSTER ACADEMICS
www.fosteracademics.com

www.fosteracademics.com

FOSTER ACADEMICS

Cataloging-in-Publication Data

Understanding cardiomyopathy / edited by Sasha Luther.
p. cm.
Includes bibliographical references and index.
ISBN 978-1-63242-929-2
1. Heart--Hypertrophy. 2. Myocardium--Diseases. 3. Heart--Diseases. 4. Heart--Size.
5. Cardiology. I. Luther, Sasha.
RC685.H9 U53 2020
616.12--dc23

Foster Academics,
118-35 Queens Blvd., Suite 400,
Forest Hills, NY 11375, USA

ISBN 978-1-63242-929-2 (Hardback)

Contents

Preface

I am honored to present to you this unique book which encompasses the most up-to-date data in the field. I was extremely pleased to get this opportunity of editing the work of experts from across the globe. I have also written papers in this field and researched the various aspects revolving around the progress of the discipline. I have tried to unify my knowledge along with that of stalwarts from every corner of the world, to produce a text which not only benefits the readers but also facilitates the growth of the field.

A group of diseases which affect the muscle of the heart is called cardiomyopathy. This includes hypertrophic cardiomyopathy, restrictive cardiomyopathy, dilated cardiomyopathy, takotsubo cardiomyopathy and arrhythmogenic right ventricular dysplasia. All these conditions are characterized by unique mechanisms and causes. Hypertrophic cardiomyopathy is usually inherited and occurs due to the heart muscle enlarging and thickening. The ventricles enlarge and weaken in dilated cardiomyopathy, while the ventricle stiffens in restrictive cardiomyopathy. Dilated cardiomyopathy may occur due to alcohol consumption, cocaine use, exposure to heavy metals and viral infections. Restrictive cardiomyopathy may occur as a result of hemochromatosis, amyloidosis and cancer treatments. The symptoms of cardiomyopathies include fainting, dizziness, fatigue, shortness of breath, arrhythmia, swelling of the lower extremities, etc. Various diagnostic procedures can be used for diagnosing a cardiomyopathy, such as ECG, echocardiogram, stress test, physical examination, etc. Depending on the type of cardiomyopathy, treatment involves medication, ablation, and the use of defibrillators, ventricular assist devices and pacemakers. In some cases, a heart transplant may also be performed. This book presents researches and studies performed by experts across the globe on cardiomyopathy. It aims to shed light on some of the unexplored aspects of cardiomyopathy and the recent researches in this condition. It is a resource guide for experts as well as students.

Finally, I would like to thank all the contributing authors for their valuable time and contributions. This book would not have been possible without their efforts. I would also like to thank my friends and family for their constant support.

Editor

1

Cardiomyopathy Caused by Mutations in Nuclear A- Type Lamin Gene

Gisèle Bonne and Antoine Muchir

Abstract

Heart disease is a major cause of morbidity and premature mortality. Cardiomyopathy is an anatomic and pathologic condition associated with muscle and electrical dysfunction of the heart, often leading to heart failure–related disability. Dilated cardiomyopathy caused by mutations in A-type lamin gene (i.e., *LMNA* cardiomyopathy) is characterized by an increase in both myocardial mass and volume. The ventricular walls become thin and stretched, compromising cardiac contractility and ultimately resulting in poor left ventricular function. Despite current strategies to aggressively manage "*LMNA* cardiomyopathy," the disorder remains a common cause of heart failure with decreased ejection fraction, and a prevalent diagnosis in individuals is referred for cardiac transplantation. Despite progress in reducing "*LMNA* cardiomyopathy"–related mortality, hospitalizations remain very frequent and rates of readmission continue to rise. It appears important and necessary to further increase our knowledge on the pathophysiology of "*LMNA* cardiomyopathy" to unveil novel molecular/cellular mechanisms to target future therapeutic approaches.

Keywords: Dilated cardiomyopathy, Genetics, *LMNA*, A-type lamins, Nuclear lamina

1. Introduction

Cardiomyopathy, a major cause of morbidity and premature mortality in developed countries, is an anatomic and pathologic condition associated with muscle and electrical dysfunction of the heart, often leading to heart failure-related disability, which is a staggering clinical and public health problem. The mechanical component of the heart is liable for pumping blood throughout the body. The electric component, as for it, produces a rhythm for the blood to be pumped correctly. Hence, both components are tightly connected and regulated. Most common symptoms of dilated cardiomyopathy are shortness of breath, leg swelling, decreased exercise tolerance, fatigue, dizziness, coughing or wheezing, weight gain, and palpitation. Given the diversity in severity of symptoms in dilated cardiomyopathy, the disease is not always diagnosed. Cardiomyopathies are a clinically heterogeneous group of cardiac muscle disorders [1]. Cardiomyopathies have historically been broken down into several major phenotypic categories. Dilated cardiomyopathy, the most common form, is a condition where the heart muscle becomes enlarged and weakened, resulting in poor left ventricular function. Despite current strategies to aggressively manage dilated cardiomyopathy, the disorder remains a common cause of heart failure with a decrease below 45% of ejection fraction and a referring for cardiac transplantation. Notwithstanding progress in reducing heart failure-related mortality, hospitalizations for heart failure remain very frequent and rates of readmissions continue to rise. It appears important and necessary to increase our knowledge on the pathophysiology of cardiomyopathies to unveil novel molecular/cellular mechanisms for future therapeutic approaches.

2. Inherited cardiomyopathies

While the most common cardiomyopathies are secondary to acquired conditions, many are inherited. Genetic mutations have been identified in 25–35% of patients presenting dilated cardiomyopathy. These mutations affect genes that encode components of a wide variety of cellular compartments and pathways, including the nuclear envelope (e.g., *LMNA, EMD*), the contractile apparatus (e.g., *MYH7, ACTC1, TPM1, TTN*), the force transduction apparatus (e.g., *MLP, DES, TNNT2*), and calcium handling (e.g., *SERCA*). The cardiac cell is composed of a complex network of proteins linking the sarcomere to the sarcolemma and the extracellular matrix, providing structural support for subcellular structures and transmitting mechanical signals within and between cells (**Figure 1**). Mutations in genes encoding proteins of the sarcolemma are disrupting the anchoring and hence abrogate the transmission of the force

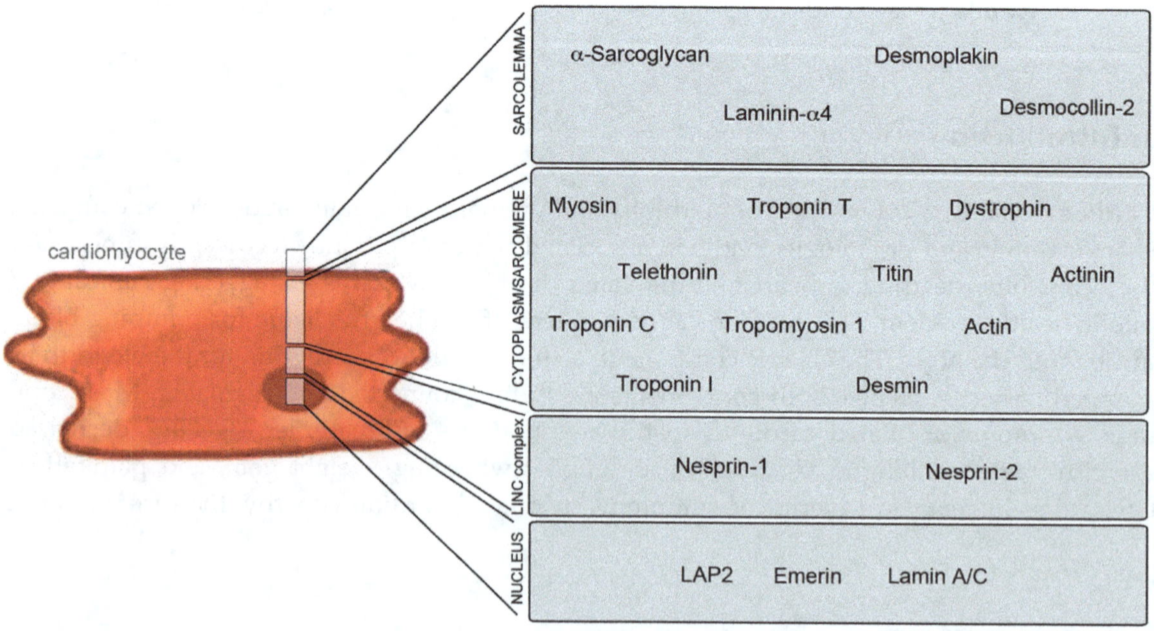

Figure 1. Cellular localizations of proteins involved in dilated cardiomyopathies.

generated by muscle contraction. Muscle contraction is due to the interaction between an actin filament and myosin heavy chain. Mutations in genes encoding contractile elements were identified as the cause of dilated cardiomyopathy. Functional units of striated muscle are called sarcomeres. Because the generated power of muscle contraction is transmitted to adjacent sarcomeres through the Z-disk, mutations in genes encoding proteins of the Z-disk causes also dilated cardiomyopathy. Part of hereditary dilated cardiomyopathies is caused by mutations in the genes encoding proteins of the nuclear envelope. Hence, disruption of the links from the sarcolemma to the sarcomere and nucleus could have a "domino effect," which leads to the disruption of systolic function and to the development of dilated cardiomyopathy.

3. *LMNA* cardiomyopathy

Among the causing genes of dilated cardiomyopathy, it has been estimated that mutations in *LMNA*, encoding nuclear lamin A/C [2], accounts for about 5–10% of familial dilated cardiomyopathy, thus representing one of the major causative genes. Affected patients often exhibit early conduction defects before left ventricle dysfunction and dilatation occur [3]. "*LMNA* cardiomyopathy" usually presents in early to mid-adulthood with symptomatic conduction system disease or arrhythmias or with symptomatic dilated cardiomyopathy (**Figure 2A**). "*LMNA* cardiomyopathy" has an intrusive clinical progression with higher rates of aggressive arrhythmias and faster course toward heart failure than most other cardiac diseases. Given the increased awareness among physicians, cardiologists are now facing difficult queries regarding patient management. These queries concern the use of defibrillators in order to avoid sudden death from aggressive ventricular arrhythmias and pharmacological interventions to improve heart failure symptoms. Once dilated cardiomyopathy is detected clinically, the management for "*LMNA* cardiomyopathy" follows the standard of care for heart failure. It is unclear whether early institution of these therapeutic agents prior to detectable cardiac dysfunction can modify the aggressive nature of "*LMNA* cardiomyopathy." There is no definitive treatment for the progressive cardiac dilatation and loss of contractility in "*LMNA* cardiomyopathy" short of heart transplantation [4].

4. A-type nuclear lamins

The *LMNA* gene, on chromosome 1q21.2-21.3, encodes nuclear A-type lamins. Lamin A and lamin C, the major somatic A-type lamins, arise via alternative splicing of pre-mRNA [5] (**Figure 3A**). Lamin A is primarily synthesized as a precursor, the prelamin A. Prelamin A has a particular C-terminal amino acid tail, which undergoes several enzymatic reactions to produce mature lamin A. Two other genes, *LMNB1* and *LMNB2*, encode lamins B1 and B2, respectively. Lamins are class V intermediate filament proteins that polymerize to form the nuclear lamina (**Figure 3B**), a fibrous network underlining the inner nuclear membrane of most eukaryotic cells (**Figure 3C**) [6–8]. The nuclear lamina is bounded to the inner nuclear membrane via interactions with integral proteins and to the chromatin. It has also been shown that lamin A/C can also interact with the cytoskeleton, through the linker of nucleoskeleton and cytoskeleton ("LINC") complex [9]. One function of the lamina is to provide structural

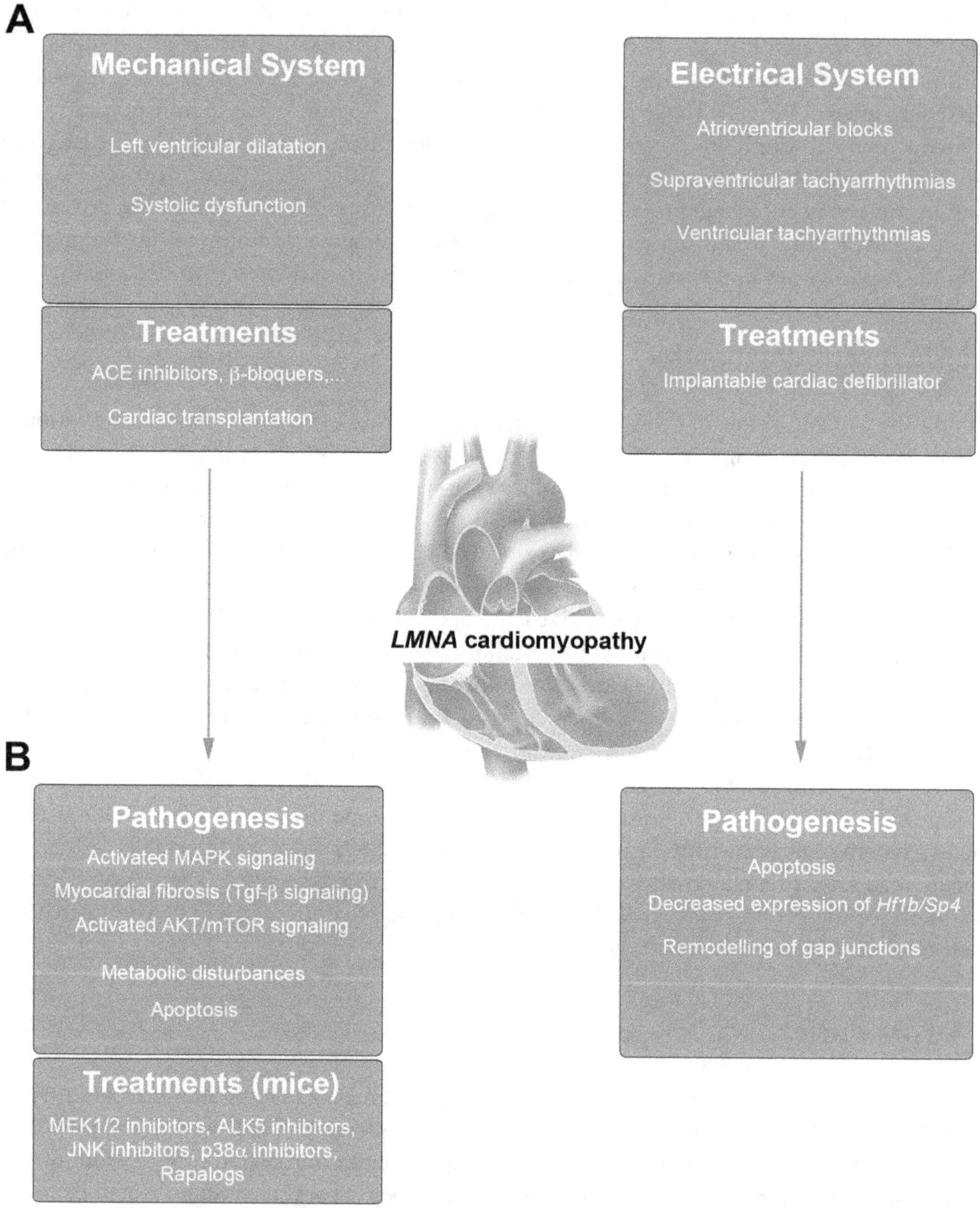

Figure 2. Cardiac symptoms of "*LMNA* cardiomyopathy (A) and pathological mechanisms (B).

support to the nucleus. Nuclear lamins have also been implicated in processes such as chromatin organization, gene regulation, DNA replication, and RNA splicing [10]. However, the specific mechanistic roles of lamins in these processes, particularly in a cell- or tissue-type–specific context, remain obscure.

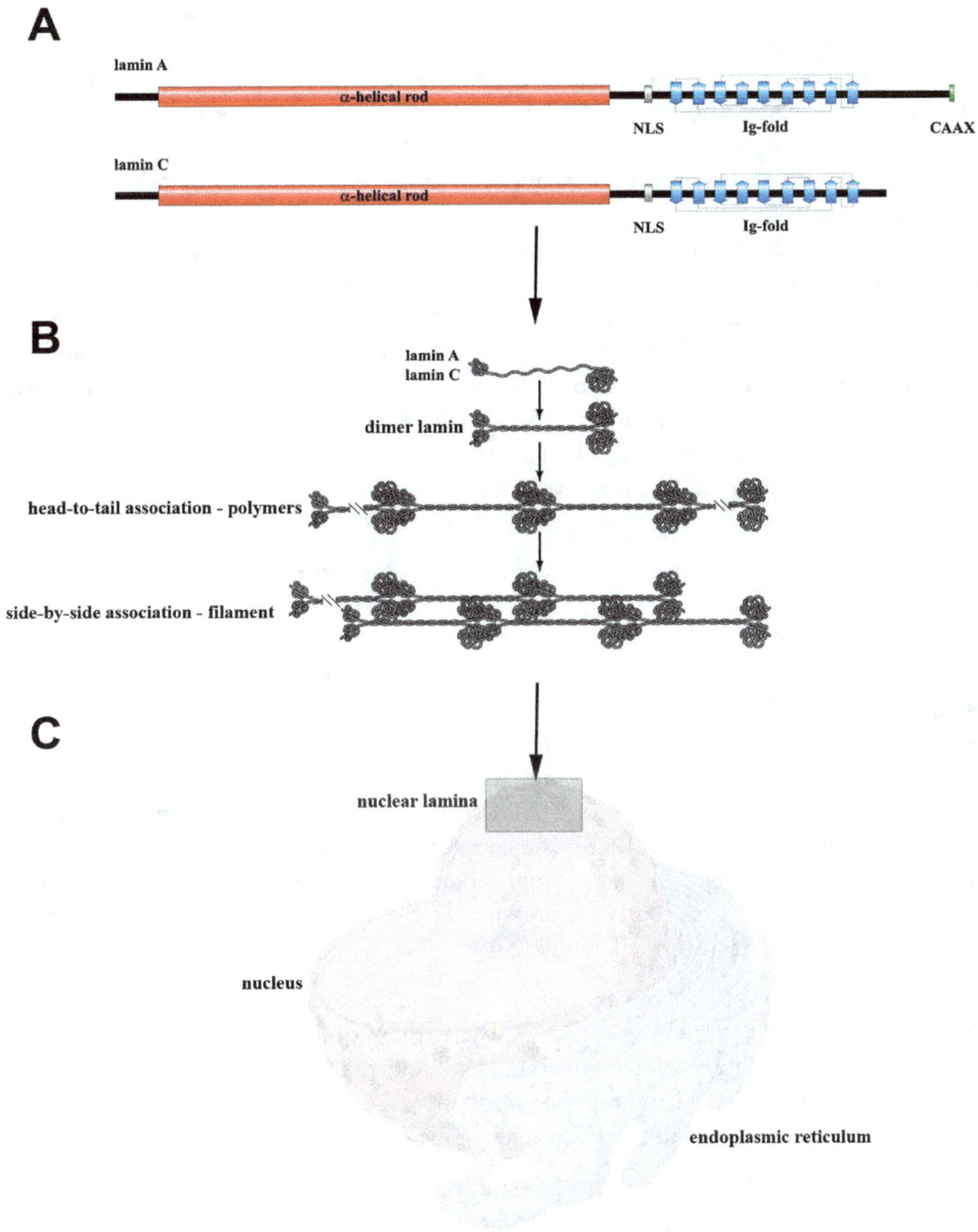

Figure 3. Nuclear lamins: structure (A), organization (B), and cellular localization (C). Modified from [10].

5. Pathogenesis

Identification of disease-causing mutations in the heart has contributed to the delineation of "*LMNA* cardiomyopathy." However, much work remains in elucidating the specific cellular mechanisms of the disease. Several hypotheses have been proposed attempting to link the pathophysiology of "*LMNA* cardiomyopathy" to known or emerging functions of lamin A/C. Among these functions include those based on that lamin A/C likely have in maintaining the mechanical integrity of cells subject to external and internal cues and signal transduction (i.e., the mechanical stress hypothesis). The "mechanical stress hypothesis" is attractive when trying to explain striated muscle diseases. It is based on the premise that the striated muscles are constantly subjected to mechanical forces and that mutations in "nucleocytoskeletal" support elements make them susceptible to damage from recurrent stress. Mouse models have been extremely helpful in deciphering crucial mechanisms, which could partially explain the pathogenesis of the disease. The development of *Lmna*$^{-/-}$ mice by Sullivan and colleagues was the first animal model of the disease [11]. Since, other models (knock-in and transgenic) have been created to study the cardiac dysfunction caused by *LMNA* mutation [12–15]. We and others reported an aberrant cardiac activation of signaling pathways in "*LMNA* cardiomyopathy" [16, 17] in mice and human, which participate to the development of contractile dysfunction (mitogen-activated protein kinase (MAPK) signaling, AKT/mTOR signaling, TGF-β signaling, etc.) [16, 18, 19] and electrical disturbances (connexin 43 remodeling, apoptosis, Hf1b expression) (**Figure 2B**).

MAPK signaling—One of the most prevalent and best-characterized responses to mechanical stress is the phosphorylation of proteins, which could be mediated by mitogen-activated protein kinase (MAPK) signaling pathway. Genes encoding proteins in MAPK signaling pathway demonstrated significantly altered expression in hearts of *Lmna* H222P mice by transcriptomic analysis [16]. We demonstrated an aberrant activation of ERK1/2, JNK, and p38α signaling, three main branches of MAPK signaling pathway involved in cellular mechanotransduction, in hearts from *Lmna* H222P mice, as early as 4 weeks of age [16, 17]. Our work proved that the activation of MAPK signaling pathway preceded the cardiac dysfunction of *Lmna* H222P mice and that it is a consequence of alterations in lamin A/C and not secondary to nonspecific effects. Accordingly, lamin A/C-deficient fibroblasts subjected to cyclic strain respond with decreased expression of the mechanosensitive genes, which are downstream targets of the MAPK pathway [20].

AKT/mTOR signaling—We showed that the *Lmna* pH222P mutation results in aberrant activation of the AKT/mTOR signaling cascade, downstream of the MAPK pathway [18]. Given that activated mTOR inhibits autophagic responses and reduces tolerance to energy deficits, the heart is therefore unable to compensate for increased energy demand and, over time, develops muscle damage and dilated cardiomyopathy.

TGF-β signaling—Cardiac fibrosis exacerbates the clinical progression of heart failure. We showed that *Lmna* H222P mice had elevated expression of TGF-β signaling as early as 12 weeks of age, which is a time that preceded development of both cardiac fibrosis and the onset of overt cardiac dysfunction [13, 19]. Our observations indicate that TGF-β is a mediator of the cardiomyopathy that develops as a result of *LMNA* mutations.

Connexin 43 remodeling—Gap junction communications describe the electrical coupling of cells through specialized cell contacts called gap junctions. In adult heart, connexin 43 is expressed in the atrial and ventricular working (contractile) myocardium. The working cardiomyocytes of the ventricle are extensively interconnected by clusters of connexin 43 located at the intercalated disks. The intercalated disks of working ventricular myocardium have a step-like configuration, with the gap junctions situated predominantly in the "horizontal" facing segments of these steps rather than the vertical segments [21, 22]. Features of gap junction organization encourage preferential propagation of the impulse in the longitudinal axis, thus contributing to the normal pattern of anisotropic spread of the impulse of healthy ventricular myocardium. The most striking form of structural remodeling connexin 43 is typically scattered in disordered fashion over the lateral surfaces in the heart from *Lmna* N195K mice (i.e., lateralization) [12].

Apoptosis—Apoptosis in all metazoan cells is mediated by caspases, a multigene family of cysteine proteases that hydrolyzes peptide bonds carboxyl to aspartic acid residues. Once activated, caspases cut cellular proteins, leading to the apoptotic demise of the cell. During the past few years, there has been accumulating evidence in both human and animal models suggesting that apoptosis may be an important mode of cell death during heart failure [23]. Myocyte apoptosis has been reported in the atrioventricular tissue from $Lmna^{+/-}$ mice [24], which could account for the evolution of electrophysiologic dysfunction.

Hf1b/Sp4—This transcription factor has been described as important for the development of the cardiac conduction system [25]. Mounkes and colleagues found that expression and localization of Hf1b/Sp4 were altered in the heart from *Lmna* N195K mice [12]. Strikingly, this study reported that Hf1b/Sp4 was not found in the ventricles and was strongly expressed in the atria in the heart from *Lmna* N195K mice, which mirror the localization in control animals. This finding needs further analysis.

The exact mechanisms by which defects in nuclear lamins cause dysregulated signaling remain to be elucidated.

6. Treatments

Advances in molecular techniques have improved the understanding of mechanisms responsible for cardiac dysfunction in "*LMNA* cardiomyopathy." It is clear that mutations in nuclear lamin A/C in cardiomyocytes can perturb cardiac function. Alterations in cardiomyocyte function initiate cascades of cellular responses that attempt to compensate for these insults. However, persistent responses at the cellular level lead to organ-wide alterations, which correlated with sudden cardiac death and heart failure. Although there exists no treatment to directly address the causes of "*LMNA* cardiomyopathy," basic studies of the processes that mediate cellular responses to cardiac stress have allowed the development of innovative treatments that address the reduction of symptoms that include drugs that decrease blood pressure (ACE inhibitors, angiotensin II receptor blockers, beta-blockers) and heart rate (beta-blockers, calcium channel blockers, digoxin) to reduce the strain on the ventricular walls. Utilization of animal and cellular models to further dissect the mechanisms of "*LMNA* cardiomyopathy" and demonstrate efficacy of drugs that specifically target disease-causing pathways holds promise that further reduction in the mortality associated with "*LMNA* cardiomyopathy" can be achieved [17–19, 26, 27].

7. Conclusion

In the past decade, there has been an extraordinary burst of researches on lamin A/C and the nuclear lamina, which has been accelerated by attempts to explain the pathogenesis of "*LMNA* cardiomyopathy." One important unanswered question is how mutations in genes expressed in most differentiated somatic cells lead to human disease affecting the cardiac tissue. Within the next several years, we will likely have more clues to answer this question, and these answers will hopefully lead to new ways to treat or prevent "*LMNA* cardiomyopathy."

Author details

Gisèle Bonne and Antoine Muchir*

*Address all correspondence to: a.muchir@institut-myologie.org

Center of Research in Myology, Paris, France

References

[1] Maron BJ, Towbin JA, Thiene G, Antzelevitch C, Corrado D, Arnett D, Moss AJ, Seidman CE, Young JB: Contemporary definitions and classification of the cardiomyopathies: an American Heart Association Scientific Statement from the Council on Clinical Cardiology, Heart Failure and Transplantation Committee; Quality of Care and Outcomes Research and Functional Genomics and Translational Biology Interdisciplinary Working Groups; and Council on Epidemiology and Prevention. Circulation. 2006;**113**:1807–1816. DOI: 10.1161/CIRCULATIONAHA.106.174287

[2] Fatkin D, MacRae C, Sasaki T, Wolff MR, Porcu M, Frenneaux M, Atherton J, Vidaillet HJ Jr, Spudich S, De Girolami U, Seidman JG, Seidman C, Muntoni F, Müehle G, Johnson W, McDonough B: Missense mutation in the rod domain of he lamin A/C gene as cause of dilated cardiomyopathy and conduction-system disease. N Engl J Med. 1999;**341**:1715–1724. DOI: 10.1056/NEJM199912023412302

[3] Meune C, Van Berlo JH, Anselme F, Bonne G, Pinto YM, Duboc D: Primary prevention of sudden death in patients with lamin A/C gene mutations. N Engl J Med. 2006;**354**:209–210. DOI: 10.1056/NEJMc052632

[4] Ben Yaou R, Gueneau L, Demay L, Stora S, Chikaoui K, Richard P, Bonne G: Heart involvement in lamin A/C related diseases. Arch Mal Coeur Vaiss. 2006;**99**:848–855.

[5] Lin F, Worman HJ: Structural organization of the human gene encoding nuclear lamin A and nuclear lamin C. J Biol Chem. 1993;**268**:16321–16326.

[6] Fisher DZ, Chaudhary N, Blobel G: cDNA sequencing of nuclear lamins A and C reveals primary and secondary structural homology to intermediate filament proteins. Proc Natl Acad Sci U S A 1986;**83**:6450–6454.

[7] McKeon FD, Kirschner MW, Caput D: Homologies in both primary and secondary structure between nuclear envelope and intermediate filament proteins. Nature 1986;**319**:463–468. DOI: 10.1038/319463a0

[8] Aebi U, Cohn J, Buhle L, Gerace L: The nuclear lamina is a meshwork of intermediate-type filaments. Nature 1986;**323**:560–564. DOI: 10.1038/323560a0

[9] Stewart CL, Roux KJ, Burke B: Blurring the boundary: the nuclear envelope extends its reach. Science 2007;**318**:1408–1412. DOI: 10.1126/science.1142034

[10] Dechat T, Pfleghaar K, Sengupta K, Shimi T, Shumaker DK, Solimando L, Goldman RD: Nuclear lamins: major factors in the structural organization and function of the nucleus and chromatin. Genes Dev. 2008;**22**:832–853. DOI: 10.1101/gad.1652708

[11] Sullivan T, Escalante-Alcade D, Bhatt H, Anver M, Bhat N, Nagashima K, Stewart CL, Burke B: Loss of A-type lamin expression compromises nuclear envelope integrity leading to muscular dystrophy. J Cell Biol. 1999;**147**:913–920.

[12] Mounkes LC, Kozlov SV, Rottman JN, Stewart CL: Expression of an LMNA-N195K variant of A-type lamins results in cardiac conduction defects and death in mice. Hum Mol Genet. 2005;**14**:2167–2180. DOI: 10.1093/hmg/ddi221

[13] Arimura T, Helbling-Leclerc A, Massart C, Varnous S, Niel F, Lacène E, Fromes Y, Toussaint M, Mura AM, Keller DI, Amthor H, Isnard R, Malissen M, Schwartz K, Bonne G: Mouse model carrying H222P-Lmna mutation develops muscular dystrophy and dilated cardiomyopathy similar to human striated muscle laminopathies. Hum Mol Genet. 2005;**14**:155–169. DOI: 10.1093/hmg/ddi017

[14] Wang Y, Herron AJ, Worman HJ: Pathology and nuclear abnormalities in hearts of transgenic mice expressing M371K lamin A encoded by an LMNA mutation causing Emery-Dreifuss muscular dystrophy. Hum Mol Genet. 2006;**15**:2479–2489. DOI: 10.1093/hmg/ddl170

[15] Cattin ME, Bertrand AT, Schlossarek S, Le Bihan MC, Jensen SS, Neuber C, Crocini C, Maron S, Lainé J, Mougenot N, Varnous S, Fromes Y, Hansen A, Eschenhagen T, Decostre V, Carrier L, Bonne G: Heterozygous Lmna delK32 mice develop dilated cardiomyopathy through a combined pathomechanism of haploinsufficiency and peptide toxicity. Hum Mol Genet. 2013;**22**:3152–3164. DOI: 10.1093/hmg/ddt172

[16] Muchir A, Pavlidis P, Decostre V, Herron AJ, Arimura T, Bonne G, Worman HJ: Activation of MAPK pathways links *LMNA* mutations to cardiomyopathy in Emery-Dreifuss muscular dystrophy. J Clin Invest. 2007;**117**:1282–1293. DOI: 10.1172/JCI29042

[17] Muchir A, Reilly SA, Wu W, Iwata S, Homma S, Bonne G, Worman HJ: Treatment with selumetinib preserves cardiac function and improves survival in cardiomyopathy caused

by mutation in the lamin A/C gene. Cardiovasc Res. 2012;**93**:311–319. DOI: 10.1093/cvr/cvr301

[18] Choi JC, Muchir A, Wu W, Iwata S, Homma S, Morrow JP, Worman HJ: Temsirolimus activates autophagy and ameliorates cardiomyopathy caused by lamin A/C gene mutation. Sci Transl Med. 2012;**4**:144ra102. DOI: 10.1126/scitranslmed.3003875

[19] Chatzifrangkeskou M, Le Dour C, Wu W, Morrow JP, Joseph LC, Beuvin M, Sera F, Homma S, Vignier N, Mougenot N, Bonne G, Lipson KE, Worman HJ, Muchir A: ERK1/2 directly acts on CTGF/CCN2 expression to mediate myocardial fibrosis in cardiomyopathy caused by mutation in the lamin A/C gene. Hum Mol Genet. 2016;ddw090. DOI: 10.1093/hmg/ddw090

[20] Lammerding J, Schulze PC, Takahashi T, Kozlov S, Sullivan T, Kamm RD, Stewart CL, Lee RT: Lamin A/C deficiency causes defective nuclear mechanics and mechanotransduction. J Clin Invest. 2004;**113**:370–378. DOI: 10.1172/JCI19670

[21] Severs NJ: Gap junction shape and orientation at the cardiac intercalated disk. Circ Res. 1989;**65**:1458–1461.

[22] Severs NJ: The cardiac gap junction and intercalated disc. Int J Cardiol. 1990;**26**:137–173.

[23] Kang PM, Izumo S: Apoptosis and heart failure: a critical review of the literature. Circ Res. 2000;**86**:1107–1113.

[24] Wolf CM, Wang L, Alcalai R, Pizard A, Burgon PG, Ahmad F, Sherwood M, Branco DM, Wakimoto H, Fishman GI, See V, Stewart CL, Conner DA, Berul CI, Seidman CE, Seidman JG: Lamin A/C haploinsufficiency causes dilated cardiomyopathy and apoptosis-triggered cardiac conduction system disease. J Mol Cell Cardiol. 2008;**44**:293–303. DOI: 10.1016/j.yjmcc.2007.11.008

[25] Nguyen-Tran VT, Kubalak SW, Minamisawa S, Fiset C, Wollert KC, Brown AB, Ruiz-Lozano P, Barrere-Lemaire S, Kondo R, Norman LW, Gourdie RG, Rahme MM, Feld GK, Clark RB, Giles WR, Chien KR: A novel genetic pathway for sudden cardiac death via defects in the transition between ventricular and conduction system cell lineages. Cell 2000;**102**:671–682.

[26] Muchir A, Shan J, Bonne G, Lehnart SE, Worman HJ: Inhibition of extracellular signal-regulated kinase signaling to prevent cardiomyopathy caused by mutation in the gene encoding A-type lamins. Hum Mol Genet. 2009;**18**:241–247. DOI: 10.1093/hmg/ddn343

[27] Wu W, Muchir A, Shan J, Bonne G, Worman HJ: Mitogen activated protein kinase inhibitors improve heart function and prevent fibrosis in cardiomyopathy caused by lamin A/C gene mutation. Circulation 2011;**123**:53–61. DOI: 10.1161/CIRCULATIONAHA.110.970673

2

Electrical Devices (Resynchronization and Defibrillators) in the Treatment of Cardiomyopathies: Indications, Present and Future of these Therapies

Miguel Ángel García García,
María de los Ángeles Rosero Arenas,
Alfonso Martínez Cornejo,
Marta Bertolo Domínguez and
Vicente Miranda Gozalvo

Abstract

Cardiomyopathies are heart diseases involving high risk of heart failure and sudden cardiac death. In this chapter, we review the use of electrical devices (cardiac resynchronization therapy and implantable cardioverter defibrillator) to reduce the progression of heart failure and prevent arrhythmogenic sudden death in patients affected with these pathologies. The future of these therapies is a more appropriate indication for primary prevention of sudden death (defibrillator) and treatment of heart failure in a broader spectrum of patients (resynchronization).

Keywords: cardiac resynchronization therapy, implantable cardioverter defibrillator, cardiomyopathy, heart failure, sudden death

1. Introduction

Cardiomyopathies (CMP) are a group of diseases that affect the cardiac muscle associated with myocardial dysfunction and can be caused by known disorders such as hypertension, ischemic heart disease, valvular disease, and so on. Other causes, such as genetic illnesses, inflammatory processes, metabolic, or toxic diseases, may also be responsible for this pathology. Its origin could also be primary, i.e., not known cause. One simple and initial classification of the CMP divides them into ischemic and nonischemic ones. In 1995, the World Health Organization (WHO)/International Society and Federation of Cardiology (ISFC) Task Force on the Definition and Classification of the Cardiomyopathies classified them into dilated, hypertrophic, restrictive, arrhythmogenic right ventricular dysplasia, and other [1]. Since these diseases can have mechanical and/or electrical dysfunction, in this chapter, we review the usefulness of electrical therapies (cardiac resynchronization therapy or/and implantable cardioverter defibrillator) to treat heart failure and arrhythmogenic sudden cardiac death associated with these diseases.

The etiology of heart failure may be predictive of long-term outcome: survival of peripartum CMP was better; medium in hypertension, myocarditis, sarcoidosis, and substance abuse; and worse in infiltrative myocardial disease –amyloidosis and hemochromatosis-, HIV disease, chemotherapy with doxorubicin, ischemic heart disease, or connective tissue disease. And in all of them, the added presence of diabetes involves an increased risk of mortality.

Heart failure is a complex clinical syndrome that causes inadequate systemic perfusion to meet the body's metabolic demands with usually increased left ventricular filling pressures. The two leading causes of death in patients with heart failure are arrhythmic or sudden cardiac death and progressive pump failure [2]. Life-threatening ventricular arrhythmias are common in patients with heart failure and CMP, and unexpected sudden cardiac death and sudden cardiac death during episodes of clinical worsening of heart failure each account for approximately one-third of deaths. Management of patients with heart failure includes several strategies: controlling contributing factors, lifestyle modification, pharmacological therapy, rehabilitation, preventive care, and electrical devices if indicated. The mode of death in patients with heart failure is more likely to be "sudden" in patients with New York Heart Association (NYHA) II-III classes and related to pump failure in patients with NYHA IV class [3].

Ventricular arrhythmias are common in heart failure and CMP. The prognosis of these arrhythmias depends on the cause of the CMP [4]. There is no preventive drug therapy to treat ventricular arrhythmias (i.e., amiodarone). However, those patients with nonsustained ventricular tachycardia may be candidates (with preliminary electrophysiological study) to an implantable cardioverter defibrillator. Patients with spontaneous sustained ventricular tachycardia are at high risk for sudden cardiac death; patients with heart failure or CMP who are survivors of sudden cardiac death due to ventricular tachycardia or ventricular fibrillation must be treated with implantable cardioverter defibrillator for secondary prevention [4, 5] (**Figure 1**).

A pacemaker placed in right ventricle can exacerbate heart failure by several mechanisms: firstly, contraction of the right ventricle before the left ventricle (interventricular dyssynchrony), and secondly the "left bundle branch block effect" causing that septum contracts before the lateral wall (intraventricular dyssynchrony); the final outcome of both phenomena results in a reduced efficiency of cardiac pump. It is likely that a pacemaker placed in right atrium and right ventricle provides benefit in heart failure, but DAVID trial, which included patients with left ventricular ejection fraction ≤40% and without indication for bradycardia showed that pacing with DDD function (dual, atrial and ventricular, pacing and sensing, and also dual, triggered and inihibited, response to sensing, according to accepted international code accepted in 2002) [6] can worsen heart failure. The same concept could be generalized to patients with CMP [7].

Therapy known as cardiac resynchronization can optimize cardiac function, symptoms, and survival in patients with heart failure with left ventricular dysfunction (with left ventricular

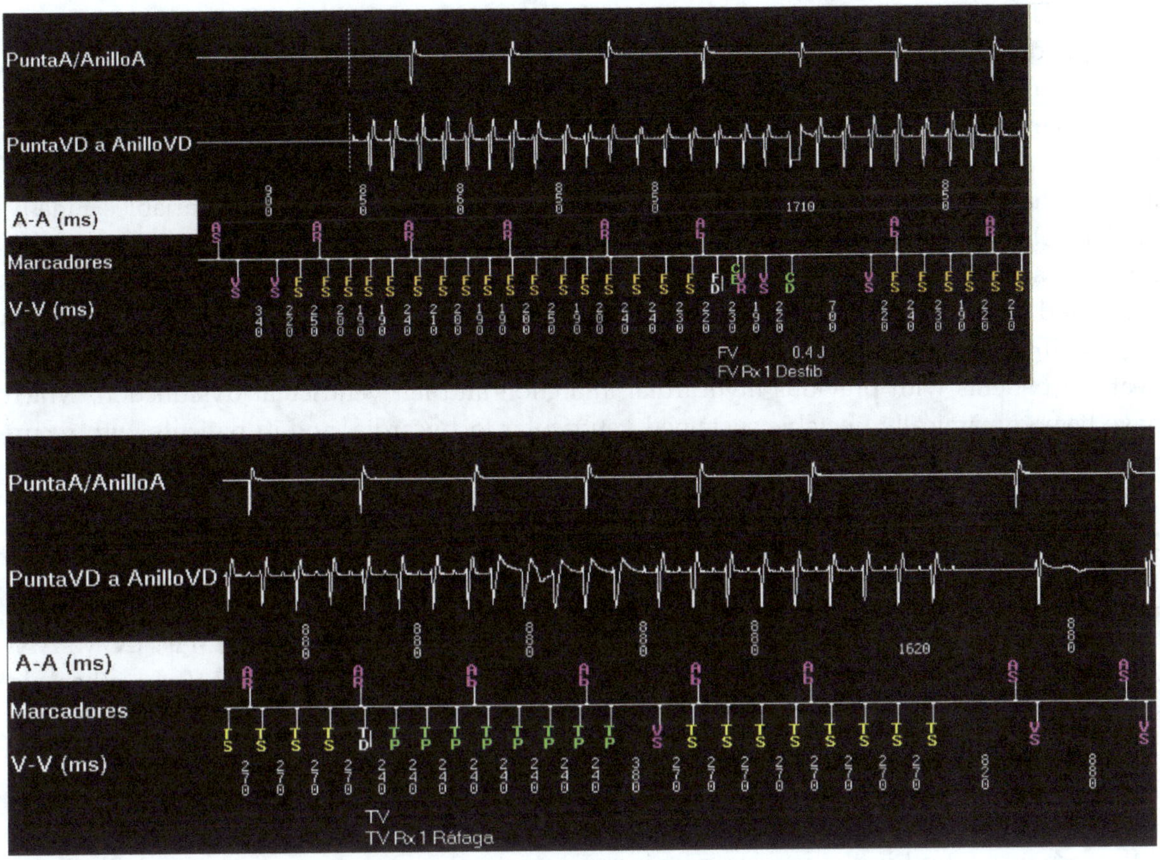

Figure 1. Endocavitary registry of two ventricular arrhythmias: ventricular tachycardia, treated with anti-tachycardia pacing (ATP), and ventricular fibrillation, treated with defibrillation (0.4 J).

ejection fraction ≤35% and wide QRS with left bundle branch block), added to optimal medical treatment. On the other hand, implantable cardioverter defibrillator can abort sudden arrhythmic deaths, thus prolonging survival in patients with cardiac disease and that patients may progress in later stages to more advanced heart failure.

2. Ischemic CMP

Risk stratification of a patient who has an acute myocardial infarction and ischemic CMP should include: identification of risk for recurrent ischemic events and identification of high risk of death (arrhythmic or non-arrhythmic of origin). Postinfarction mortality has decreased by optimizing the initial therapy (reperfusion) and secondary prevention measures [4].

2.1. Role of implantable cardioverter defibrillator

Several works (VALIANT [8]) described an increased risk of sudden cardiac death in patients with postinfarction left ventricular failure; the rate of sudden cardiac death or resuscitated cardiac arrest was 1.4 % in the first month, with a rate of 2.3% if left ventricular ejection fraction <30%), but the frequency of use of reperfusion therapy and beta-blockers was low. Two studies

(DINAMIT [9] and IRIS [10]) showed no improvement in survival after implantable cardioverter defibrillator placement between 31 and 40 days post infarction. Several risk factors are associated with threatening arrhythmia: low ejection fraction of left ventricle or history of heart failure, ventricular tachycardia induced in the electrophysiologic study, spontaneous ventricular premature beats and nonsustained ventricular tachycardia seen in the 24-hour Holter, and other. On the other hand, reperfusion therapy has decreased the predictive value of these variables. Finally, implantable cardioverter defibrillator should be recommended in patients with a left ventricular ejection fraction ≤30% (MADIT II criteria) or with ischemic CMP, left ventricular ejection fraction ≤35%, and NYHA II or III heart failure (SCD-HEFT criteria) [11] (**Figure 2**). In recent guidelines [12, 13], implantable cardioverter defibrillator is an effective therapy to reduce sudden cardiac death in patients with previous myocardial infarction and left ventricular dysfunction, which have hemodynamically unstable sustained ventricular tachycardia, and in patients with recurrent ventricular tachycardia and normal/near normal left ventricular function.

2.2. Role of cardiac resynchronization therapy

The usefulness of resynchronization is demonstrated in patients with ischemic CMP. In several pivotal studies, which demonstrated the utility of resynchronization (CARE-HF, COMPANION, etc), there was a significant percentage of patients with ischemic CMP. In other old studies [14], patients with ischemic CMP may respond less favorably to resynchronization compared with patients with idiopathic dilated CMP. In recent years, studies comparing the effectiveness of this therapy in ischemic vs dilated CMP have been developed [15]; estimated survival at 4 years were 55% for ischemic and 77% for dilated CMP, and no significant difference was found in the incidence of inappropriate implantable cardioverter defibrillator shocks between both groups. Patients with implantable cardioverter defibrillator functionality remained at higher risk for death after controlling for pre-implant variables (hazard ratio (HR), 1.6). So, patients with dilated CMP experienced greater improvement in left ventricular systolic function and reverse remodeling than those with ischemic CMP, which means sustaining a greater survival benefit.

Another study [16] showed that after atrioventricular node ablation along with biventricular pacemaker placement, in patients with heart failure and refractory atrial fibrillation, echocardiographic reverse remodeling was lower in patients with ischemic compared with dilated CMP [16], with a greater number of hospitalizations due to heart failure in this first group and less improvement of left ventricular ejection fraction.

Finally, a combination of resynchronization + surgery in dilated ischemic CMP could be useful: optimization of ventricular function by myocardial revascularization with synchronized contraction of papillary muscle by biventricular pacing could improve the abnormal conformation/shape of the left ventricle, responsible for the functional mitral regurgitation. Therefore, preoperative assessment of myocardial viability and synchronism of the papillary muscles is the key to the success of this intervention.

Recent clinical guidelines [17] show greater benefit of CRT in several subgroups: women, QRS ≥150 ms, and nonischemic CMP. Despite the lower efficacy against nonischemic patients, the implant in these patients is recommended.

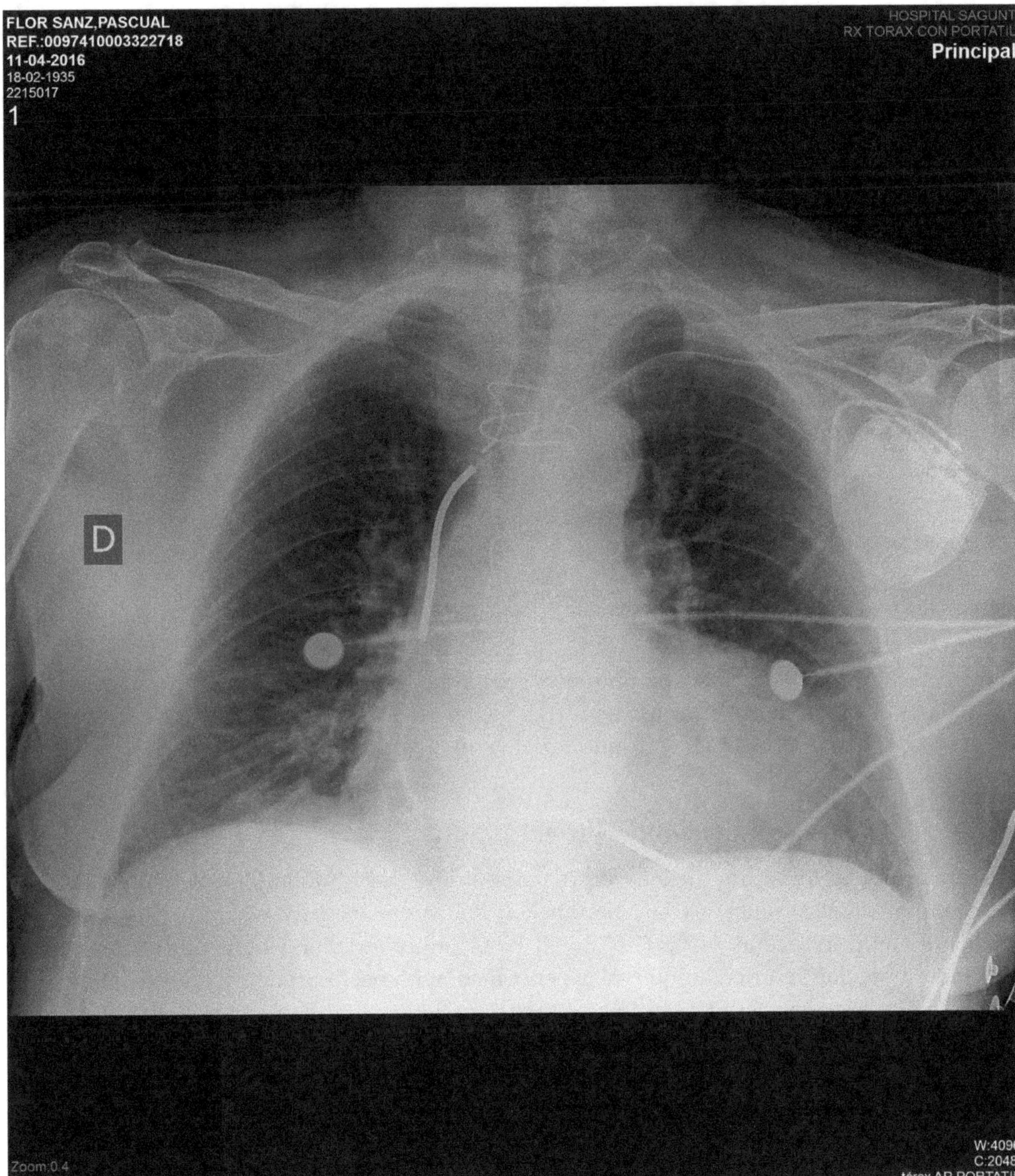

Figure 2. Monocameral implantable cardioverter defibrillator in a patient with ischemic dilated cardiomyopathy.

3. Myocarditis

It is an inflammatory disease of the myocardium, characterized from a histopathologic point of view by inflammatory infiltrates within the myocardium associated with degeneration and necrosis, with a nonischemic origin. The most common etiology is infectious, followed by immune (drugs, autoimmune diseases, etc) and toxic (drugs, metals, radiation, etc). Acute myocarditis can lead to chronic myocarditis or dilated CMP up to 10% of cases [18, 19]. In patients with sudden cardiac death, sustained ventricular tachycardia, ventricular fibrillation, and/or dilated CMP with ventricular dysfunction, the decision to implant and implantable cardioverter defibrillator should be based on the same indications as in other CMP, according to clinical practice guidelines [13]. It seems reasonable to delay the placement of an implantable cardioverter defibrillator until the resolution of the acute episode, meanwhile can be raised using a vest defibrillator as a bridge in high-risk patients [20]. Once dilated CMP has been developed, implantation of a cardiac resynchronization therapy device is recommended in patients with severe depression of left ventricular systolic function (<35%) and left bundle block in functional class II–IV [21].

In clinical guidelines [12, 13], implantable cardioverter defibrillator is indicated if inflammatory infiltrates persist in biopsies and if there is abnormal fibrosis in magnetic resonance; these elements are risk factors for sudden cardiac death.

4. Hypertrophic CMP

Patients with hypertrophic CMP can develop left ventricle outflow tract gradient/obstruction, diastolic dysfunction, myocardial ischemia, mitral regurgitation, and systolic dysfunction (in advanced stages) [22]. Therapeutic options to decrease the pressure gradient are as follows: drugs (beta-blockers or calcium antagonists), septal resection surgery, septal percutaneous reduction with ablation with alcohol, and atrial ventricular permanent pacing.

4.1. Role of cardiac resynchronization therapy

The aim consists of reducing the left ventricular outflow tract gradient, probably related with heart failure, classically using DDD pacemaker, and more recently with cardiac resynchronization therapy. In several works (1970s and 1980s), right atrial and right ventricular pacing, with short auricular-ventricular interval is performed, with positive effects: pre-excitation from right ventricular apex—with paradoxical septal movement and ejection speed reduction, delayed septal contraction—with systolic anterior motion of mitral valve improvement, and reduction of mitral regurgitation and subaortic gradient; a critical issue is to maintain constant ventricular and auricular capture. However, the success of the therapy lies in optimized individual programming of stimulation parameters to maintain atrial ventricular synchrony. The maintained benefit in functional status of sequential atrial ventricular pacing has been demonstrated in long series of cases (median follow-up of 8.5 years) [23]. Lenarczyk et al. [24] shows in his preliminary study a decrease in outflow tract gradient and improvement of the functional status. In several series, we can see a symptomatic benefit and an improvement of exercise capacity, although evolution is erratic. In recent guidelines for the treatment of hypertrophic CMP [25], cardiac resynchronization therapy is recommended in the following situations: sequential conventional pacing for reducing gradient or facilitating medical treatment if gradient ≥50 mmHg, sinus rhythm and refractory symptoms to medical treatment with contraindication to myectomy or septal ablation, with high risk to develop atrial ventricular block after it; resynchronization is also indicated in patients who meet indications of bicameral implantable cardioverter defibrillator to make sequential pacing.

We are waiting for the results of the study TRICHAMPION (clinicaltrials.gov NCT01614717): triple chamber pacing in hypertrophic obstructive cardiomyopathy patients. This is a prospective, randomized, single blind trial including N = 80 patients with atrial pacing only in back-up versus atrial biventricular pacing for 1 year. Expected preliminary results will be in 2016.

Recent clinical guidelines [17] show, in the absence of current clinical trials, the option of considering cardiac resynchronization therapy in individual patients with left ventricular failure data and asynchrony. And for patients with left ventricular outflow tract obstruction and treated with dual chamber pacemaker or implantable cardioverter defibrillator, you must schedule a short atrial ventricular interval for maximum apical right ventricle pre-excitation without altering left ventricle diastolic filling.

4.2. Role of implantable cardioverter defibrillator

Hypertrophic CMP is the most frequent cause of sudden cardiac death in adults under 35 years; annual mortality is 1% and half of it is sudden cardiac death [26, 27]. In the Spanish Implantable Cardioverter Defibrillator registry [28], 6% of carriers of this device had a previous diagnosis of hypertrophic CMP. Unfortunately, sudden cardiac death could be the first manifestation of this entity, so it is necessary a risk stratification. However, although implantable cardioverter defibrillator is recommended for high-risk patients with hypertrophic CMP, there is no agreement on its general use. In European centers, a conservative approach has been adopted: in primary prevention, there is indication to implant an implantable cardioverter defibrillator if at least two risk factors are present [27]; but that does not mean it is accompanied by theoretical high risk. It can be seen at an annual rate of 11.1% adequate treatment in secondary prevention and 1.6% in primary prevention.

In several series [29], differences are observed in the placement criteria (**Table 1**) between hospitals and even populations of each center. It is remarkable that patients with an episode of resuscitated sudden cardiac death or sustained ventricular tachycardia had fewer risk factors than those with implantable cardioverter defibrillator for primary prevention (1.94 vs 2.96). The main factors associated with appropriate therapies were history of resuscitated sudden death and sustained ventricular tachycardia. These data reflect the difficulty in identifying patients at risk and make adequate primary prevention. The history of sustained ventricular tachycardia or ventricular fibrillation makes unnecessary to look for other risk factors. On the other hand, the presence of ventricular aneurysm, myocardial infarction, or systolic dysfunction may indicate the need for this therapy.

The current selection criteria do not predict in a reliable manner the occurrence of sudden cardiac death or ventricular arrhythmias. On the other hand, the quantification of fibrosis or genetic study may help proper selection of candidates for implantable cardioverter defibrillator for primary prevention. This becomes more important if we consider the associated complications in the primary prevention group (unnecessary electric shocks, battery replacements, etc). A new algorithm [30] can give greater discriminatory power than previous ones.

• Resuscitated SD
• Sustained VT
• Family history of SD
• Causeless recurrent syncope (without apparent cause)
• Ventricular hypertrophy (≥30 mm)
• Subaortic gradient (left ventricular outflow tract, LVOT >30 mmHg at rest)
• Abnormal response to exertion in less than 45 years (inability to increase 25 mmHg systolic arterial pressure)
• NSVT in Holter ECG (three or more ventricular beats, followed by more than 120 beats/min and less than 30 s in length)

Table 1. Checked risk factors of sudden death. SD, sudden death. VT, ventricular tachycardia. NSVT, non sustained VT.

Recent clinical guidelines [12, 13] recommend, in the absence of clinical trials, the use of implantable cardioverter defibrillator for secondary prevention in patients with aborted cardiac arrest or sustained ventricular tachycardia associated with a high risk of subsequent lethal arrhythmia. Also, recommendations for implantable cardioverter defibrillator therapy for primary prophylaxis are based on the 5-year SCD risk calculated using the HCM Risk-SCD model and taking into account the age and general health of the patient.

5. Dilated MCP

The etiology of this CMP is varied: idiopathic 50% (**Figure 3**), myocarditis 9%, ischemic CMP 7%, infiltrative disease 5%, and other (peripartum, arterial hypertension, treatment with doxorubicin, etc.

Chagas disease: It is a protozoal infection due to *Tripanosoma cruzi*. It is the leading cause of dilated CMP in Central/South America and is the leading cause of cardiovascular death in patients between 30 and 50 years old. Cardiac involvement is manifested as arrhythmias, heart failure, and thromboembolic phenomena. In these countries it is a major cause of sudden cardiac death. Nonsustained ventricular tachycardia, NYHA functional class, and left ventricular ejection fraction are predictors of mortality, with a 16% survival at 36 months in patients with NYHA class IV and left ventricular ejection fraction <35% despite optimal medical treatment [31]. With similar indications to previous trials (severe heart failure despite optimal medical treatment, QRS > 120 ms, left ventricular ejection fraction <35%, and left ventricular end-diastolic diameter >55 mm assessed by Doppler echocardiography), improved NYHA functional status is obtained, with increase in left ventricular ejection fraction and reduction in left ventricular end diastolic diameter; 33% of patients do not respond to cardiac resynchronization therapy, probably by the advanced NYHA class.

Pharmacological treatment has little benefit, and recurrence rates of severe arrhythmia are close to 100%. Mortality is high—40% at 1 year, with frequent need for implantable cardioverter defibrillator implantation when evolves to dilated CMP [32]. Recent guidelines

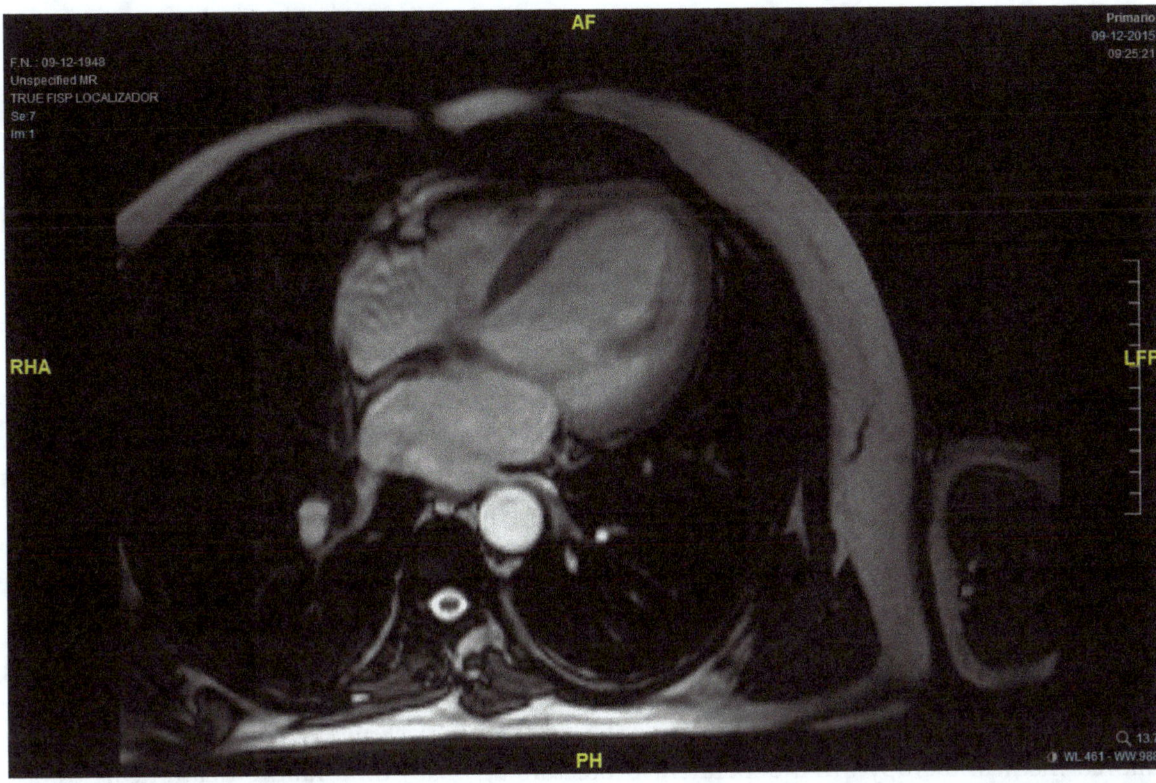

Figure 3. MR image of a patient with idiopathic dilated cardiomyopathy, with increased ventricular dimensions with a homogeneous myocardial uptake signal.

[11, 12] say that implanted cardioverter defibrillator should be considered in patients with left ventricular ejection fraction <40% when they are expected to survive >1 year with good functional status

Stress CMP (*takotsubo*) does not seem to be an indication for treatment with cardiac resynchronization therapy even in cases with refractory heart failure (usual indication of these devices in ambulatory patients).

Cardiac involvement in *Becker muscular dystrophy* varies from myocardial hypertrophy with preserved systolic function to severe left ventricular dilatation with anomalies in contractility by anomalies in contractility and severe depression of systolic function. Cardiac resynchronization therapy implantation depends on the baseline condition and comorbidities of patients. Few cases have been described [33].

Peripartum: It is a rare form of nonischemic CMP defined as heart failure secondary to left ventricular systolic dysfunction with a left ventricular ejection fraction <45% toward the end of pregnancy or in the months following delivery, where no other cause of heart failure can be found. The treatment of peripartum CMP is similar to that employed for other types of heart failure with left ventricular dysfunction; however, modifications to standard therapy are often necessary to ensure the safety of the mother and the unborn or breastfeeding child. The time to potential recovery from severe remodeling of ventricular function is difficult to predict [34]. In general, severely reduced left ventricular ejection fraction is linked to a higher risk of life-threatening ventricular tachyarrhythmic events, and implantation of a defibrillator is often recommended. An alternative for these patients can be the wearable cardioverter/defibrillator, with temporary protection during a phase of high arrhythmic risk [35]. An elevated incidence of ventricular fibrillation episodes during an early phase of peripartum CMP in patients with severely reduced left ventricular ejection fraction and heart failure symptoms and uninterrupted vest defibrillator wearing for up to 6 months can protect these young mothers from dying suddenly and yield important information about a potential permanent risk that will indicate implantable cardioverter defibrillator implantation. Recent guidelines [12, 13] point that implantation of an implantable cardioverter defibrillator in patients with ventricular arrhythmia or low left ventricular ejection fraction should follow standard guidelines; the high rate of spontaneous recovery of dilated CMP after delivery must be considered when decisions are made.

Amyloid CMP: The efficacy and safety of implantable cardioverter defibrillator are uncertain. Sudden cardiac death is common in patients with cardiac amyloidosis, but electromechanical dissociation seems to be a significant cause of sudden death [36]. In recent guidelines [12, 13], implantable cardioverter defibrillator should be considered in patients with ventricular arrhythmia causing hemodynamic instability who are expected to survive >1 year with good functional status.

Idiopathic dilated CMP: Several observational registries [37] show that early diagnosis and tailored medical therapy are independent protectors against pump-failure death/heart transplant, and lower left ventricular ejection fraction is a predictor of sudden death, while implantable cardioverter defibrillator has a protective role.

Any observational study [38] shows the usefulness of cardiac resynchronization therapy in patients with *dilated CMP of valvular origin after corrective valve surgery* (an underrepresented population in randomized controlled trials). In patients with left bundle branch block, wide QRS (161 ms), and advanced functional class (III 82% - IV), there is a functional improvement in class and better data in left ventricular remodelation and asynchrony.

5.1. Role of cardiac resynchronization therapy

The usefulness of resynchronization has been recorded in clinical trials that included patients with severe depression of left ventricular systolic function, complete left bundle brain block, and heart failure syndrome. One important issue has been described recently: the relationship between QRS duration and left ventricular remodelation. Several factors that help to predict response to cardiac resynchronization replacement have been identified: systolic pulmonary artery pressure, renal function, left ventricular dyssynchrony, inappropriate left ventricular electrode position, ischemia, and 6-minute walking distance; but it remains unclear if QRS duration, measured before cardiac resynchronization therapy, can predict its effectiveness (conflicting results, with data pointing to one direction and to the opposite [39]). And patients with nonischemic CMP are more likely to benefit from cardiac resynchronization therapy compared to patients with ischemic CMP. According to the reduction of left ventricular end-diastolic diameter 6 months after cardiac resynchronization therapy, patients were divided into responder and nonresponder; measured parameters were not statistically different before resynchronization. After 6 months, responders exhibited significant reversal of their left ventricular remodeling, with improved left ventricular ejection fraction and exercise tolerance, and a shorter QRS compared to nonresponders; the preoperative parameters were not predictive of the ultimate response of patients to resynchronization. Zhang [39] also shows that QRS duration change correlated with reduction in left ventricular end-diastolic diameter; QRS duration that can easily measured before and after resynchronization may be a predictive factor of response to cardiac resynchronization therapy in patients with heart failure due to dilated CMP. In a Spanish work, it is exposed that early normalization of ejection fraction after resynchronization is long-term maintained and identify better clinical and arrhythmic prognosis [40].

Cardiac resynchronization therapy is not strongly recommended for patients with narrow QRS. There are some described cases of CRT implant in patients with dilated CMP and narrow QRS in which it was obtained a dramatic response optimizing the atrioventricular delay, remembering the importance of atrioventricular optimization for successful resynchronization.

In addition, early normalization of left ventricular function in idiopathic dilated CMP is held long term after resynchronization device implant and indicates an improvement in prognosis from clinical and arrhythmic points of view. A decrease in cardiovascular mortality is observed, and also there is a decrease of arrhythmic events; this finding is consistent as described by García Lunar et al. [41]. The question is whether resynchronization device must be associated with implantable cardioverter defibrillator over time or even this mixed device (resynchronization + defibrillator) must be replaced by a resynchronization device only, especially if patient has inappropriate therapies.

It is stated in clinical guidelines [17] that the benefit is greater in patients with wider QRS and left bundle branch block and in women and non-ischemic cardiomyopathy, intermediate in men with ischemic cardiomyopathy; and lesser, or even non-responsive, in patients with narrow QRS and without left bundle block.

5.2. Role of implantable cardioverter defibrillator

Life-threatening ventricular arrhythmias are common in patients with heart failure and CMP, and their presence may lead to sudden death. These devices may have a primary and secondary indication. Secondary prevention with implantable cardioverter defibrillator is planned in patients with heart failure and CMP, also dilated CMP, who survive to an episode of sudden cardiac death. This indication is based on the results of several studies, AVID (entry criteria: left ventricular ejection fraction <40%), CASH, and CIDS. Some studies show a greater benefit of defibrillators in younger patients [42], whereas other studies did not found such differences [43, 44]. Also, there are studies focused on primary prevention in nonischemic dilated CMP; the trials CAT [45] and AMIOVIRT [46] showed a nonsignificant trend to decreased mortality, due to its methodological limitations. Other trials (DEFINITE, SCD-HeFT y COMPANION) did show reduction in mortality. At the view of these results and the results of a recent meta-analysis, primary prevention with implantable cardioverter defibrillator in patients with dilated CMP, left ventricular ejection fraction ≤35%, and NYHA II-III is recommended. The ability to induce ventricular arrhythmias is not predictive of sudden cardiac death in patients with nonischemic CMP; thus, electrophysiology testing does not have a role in risk stratification of these patients [5] (**Figure 4**).

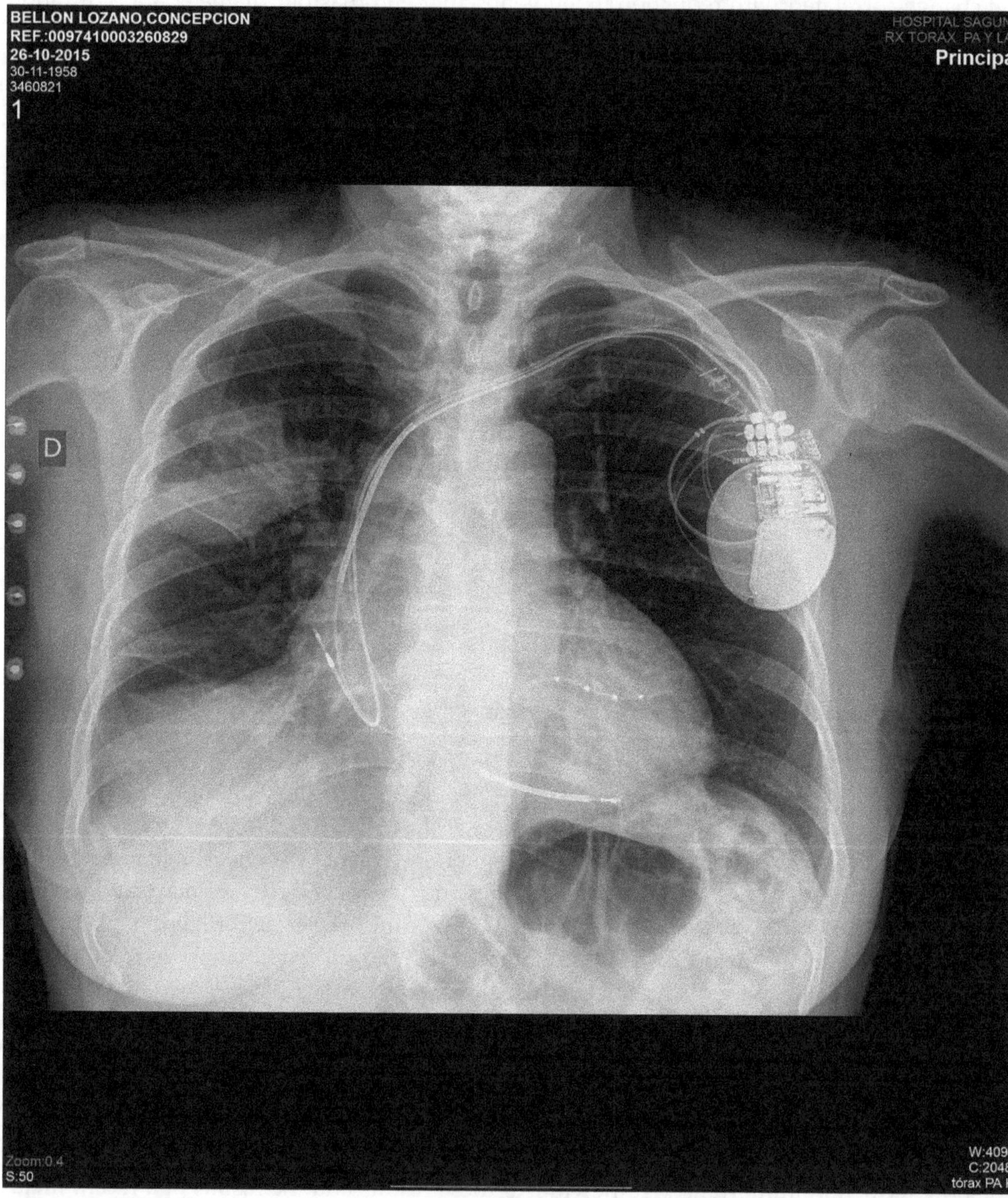

Figure 4. Cardiac resynchronization therapy in the same patient with idiopathic dilated cardiomyopathy. An alveolar condensation in the medium lobe compatible with nosocomial pneumonia (coincident with device implantation) can be seen.

As we have said before, in recent guidelines [12, 13], implantable cardioverter defibrillator is recommended, as secondary prophylaxis, in patients with hemodynamically nontolerated ventricular tachycardia/ventricular fibrillation, who are expected to survive for >1 year with good functional status. And for primary prophylaxis, defibrillator is recommended in patients with symptomatic heart failure (NYHA class II–III) and left ventricular ejection fraction ≤35% despite ≥3 months of treatment with optimal medical treatment who are expected to survive for >1 year with good functional status.

6. Restrictive CMP

This is the least frequent in the group of CMP and the only one for which the WHO/ISFC Task Force 81 does not offer specific diagnostic criteria. The diagnosis is based on clinical signs of heart failure due to a restriction on the diastolic filling of the heart with preserved systolic function and in the absence of hypertrophy or ventricular dilation. Amyloidosis, mucopolisacaridosis, and Löeffler's endocarditis are the more frequent causes. Treatment does not follow standard treatment guidelines as in other cases of cardiomyopathies and is based on a careful management of diuretics and vasodilators. The management of restrictive CMP is difficult because the underlying processes usually do not respond to intervention and is mostly palliative. In several cases, there has been an indication of implantable cardioverter defibrillator to prevent sudden cardiac death in high-risk patients; recent guidelines [12, 13] make a similar recommendation to other diseases with poor prognosis and state that defibrillators are recommended in patients with sustained ventricular arrhythmia causing hemodynamic instability who are expected to survive >1 year with good functional status to reduce the risk of sudden cardiac death. In relation to its pathophysiology, there is no indication to resynchronization. In most cases of restrictive CMP, caused by amyloidosis or other infiltrative diseases, there is a very poor prognosis, except in the case that the patient will receive a heart transplant. In patients with sarcoidosis, defibrillator implantation is recommended if left ventricular ejection fraction is <35%, maintained after a period of immunosuppression, and considered in patients with induced ventricular tachycardia in electrophysiology test and with late gadolinium enhancement in cardiac gammagraphy, although the left ventricular function is normal [47].

7. Arrhythmogenic right ventricular cardiomyopathy (ARVC)

It is a CMP, a hereditary disease of the desmosomal proteins, and is associated with sudden cardiac death; there is a fibrofatty replacement of the right ventricle myocardium that initially produces typical regional wall motion abnormalities that later become global and finally leads to right ventricular dilatation [48]. Its mechanism is re-entrant arrhythmias.

7.1. Role of implantable cardioverter defibrillator

Selection of patients for defibrillator is controversial. Natural history of the disease suggests several risk factors for sudden cardiac death: marked right ventricle dilatation, left ventricular involvement with left ventricular reduced function, occurrence of prior hemodynamically unstable rapid sustained monomorphic ventricular tachycardia or ventricular fibrillation, and history of syncope; T-wave inversions could be a predictor of any ventricular arrhythmia in follow-up and a younger age; probably, the major risk for death was reduced left ventricular function [49]. Inducible sustained monomorphic ventricular tachycardia did not predict the presence of the same arrhythmia in the follow-up (although Bhonsale et al. found a relationship in their work [50]). When defibrillator is placed, anti-tachycardia pacing is highly successful in terminating sustained monomorphic ventricular tachycardia and should be programmed for all sustained monomorphic ventricular tachycardia, regardless of heart rate. Some authors comment that defibrillator implant with primary prevention has an excessively low rate of appropriate therapies, and the criteria for risk stratification have little predictive power; for these reasons, there should be revised. New genetic techniques help us to classify left ventricular hypertrophy in some patients as Fabry disease or other metabolopathies, with different prognosis and risk of sudden death than primary hypertrophic CMP. In addition, some registries have short (3.3 years) follow-up, and there have been appropriate therapies 9–10 years after the implant; given the youth of these patients and the long at-risk period, it is

Predictor variable	Definition	Coding
Age	Age at evaluation [30]	Continuous, years
Family history of SCD	History of sudden cardiac death in one or more first degree relatives under 40 years of age or SCD in a first degree relative with confirmed HCM at any age (post-or ante-mortem diagnosis) [13, 22, 28, 29]	Binary (yes = 1/no = 0)
Maximal wall thickness	The greatest thickness in the anterior septum, posterior septum, lateral wall, and posterior wall of the LV, measured at the level of the mitral value, papillary muscles, and apex using parasternal short-axis plane using 2D echocardiography at the time of evaluation [15, 17, 20, 23, 24, 26]	Continuous, mm
Fractional shortening	(LV end-diastolic dimension-LV end-systolic dimension)/LV end-diastolic dimension measured by M-Mode or 2D echocardiography at time of evaluation [23]	Continuous, %
Left atrial diameter	Left atrial diameter determined by M-Mode or 2D echocardiography in the parasternal long-axis plane at the time of evaluation [30]	Continuous, mm
Maximal left ventricular outflow tract gradients	The maximum LV outflow gradient determined at rest and with Valsalva provocation (irrespective of concurrent medical treatment) using pulsed and continuous wave Doppler from the apical three- and five-chamber views. Peak outflow tract gradients were determined using the modified Bernoulli equation: Gradient = 4*V* [2], where *V* is the peak aortic outflow velocity [13, 18, 22, 27, 28]	Continuous, mmHg
Nonsustained ventricular tachycardia	≥3 consecutive ventricular beats at a rate of ≥120 bpm and <30 s in duration on Holter monitoring (minimum duration 24 hours) at or prior to evaluation [13, 17, 28, 29]	Binary (yes = 1/no = 0)
Unexplained syncope	History of unexplained syncope at or prior to evaluation [13, 20, 25, 28, 30]	Binary (yes = 1/no = 0)

Table 2. HCM Risk-SCD tool. HCM, hypertrophic CMP. SCD, sudden cardiac death. LV, left ventricle.

very important to perform long follow-up periods. The number of inappropriate therapies can decrease with better diagnostic algorithms. Recent guidelines for management of this disease [51] highlight several elements; the most important, little usefulness of algorithms based on binary variables that do not take into account the magnitude of each risk factor, with poor discriminatory power between high and low risk. Therefore, it is recommended to use the HCM Risk-SCD tool (**Table 2**) [30]. Recent guidelines [12, 13] state that defibrillator implantation is recommended in patients with a history of aborted sudden cardiac death and hemodynamically poorly tolerated ventricular tachycardia (secondary prevention) and should be considered in patients who have hemodynamically well-tolerated sustained Ventricular tachycardia or have one or more recognized risk factors for ventricular arrhythmia with a life expectancy >1 year.

7.2. Role of cardiac resynchronization therapy

It has been described as any case of mixed defibrillator-resynchronization device in special circumstances. In advanced cases of this disease, with low voltages in electrical signal from right ventricle, there can be difficult to detect ventricular tachyarrhythmias. The advanced degree of atrioventricular block indicates permanent cardiac pacing. There must be a catheter in coronary sinus for sensing and pacing, and another catheter in right ventricle as backup if left ventricle catheter capture fails, taking into account the high degree of atrioventricular block.

Acknowledgements

The authors thank Leyre Cendrero and Omar Ferrús, technical consultants of Medtronic Company; Ricardo Ruiz and Francisco Javier Chorro, from Cardiology Department of Hospital Clínico, Valencia; and Vicent López and all staff in Intensive Care Unit of Hospital Sagunto, for their help in the preparation of this work.

Author details

Miguel Ángel García García[1*], María de los Ángeles Rosero Arenas[2], Alfonso Martínez Cornejo[1], Marta Bertolo Domínguez[3] and Vicente Miranda Gozalvo[4]

*Address all correspondence to: mangelesymangel@hotmail.com

1 Intensive Care Unit, Sagunto Hospital, Valencia, Spain

2 Centro de Salud (Health Facility) Cheste, Valencia, Spain

3 Radiology Department, Sagunto Hospital, Valencia, Spain

4 ERESA/Radiology Department, Sagunto Hospital, Valencia, Spain

References

[1] Richardson P, McKenna W, Bristow M et al. Report of the 1995 World Health Organization/International Society and Federation of Cardiology Task Force on the Definition and Classification of Cardiomyopathies. Circulation. 1996; 93: 841–842.

[2] The SOLVD Investigators. Effect of enalapril on survival in patients with reduced left ventricular ejection fractions and congestive heart failure. N Engl J Med 1991; 325: 293–302.

[3] Marine JE, Russo AM. Primary prevention of sudden cardiac death in heart failure and cardiomyopathy. In: UpToDate, Post TW(Ed), UpToDate, Waltham, MA. (Accessed on April 07, 2016).

[4] Podrid PJ, Ganz LI. Incidence of and risk stratification for sudden cardiac death after acute myocardial infarction.

[5] Podrid PJ. Ventricular arrhythmias in heart failure and cardiomyopathy. In: UpToDate, Post TW(Ed), UpToDate, Waltham, MA. (Accessed on April 18, 2016).

[6] Bernstein AD, Daubert JC, Fletcher RD et al. The revised NASPE/BPEG generic code for antibradycardia, adaptative-rate, and multisite pacing. North American Society of Pacing and Electrophysiology/British Pacing and Electrophysiology Group. Pacing Clin Electrophysiol 2002; 25: 260–264.

[7] Saxon LA. Overview of cardiac pacing in heart failure. In: UpToDate, Post TW(Ed), UpToDate, Waltham, MA. (Accessed on April 18, 2016).

[8] Pfeffer MA, McMurray JJ, Velazquez EJ et al. Valsartan, captopril, or both in myocardial infarction complicated by heart failure, left ventricular dysfunction or both. N Engl J Med 2003; 349: 893–906.

[9] Höhnloser SH, Kuck KH, DorianP et al. Prophylactic use of an implantable cardioverter-defibrillator after acute myocardial infarction. N Engl J Med 2004; 351: 2481–2488.

[10] Steinbeck G, Andresen D, SeidlK et al. Defibrillator implantation early after myocardial infarction. N Engl J Med 2009; 361: 1427–1436.

[11] Bardy GH, Lee KL, Mark DB et al. Amiodarone or an implantable cardioverter-defibrillator for congestive heart failure. N Engl J Med 2004; 352: 225.

[12] Zipes DP, Camm AF, Borggrefe M et al. ACC/AHA/ESC 2006 Guidelines for management of patients with ventricular arrhythmias and the prevention of sudden cardiac death. J Am Coll Cardiol 2006; 48: e247–e346.

[13] Priori SG, Blomström-Lundqvist C, Mazzanti A et al. 2015 ESC Guidelines for the management of patients with ventricular arrhythmias and the prevention of sudden cardiac death. Eur Heart J 2015; 36:2793–2867.

[14] Molhoek SG, Bax JJ, van ErvenL et al. Comparison of benefits from cardiac resynchronization therapy in patients with ischemic cardiomyopathy versus idiopathic dilated cardiomyopathy. Am J Cardiol 2004; 93: 860–863.

[15] McLeod CJ, Shen WK, Rea RF et al. Differential outcome of cardiac resynchronization therapy in ischemic cardiomyopathy and idiopathic dilated cardiomyopathy. Heart Rhythm 2011; 8: 377–382.

[16] Sohinki D, Ho J, Srinivasan N et al. Outcomes after atrioventricular node ablation and biventricular pacing in patients with refractory atrial fibrillation and heart failure: a comparison between non-ischaemic and ischaemic cardiomyopathy. Europace 2014; 16: 880–886.

[17] The Task Force on cardiac pacing and resynchronization therapy of the European Society of Cardiology (ESC). Developed in collaboration with the European Heart Rhythm Association (EHRA), Brignole M, Auricchio A, Baron-Esquivias et al. 2013 ESC Guidelines on cardiac pacing and cardiac resynchronization therapy. Rev Esp Cardiol (Engl Ed). 2014 Jan;67(1):58.

[18] Baughman KL. Diagnosis of myocarditis: death of Dallas criteria. Circulation 2006; 113: 593–595.

[19] D'Ambrosio A, Patti G, Manzoli A et al. The fate of acute myocarditis between spontaneous improvement and evolution to dilated cardiomyopathy: a review. Heart 2001; 85: 499–504.

[20] Chung MK. The role of the wearable cardioverter defibrillator in clinical practice. Cardiol Clin 2014; 32: 253–270.

[21] Dickstein K, Vardas PE, Auricchio A et al. 2010 Focused update of ESC guidelines on device therapy in heart failure: an update of the 2008 ESC guidelines for the diagnosis and treatment of acute and chronic heart failure and the 2007 ESC guidelines for cardiac and resynchronization therapy. Eur J Heart Fail 2010; 12: 1143–1153.

[22] Maron MS. Hypertrophic cardiomyopathy: clinical manifestations, diagnosis and evaluation. In: UpToDate, Post TW (Ed), UpToDate, Waltham, MA. (Accessed on April 07, 2016).

[23] Jurado Román A, Montero Cabezas JM, Rubio Alonso B et al. Sequential Atrioventricular Pacing in Patients With Hypertrophic Cardiomyopathy: An 18-year Experience. Rev Esp Cardiol(Engl Ed). 2016 Apr;69 (4):377-83.

[24] Lenarczyk R, Wozniak R, Kowalski O et al. Effect of cardiac resynchronization on gradient reduction in patients with obstructive hypertrophic cardiomyopathy: preliminary study. Pacing Clin Electrophysiol 2011; 34: 1544–1552.

[25] Authors/Task Force members, Elliott PM, Anastasakis A, Borger MA et al. 2014 ESC Guidelines on diagnosis and management of hypertrophic cardiomyopathy: the Task Force for the Diagnosis and Management of Hypertrophic Cardiomyopathy of the European Society of Cardiology (ESC). Eur Heart J. 2014 Oct 14;35(39):2733-79.

[26] Maron BJ. Prevention of sudden death with the implantable defibrillator in hypertrophic cardiomyopathy. Rev Esp Cardiol. 2006 Jun;59:527-30.

[27] Maron BJ. Hypertrophic cardiomyopathy: a systematic review. JAMA. 2002 Mar 13;287:1308-20.

[28] Peinado R, Arenal A, Arribas F et al. Spanish implantable cardioverter-defibrillator registry. First official report of the spanish society of cardiology working group on implantable cardioverter-defibrillators (2002-2004). Rev Esp Cardiol. 2005;58:1435-49.

[29] Marín F, Gimeno JR, Payá E et al. The implantable cardioverter-defibrillator and hypertrophic cardiomyopathy. Experience at three centers. Rev Esp Cardiol. 2006 Jun;59(6):537-44.

[30] O'Mahony C, Jichi F, Pavlou M et al. A novel clinical risk prediction model for sudden cardiac death in hypertrophic cardiomyopathy (HCM Risk-SCD). Eur Heart J 2014; 35: 2010–2020.

[31] Rassi A Jr, Rassi A, Rassi SG et al. Predictors of mortality in chronic Chagas disease: a systematic review of observational studies. Circulation 2007; 115: 1101–1108.

[32] Muratore C, Rabinovich R, Iglesias R et al. Implantable cardioverter defibrillators in patients with Chagas' disease: Are they different from patients with coronary disease? Pacing Clin Electrophysiol 1997; 20: 194–197.

[33] Andrikopoulos G, Kourouklis S, Trika C et al. Cardiac resynchronization therapy in Becker muscular dystrophy. Hellenic J Cardiol 2013; 54: 227–229.

[34] Tsang W, Bales AC, Lang RM. Peripartum cardiomyopathy: treatment and prognosis. In: UpToDate, Post TW(Ed), UpToDate, Waltham, MA. (Accessed on April 07, 2016).

[35] Duncker D, Haghikia A, Konig T et al. Risk for ventricular fibrillation in peripartum cardiomyopathy with severely reduced left ventricular function value of the wearing cardioverter/defibrillator. Eur J Heart Fail 2014; 16: 1331–1336.

[36] McKenna WJ. Treatment of amyloid cardiomyopathy. In: UpToDate, Post TW(Ed), UpToDate, Waltham, MA. (Accessed on April 07, 2016).

[37] Merlo M, Pivetta A, Pinamonti B et al. Long-term prognostic impact of therapeutic strategies in patients with idiopathic dilated cardiomyopathy: Changing mortality over the last 30 years. Eur J Heart Fail 2014; 16: 317–324.

[38] Macías A, Gavira JJ, Castaño S et al. Cardiac resynchronization therapy and valvular cardiomyopathy after corrective surgery. Rev Esp Cardiol 2008; 61: 1088–1091.

[39] Zhang J, Zhang Y, Zhou X et al. QRS duration shortening predicts left ventricular reverse remodeling in patients with dilated cardiomyopathy after cardiac resynchronization therapy. Acta Cardiol 2015; 70: 307–313.

[40] Cabrera-Bueno F, Alzueta J, Fernández-Pastor J et al. Premature normalizing of ejection fraction after resynchronization inidiopathic dilated cardiomyopathy is maintained long-term and identifies the best clinical arrhythmic prognosis Cardiocore 2015; 50: 71–75.

[41] García Lunar I, Castro Urda V, Toquero Ramos J et al. Ventricular arrhythmias in super-responders to cardiac resynchronization therapy. Rev Esp Cardiol (Engl Ed). 2014;67:883-9.

[42] Healey JS. Hallstrom AP, Kuck KH et al. Role of the implantable defibrillator among elderly patients with a history of life-threatening ventricular arrhythmias. Eur Heart J 2007; 28: 1746 - 9.

[43] Huang DT, Sesselberg HW, McNittS et al. Improved survival associated with prophylactic implantable defibrillators in elderly patients with prior myocardial infarction and depressed ventricular function: a MADIT-II substudy. J Cardiovasc Electrophysiol 2007; 18: 833 – 8.

[44] Duray G, Richter S, Manegold J et al. Efficacy and safety of ICD therapy in a population of elderly patients treated with optimal background medication. J Interv Card Electrophysiol 2005; 14: 169 - 73.

[45] Strickberger SA, Hummel JD, Bartlett TG et al. Amiodarone versus implantable cardioverter-defibrillator: randomized trial in patients with nonischemic dilated cardiomyopathy and asymptomatic nonsustained ventricular tachycardia—AMIOVIRT. J Am Coll Cardiol 2003; 41: 1707 - 12.

[46] Bänsch D, Antz M, Boczor S et al. Primary prevention of sudden cardiac death in idiopathic dilated cardiomyopathy: the Cardiomyopathy Trial (CAT). Circulation 2002; 105: 1453 – 8.

[47] Birnie DH, Sauer WH, Bogun F et al. Diagnosis and management of arrhythmias associated with cardiac sarcoidosis. Heart Rhythm 2014; 11: 1304–1323.

[48] McKenna WJ. Clinical manifestations and diagnosis of arrhythmogenic right ventricular cardiomyopathy. In: UpToDate, Post TW(Ed), UpToDate, Waltham, MA. (Accessed on April 07, 2016).

[49] Link MS, Laidlaw D, Polonsky B et al. Ventricular arrhythmias in the North American Multidisciplinary Study of Arrhythmogenic right ventricular cardiomyopathy. Predictors, characteristics and treatment. J Am Coll Cardiol 2014; 64: 119 - 25.

[50] Bohnsale A, James CA, Tichnell C et al. Incidence and predictors of implantable cardioverter-defibrillator therapy in patients with arrhythmogenic right ventricular dysplasia/cardiomyopathy undergoing implantable cardioverter-defibrillator implantation for primary prevention. J Am Coll Cardiol 2011; 58: 1485 - 96.

[51] McKenna WJ. Arrhythmogenic right ventricular cardiomyopathy: treatment and prognosis. In: UpToDate, Post TW(Ed), UpToDate, Waltham, MA. (Accessed on April 07, 2016).

3

Heart Failure with Preserved Ejection Fraction

Hakan Altay and Seckin Pehlivanoglu

Abstract

Heart failure with preserved ejection fraction (HFpEF) is now recognized as a major and growing public health problem worldwide. This heart failure subtype disproportionately affects women and the elderly and is commonly associated with other cardiovascular comorbidities, such as hypertension, diabetes and chronic kidney disease. There are uncertainties and debates regarding the definition, diagnosis and pathophysiology with the consequence that all outcome trials performed so far cannot yield an effective treatment as in heart failure with reduced ejection fraction (HFrEF). Here we present an overview of epidemiology, pathophysiology, diagnosis and therapeutic approaches emerging from large outcome clinical trials.

Keywords: heart failure, ejection fraction, diastolic, diagnosis, treatment

1. Introduction

Heart failure (HF) is a clinical syndrome of dyspnea, fatigue and fluid retention secondary to impaired cardiac function [1]. Cardiac function may be impaired structurally or functionally with resultant decreased ejection or filling capacity both of which can reduce cardiac output and/or increase intracardiac pressures at rest or during exercise. Systolic dysfunction leading to reduced left ventricular ejection fraction (LVEF) (LVEF < 40%) had long been believed to be the predominant cause of heart failure. However, HF remains to be a growing health problem in the community despite recent improvements in the management of HF with reduced ejection fraction (HFrEF). Another subset of heart failure which occurs in the setting of normal or near normal left ventricular ejection fraction (LVEF > 50%) has been evolving for the last two decades. This distinct HF subtype has been called HF with preserved ejection fraction (HFpEF). Once included in HFpEF, the newly defined HF with midrange EF (HFmrEF) comprises the HF patients with EF between 40 and 50% [2]. HFmrEF will be discussed in the context of HFPEF because most of the trials and epidemiological studies to date have included patients with EF > 40%.

Current data indicate that at least half of the HF population has a normal or near-normal LVEF [3]. Even more striking is the finding that the percent of patients with HFpEF appears to be increasing in relation to the percent that have HFrEF [4]. One of the reasons for this shift in the ratio between HFpEF and HFrEF is related to the greater availability of therapeutic interventions that limit myocardial damage (particularly, in the setting of an acute myocardial infarction), hence reducing incidence of HFrEF. Another important reason for this increase in prevalence of HFpEF is increasing number of obese and elderly patients. It is also worth mentioning that there is an increased number of patients with possible misdiagnosis of HFpEF who have otherwise alternative causes for their symptoms such as obesity, lung disease and myocardial ischemia [5].

In the past, HFpEF was thought to be a benign condition, but now it is well known that it causes substantial morbidity and mortality [6]. Despite being an enormous and dreadful problem of this era, there has been little progress in developing effective treatments that will alter the natural history of the condition. Contemporary medicine can offer nothing but only diuretic for treatment. This is partly due to an incomplete understanding of the disease and partly due to the huge diversity of clinical phenotype.

2. Epidemiology

Over 90% of patients with HFpEF are aged ≥60 years at the time of diagnosis making it obvious that this is a disease of elderly [7]. The prevalence in the community has varied from 1.1% to 5.5% of the general population [8]. This wide variation is primarily attributed to the different cutoff values of normal EF in different studies. Moreover, the prevalence has been found to vary with age and gender. A large community-based study found that the prevalence of HFpEF increased from 0% in males to 1% in females in the age group of 25–49 years to 4–6% in males and 8–10% in females above 80 years, indicating a dramatic rise in the prevalence with increasing age but additionally a higher prevalence among females as compared to age-matched males [9]. The demographic characteristics present in patients with HFpEF differ significantly from those in patients with HFREF. Compared with those with HFrEF, patients with HFpEF are older, more often female, more often have hypertensive heart disease and less often have ischemic heart disease [10]. There is a similar prevalence of DM but remarkably higher prevalence of obesity in patients with HFpEF compared to HFrEF. Atrial fibrillation (AF) is also more prevalent in HFpEF [11]. HFpEF patients also have a higher burden of both cardiovascular and non-cardiovascular comorbid diseases. **Table 1** summarizes various comorbidities usually seen in association with HFpEF. Comorbid conditions especially renal insufficiency and atrial fibrillation may be less common in randomized controlled trials than hospital-based registries due to exclusion criteria.

Whether overall mortality rates differ between patients with HFpEF and HFrEF is not clear. Some community-based epidemiological studies have shown that the annual mortality rate is

Comorbid conditions	Frequency
Hypertension	60–80%
Ischemic heart disease	35–70%
Diabetes	20–45%
Atrial fibrillation	15–40%
COPD	31%
Renal insufficiency	26%

COPD: Chronic obstructive pulmonary disease.

Table 1. Comorbid conditions seen in association with HFPEF.

same and approaches 15% for both groups of patients [4]. Conversely, data from randomized clinical trials suggest that patients with HFpEF have a lower annual mortality (approaching 5%) than patients with HFrEF. The lower mortality rate detected in the randomized trials can be explained by strict exclusion of comorbid diseases [12]. When the data from I-PRESERVE (The Irbesartan in Heart Failure With Preserved Ejection Fraction Study) trial was analyzed with respect to mode of death in HFpEF, it was seen that cardiovascular (CV) diseases (60%) are the leading cause of death including sudden cardiac death (26%), HF (15%), myocardial infarction (5%) and stroke (9%) followed by non-CV causes (30%) and unknown (10%) [13]. Compared with HFrEF [14], HFpEF patients have more non-cardiovascular (30% vs. 15%), fewer sudden (26% vs. 40%) and fewer heart failure deaths (15% vs. 35%). In parallel with I-PRESERVE trial results, the cause-specific mortality estimates show that the non-cardiovascular causes of death constitute nearly 30 to 50% of all deaths in HFpEF patients while only 15–18% in HFrEF patients [15]. The older age and high burden of comorbidities can explain the higher non-cardiovascular mortality in HFpEF patients. Large HFpEF trials showed that the patients with HFpEF have lower hospitalization rates than those with HFrEF [16]. Furthermore, HFrEF patients have nearly 1% absolute higher in-hospital mortality rate than HFpEF patients [17].

3. Pathophysiology

In contrast to HFrEF patients who have main abnormalities in systolic function, left ventricular dilation and eccentric remodeling, patients with HFpEF have main abnormalities in diastolic function, normal left ventricular size and concentric hypertrophy. Normal LVEF does not imply normal cardiac output. In HFrEF, decreased cardiac output can be explained more easily with reduced ejection fraction and subsequent reduced stroke volume. HFpEF patients also exhibit a low cardiac output that is comparable to that seen in HFrEF patients. The pathophysiological abnormality leading to decreased cardiac output in HFpEF is more complex and since HFpEF is a heterogeneous clinical diagnosis, it encompasses a variety of underlying pathophysiological processes.

HFpEF is caused by the complex interplay of multiple impairments in ventricular diastolic function, adverse cardiac remodeling, stiffening of the ventricles, pulmonary hypertension, atrial dysfunction and abnormal ventricular-vascular coupling related to stiffening of the vasculature and hence decreased vascular compliance, endothelial dysfunction, impaired vasodilatation and coronary ischemia, impaired renal handling of salt and fluid and impairment of heart rate (HR) reserve [18]. Left ventricular diastolic dysfunction is the result of myocardial hypertrophy, fibrosis and/or altered myocyte calcium handling (delayed calcium uptake by the myocyte sarcoplasmic reticulum and calcium efflux from the myocyte) [19]. The pathophysiology of diastolic dysfunction includes delayed relaxation, impaired LV filling and/or increased stiffness. A slowing of the normal diastolic relaxation of the ventricle can in turn increase the left ventricular and left atrial pressures [20].

There are a number of causes, which lead to HFpEF. Age seems to be the dominant risk factor for HFpEF. Heart failure with preserved EF is exclusively a disease of elderly. As one ages, there is an increased collagen deposition with a reduction in the amount of elastin, which can lead to increased stiffness of the heart and blood vessels leading to ultimate HFpEF. Chronic hypertension, which is highly prevalent in HFpEF, leads to left ventricular hypertrophy and increased connective tissue content, both of which decrease cardiac compliance. Due to decreased compliance, in HFpEF LV functions on a steeper diastolic pressure-volume relationship compared with the normal ventricle. This leads to decreased LV end-diastolic volumes and a compensatory rise in LV filling pressure to maintain cardiac output. This high LV filling pressures lead to fluid accumulation in the lungs, which cause dyspnea, which is the common symptom of heart failure. As well as leading to symptoms of dyspnea, elevation in LV filling pressures produces secondary pulmonary hypertension and atrial remodeling that can predispose a patient to the development of right ventricular (RV) dysfunction and atrial fibrillation, respectively. Although epicardial coronary artery disease causing ischemic heart disease is less common in patients with HFpEF compared to HFrEF, subendocardial ischemia related to increased left ventricular diastolic pressures in a left ventricle with concentric remodeling is more common in patients with HFpEF. Multiple studies have shown an association between endothelial dysfunction and HFpEF and endothelial dysfunction was suggested to be as a prominent determinant of HFpEF [21]. Vascular stiffness is also an important contributor to pathophysiological process that leads to HFpEF. As a result of ventricular-arterial uncoupling, cardiac output decreases. Regardless of EF, ultimate decrease in cardiac output causes activation of neurohormonal mechanisms that lead to activation of vasoconstriction, salt and water retention and increased diastolic filling pressures [22]. HFpEF patients display neurohormonal profiles similar to HFrEF, with elevated circulating neurohormones, such as natriuretic peptides and norepinephrine [23].

Chronotropic incompetence (CI) is a potential pathophysiological factor in HFpEF, contributing to reduced exercise capacity. The increase in heart rate as a result of an activity or exercise is one of the two main contributors of increased cardiac output to meet the excess need of energy consumption. Moreover, the increase in HR is the strongest contributor to the ability to perform sustained aerobic exercise [24]. Phan et al. have shown that CI can be seen in patients with HFpEF during maximal exercise [25]. In this study, the prevalence of CI was 35% in HFpEF subjects. Chronotropic incompetence may be a significant contributor to severe, symptomatic exercise intolerance, which is the most common symptom in HFpEF. Atrial fibrillation (AF) is also common in patients with diastolic dysfunction and contributes to the pathophysiology of HFpEF. AF eliminates the late diastolic atrial contribution to LV filling, upon which patients with diastolic dysfunction are dependent and is poorly tolerated leading to both pulmonary edema and decreased cardiac output.

4. Diagnosis

The diagnosis of HFpEF is more challenging than the diagnosis of HFrEF. Part of the challenge is the fact that the HFpEF is a heterogeneous clinical entity, whose manifestations and outcomes remain difficult to be predicted. In essence, it's a diagnosis of exclusion. According to the recent ESC 2016 HF guideline [2], for the diagnosis of HFpEF, three essential criteria should be met. **Table 2** shows these criteria for diagnosis of HFpEF. As in HFrEF, HFpEF is a clinical diagnosis. Symptoms are often nonspecific and do not, therefore, help discriminate between HFpEF and HFrEF. Exercise dyspnea may be the only symptom with no detectable sign especially in the early stages of HFpEF. Exercise dyspnea is particularly difficult to interpret in elderly and in obese, comprising most of the HFrEF population. Objective evidence of reduced exercise capacity provided by cardiometabolic exercise testing with measurement of peak exercise oxygen consumption (VO_{2max}) or by the 6 min walking test can be used for judgment of exercise dyspnea in the context of HF symptom. Signs of congestive HF such as lung crepitations, pulmonary edema, jugular venous distention and ankle edema may not always be present, especially in the early stages. The "presence of signs or symptoms of congestive heart failure" as the first criterium for the diagnosis of HFpEF is therefore put instead of the "presence of signs and symptoms of congestive heart failure" [2].

Once a clinical diagnosis of HF has been made, the presence of HFpEF can be established by confirming a normal or near-normal LVEF, often by an echocardiogram. Echocardiography is an essential tool in evaluating patients with unexplained dyspnea. Bearing in mind that HFpEF is a diagnosis of exclusion, echocardiography should first provide information about the left ventricular systolic performance (commonly assessed using ejection fraction), valvular disease and pericardial disease. After exclusion of other possible explanations for HF, echocardiography should provide evidence of structural heart disease such as left ventricular hypertrophy, left atrial enlargement and pulmonary hypertension. Diastolic dysfunction can also be diagnosed further using the Doppler echocardiography (based on mitral inflow

1) Symptoms and/or signs of congestive heart failure
2) Non-dilated left ventricle (LV end-diastolic volume index (LVEDVI) < 97 mL/m²) with preserved ejection fraction (≥50%)
3) a) Elevated levels of natriuretic peptides b) At least one additional criterion i) Relevant structural heart disease (LVH and/or LAD) ii) Diastolic dysfunction

BNP, B-type natriuretic peptide; HFPEF, heart failure with preserved ejection fraction; LAD, left atrial dilation; LV, left ventricular; LVH, left ventricular hypertrophy.
a Signs may not be present in the early stages of HF (especially in HFpEF) and in patients treated with diuretics.
b BNP > 35 pg/ml and/or NT-proBNP > 125 pg/mL.

Table 2. Criteria for the diagnosis of HFPEF.

velocities). It is graded based on the ratio of the early, E, to late diastolic, inflow velocity, A (mild, moderate and severe) [26]. Grade I is abnormal relaxation pattern (E < A), grade II is pseudonormal pattern (E > A), grade III is restrictive pattern (E >> A) and grade IV is irreversible restrictive pattern [27]. The pseudonormal stage (grade II), which refers to a situation when filling pressures are elevated but the mitral inflow pattern appears normal, is creating a state of confusion. Assessment of pulmonary vein flow (PVF) velocity waveforms provide information complementary to that obtained from transmitral flow (TMF) patterns. Therefore, PVF pattern can be used to differentiate a normal from a pseudonormal TMF pattern. Grade III and grade IV diastolic dysfunctions are called restrictive filling dynamics. These are both severe forms of diastolic dysfunction and patients tend to have advanced HF symptoms at this stage.

Elevated LV filling pressures are the main and essential physiologic consequence of diastolic dysfunction. In the presence of symptoms and/or signs of HF and normal or near-normal EF, high LV filling pressures help a lot to put the diagnosis of HFpEF. Pulsed-Doppler-derived TMF is largely influenced by preload. Left ventricular filling pressures can also be estimated by myocardial tissue-Doppler-derived early diastolic annular velocity, designated E′ which is, to a large extent, regarded as a preload-independent index of diastolic performance. The use of tissue Doppler imaging-derived indices that correct for the influence of myocardial relaxation on the load-dependent early diastolic mitral flow E/E′ ratio (i.e., the ratio of mitral inflow, E, to early diastolic annular velocity, E′) as a means of estimating LV filling pressure is more reliable. Therefore, noninvasive diagnostic evidence of diastolic LV dysfunction is preferably derived from myocardial TD. If myocardial TD yields values E/E′ > 15, it puts diagnosis of high LV filling pressure. When the ratio is lower than 8, LV filling pressures are considered low. If TD yields an E/E′ ratio suggestive of LV diastolic dysfunction but not diagnostic (15 > E/E′ > 8), then additional echo variables are required for diagnostic evidence of LV diastolic dysfunction, which include Doppler flow profile of mitral valve or pulmonary veins, measurement of LV mass index (LVMi) or left atrium volume index (LAVi), electrocardiographic evidence of atrial fibrillation, or high levels of BNP or NT-proBNP. No single echocardiography variable is sufficiently accurate to be used in isolation to make a diagnosis of LV diastolic dysfunction. Therefore, a comprehensive echocardiography examination incorporating all relevant two- dimensional and Doppler data is recommended [2]. Invasive method of measuring filling pressure is more precise and yields higher diagnostic performance but not practical. Invasive diagnostic evidence of diastolic LV dysfunction can be obtained by LV end-diastolic pressure (LVEDP) or pulmonary capillary wedge pressure (PCWP). Filling pressures are considered elevated when the mean PCWP is >12 mm Hg or when the LVEDP is >16 mm Hg.

It is noteworthy that diastolic dysfunction is not always present in HFpEF, being observed by echocardiography in only two-thirds of patients at rest [28]. However, many patients with HFpEF display elevated LV filling pressures only during the stress of exercise, indicating an earlier stage of disease [29]. In such patients, the diagnosis of HFpEF could only be made using exercise hemodynamic evaluation using supine bicycle diastolic stress test. After stress, an increase in E/E′ and tricuspid regurgitation (TR) velocity indicating a high pulmonary artery systolic pressure can truly put the diagnosis of HFpEF [2].

Biomarkers have been recently used in the diagnostic workup of HF. BNP is synthesized and released upon LV wall stretch from increased pressure or volume. The plasma levels of BNP are raised in HF regardless of EF. However, natriuretic peptides (NPs) are less elevated in HFpEF compared to HFrEF. NPs are an important aid for the diagnosis of HF, especially in the non-acute setting when echocardiography is not immediately available. In the Breathing Not Properly study, BNP levels at the time of emergency admission were significantly elevated in HFpEF, when compared to other causes of dyspnea (median 413 vs. 34 pg/ml, $p < 0.001$) but significantly lower than in patients with HFrEF (median 413 vs. 821 pg/ml, $p < 0.001$) [30]. Many patients with HFpEF display elevated filling pressures only during exercise. This intermittent nature of pressure elevation is likely to explain the reduced BNP level observed in patients with HFpEF [31].

5. Challenges in the diagnosis of HFpEF

Diagnosis of HFpEF is more difficult than the diagnosis of HFREF because it is largely one of the exclusions, i.e., potential noncardiac causes of patients' symptoms (lung disease, anemia, chronic kidney disease, or obesity) that must first be eliminated. For most patients with a diagnosis of heart failure but preserved left ventricular systolic function based on symptoms and signs of HF which are highly nonspecific and normal EF, the diagnosis of HFpEF is rarely needed [5]. Before ascribing symptoms to HFpEF for which there is no evidence-based treatment, we should thoroughly investigate patient for other possible treatable causes of dyspnea with calculation of body mass index, pulmonary function testing, exercise electrocardiography and probably stress echocardiography.

The diagnostic criteria put forward for HFpEF has some important pitfalls. In HFpEF, exertional dyspnea is frequently the earliest symptom due to increased LV filling pressures ensuing some degree of pulmonary congestion. Since many patients with HFPEF present with dyspnea and no signs of fluid overload, exertional dyspnea was considered sufficient clinical evidence to suggest the presence of clinical heart failure in the recent guidelines [2]. Keeping in mind that dyspnea is a ubiquitous complaint especially in elderly and obese who represent a large proportion of HFpEF patients and other comorbid conditions such as chronic obstructive pulmonary disease and renal insufficiency which are usually present concomitant with HFpEF, dyspnea cannot be a reliable diagnostic criteria without objective evidence of reduced exercise performance provided by metabolic exercise testing. Meanwhile, because early signs and symptoms of HFpEF such as exercise dyspnea may also be the presenting symptoms of other alternative conditions or diseases, delayed diagnosis has also been a matter.

Diastolic dysfunction as assessed noninvasively by echocardiography is highly prevalent in elderly population who has no symptoms attributable to HF. This condition suggests some controversy regarding the accuracy of noninvasive measures of diastolic function by echocardiography [32]. Assessment should take into consideration patients' ages and heart rates (mitral E, E/A ratio and annular e′ decrease with increasing heart rate). Specifically, in older individuals without histories of cardiovascular disease, caution should be exercised before concluding that grade I diastolic dysfunction is present. Because the majority of subjects aged over 60 years without histories of cardiovascular disease have E/A ratios, <1 and E deceleration time (EDT) > 200 ms, such values in the absence of further indicators of LV dysfunction (e.g., LV hypertrophy and LA enlargement), can be considered normal for age. In other words, echocardiogram suggesting diastolic dysfunction on the basis of an abnormal E/A ratio is not diagnostic and represents insufficient investigation. Second, the echocardiographic markers of diastolic dysfunction may be absent in a significant proportion of patients diagnosed with HFpEF.

Natriuretic peptides could give inconclusive results in a number of situations. In normal individuals, the concentration of NT-proBNP rises with age and is higher in women than in men [33]. Therefore, age-stratified cutoff points for NT-proBNP (≥450 for ages < 50 years, ≥900 for 50–75 years and ≥1800 pg/mL for >75 years) were shown to perform the best diagnostic performance for rule in acute HF setting [34]. Beyond HF, a number of cardiopulmonary disorders are also associated with elevated BNP or NT-proBNP values: acute coronary syndrome, myocarditis, valvular heart disease, hypertrophic cardiomyopathy, cardiotoxic drugs, atrial fibrillation, or flutter and right ventricular dysfunction in the setting of significant pulmonary disease (pulmonary hypertension, pulmonary embolism). Other conditions that are associated with higher BNP or NT-proBNP levels may be related to comorbidities such as advanced age, renal dysfunction, stroke, sepsis and other high output states. It should be kept in mind that plasma levels of BNP rise independently of LV filling pressures once glomerular filtration rate falls below 60 mL/min because renal dysfunction is highly prevalent in HFpEF population. AF also confounds the utility of BNP for diagnosing HFpEF [35, 36].

6. Treatment

Prevention of HFpEF through treatment of risk factors (e.g., hypertension, diabetes and coronary artery disease) especially at early stages is effective and still the most important part of management of HFpEF since specific treatments are yet to be discovered [37]. Hypertension antedates the development of HFpEF in nearly 90% of the cases and it confers a two- to threefold increased risk of developing HFpEF [38]. Therefore, strict control of hypertension will inevitably prevent development of HFpEF. Improving cardiorespiratory fitness among low-fit sedentary individuals by exercise training could be another preventive approach against HFpEF. And, targeting obesity in the early childhood will also prevent development of HFpEF in the future.

As a non-pharmacologic therapy, exercise training has clearly been shown to benefit cardiorespiratory health in patients with HFrEF. Recent studies have addressed the effects of exercise training in patients with HFpEF. Although the effects on HF-related mortality and hospitalizations were not studied, these reports showed that moderate supervised exercise program had positive effects on the quality of life, exercise tolerance but not left ventricular EF [39, 40]. No pharmacologic therapy has been shown to be effective in improving outcomes in patients with heart failure with HFpEF. There is no single explanation for the negative results of past HFpEF trials. Potential contributors include an incomplete understanding of HFpEF pathophysiology, inadequate diagnostic criteria, recruitment of patients without true HF or at early stages of the syndrome, poor matching of therapeutic mechanisms and primary pathophysiological processes, suboptimal study designs, inadequate statistical power, or patient heterogeneity [41]. Another possible explanation is the fact that non-cardiovascular mortality is higher in HFpEF than HFrEF highlighting one of the difficulties in the development of an effective therapeutic strategy in the overall patients with HFpEF.

The treatment recommendations from the American Heart Association have set four goals in the management of these patients: (a) control of hypertension, (b) control of heart rate especially in the patients with atrial fibrillation, (c) control of pulmonary and peripheral edema and (d) prevention of myocardial ischemia [1]. 2013 ACC/AHA Guideline on HF had only two class I recommendations for HFpEF treatment. One of them is the use of diuretics in order to reduce volume overload and improve dyspnea. The second one is the control of blood pressure. The guideline also recommends revascularization in patients whom symptoms or demonstrable ischemia are thought to contribute HF symptoms as class II recommendation. Management of AF is another class II recommendation of the American guideline. The guideline does not underscore rhythm control or rate control in HFpEF since there was no specific trial comparing these two strategies in HFpEF until now. The recent 2016 European Society of Cardiology (ESC) Guideline could not make any further recommendations on top of 2013 American guideline in this regard except recommending screening patients with HFpEF for both cardiovascular and non-cardiovascular comorbidities, which then should be treated accordingly [2].

Table 3 summarizes the major clinical trials that have evaluated the efficacy of various therapeutic drugs in patients with HFpEF. The renin-angiotensin-aldosterone system (RAAS) is involved in many of the pathophysiological processes associated with this disease (including hypertension, left ventricular hypertrophy, myocardial fibrosis and vascular dysfunction) and inhibitors of this system can prevent neurohormonal activation and prevent ventricular remodeling [22]. RAAS blockers have been long time investigated whether they could be effective therapeutic option for these patients. Three large trials have evaluated inhibitors of the RAAS in patients with HFpEF but none of them proved to be beneficial. The Candesartan in Heart Failure: Assessment of Reduction in Mortality and Morbidity (CHARM)-preserved trial evaluated the effect of candesartan on elderly patients with HFpEF [42]. Candesartan showed no significant reduction of cardiovascular death but showed significant reduction in HF hospitalization. The Perindopril in Elderly People with Chronic Heart Failure (PEP-CHF) trial was a randomized placebo-controlled trial which evaluated the effect of perindopril on patients with HFpEF [43]. At the end of the study, perindopril showed no significant effect on mortality, but showed significant benefit in unplanned HF hospitalization in 1 year. The Irbesartan in Heart Failure with Preserved Ejection Fraction Study (I-PRESERVE) investigated the effect of the angiotensin-receptor blocker irbesartan on mortality and cardiovascular morbidity in patients with HFpEF [44]. Treatment with irbesartan did not reduce the risk of death or hospitalization for cardiovascular causes among HFpEF patients nor did it improve any of the secondary clinical outcomes, including disease-specific quality of life.

The Study of the Effects of Nebivolol Intervention on Outcomes and Rehospitalization in Seniors (SENIORS) with Heart Failure, which consist of both HFrEF and HFpEF patients,

Trial	Year	Intervention	No. of subjects	Key inclusion criteria	Key exclusion criteria	Outcome(s)	Findings
CHARM-preserved	2003	Candesartan versus placebo	3023	Age > 18 years LVEF > 40% NYHA class II–IV	Persistent systolic or diastolic hypertension	Hospitalization Mortality	No effect on mortality Slight reduction in HF hospitalization
PEP-CHF	2006	Perindopril versus placebo	846	>40%		Rehospitalization at 1 year Mortality	No effect on mortality Decreased 1 year rehospitalization and increased exercise capacity
SENIORS	2006	Nebivolol versus placebo	752	>35%		CV-related hospitalization Mortality	No effect on mortality or hospitalization in patients with EF > 40%
I-PRESERVE	2008	Irbesartan versus placebo	4128	Age > 60 years LVEF > 45% NYHA class II–IV and HF hospitalization < 6 months or NYHA class III/IV and abnormal CXR, ECG, or echocardiogram	AF with resting heart rate > 120 beats/min Cor pulmonale Clinically significant pulmonary disease Significant valvular disease Hb < 11 g/dl BP > 160/95 mm Hg despite therapy	Mortality Hospitalization	No effect on mortality or CV hospitalization
ALDO-DHF	2013	Spironolactone versus placebo	422	Age > 50 LVEF > 50% NYHA class II or III Echo evidence of diastolic dysfunction (grade ≥I) Atrial fibrillation at presentation, maximum exercise capacity (peak VO_2) < 25 mL/kg/min	Significant CAD Significant pulmonary disease GFR < 30 ml/min MI or CABG in past 3 months	Improvement in diastolic function (E/e′) And maximal exercise capacity (VO_2)	Improved diastolic function Induced reverse remodeling Improved neuroendocrine activation but not improve heart failure symptoms or quality of life and slightly reduced 6 min walk distance

Trial	Year	Intervention	No. of subjects	Key inclusion criteria	Key exclusion criteria	Outcome(s)	Findings
TOPCAT	2014	Spironolactone versus placebo	3445	Age > 50 LVEF > 45% ≥1 HF hospitalization in the previous 12 months or BNP ≥100 pg/mL or NT-proBNP ≥360 pg/mL Controlled systolic blood pressure asystolic blood pressure < 140 mm Hg or 140 to 160 mm Hg if on ≥3 antihypertensive medications	COPD Infiltrative of hypertrophic CMP Significant valve disease AF with resting heart rate >90 beats/min GFR < 30 ml/min MI or CABG in past 3 months PCI in past 30 days	Death from cardiovascular causes Aborted cardiac arrest Hospitalization for HF	No effect on cardiovascular death Reduced HF hospitalization Induced an increase in serum creatinine and potassium levels
PARAMOUNT	2012	LCZ 696 versus valsartan	301	Age > 40 years EF > 45%, NYHA class II and III, Elevations of NT-proBNP > 400 pg/ml	LVEF < 45% Isolated right heart failure owing to pulmonary disease Dyspnea from non cardiac causes GFR < 30 ml/min Primary valvular or myocardial diseases Coronary or cerebrovascular diseases needing revascularization within 3 months	Reduction in NT-proBNP at 12 weeks NYHA functional class and LA dimension at 36 weeks	Reduced natriuretic peptides at 12 weeks Improved NYHA class and improved left atrial dimensions at 36 weeks

Trial	Year	Intervention	No. of subjects	Key inclusion criteria	Key exclusion criteria	Outcome(s)	Findings
RELAX HF	2013	versus placebo	**216**	LVEF > 45% NYHA II–IV Previous hospitalization for HF Increased pro NT-pro BNPİ or invasively measured high filling pressure Peak $VO_2 < 60\%$	Any obstacle for exercise testing Need for nitrate therapy Primary pulmonary Arteriopathy Primary valve disease Other causes of dyspnea	Exercise capacity Clinical status	No effect on exercise capacity or clinical status

All abbreviations are explained in the text of the manuscript.

Table 3. Major clinical trials in patients with HFPEF.

showed that a beta1-blocker with nitric oxide-potentiating vasodilatory effect, nebivolol, reduces hospitalization in older HF patients with preserved and reduced EF but had no effect on mortality [45]. Preserved EF was considered as EF > 35% which constitutes 35% of the overall study population. The proportion of patients with truly preserved EF (>50%) was very small. Therefore, although the overall study suggests a modest benefit of nebivolol, the results can't be extrapolated to true HFpEF patients.

The mineralocorticoid receptor antagonists spironolactone and eplerenone have been shown to reduce total and cardiovascular mortality across the spectrum of HFrEF and in patients with acute myocardial infarction complicated by left ventricular dysfunction and heart failure [46–48]. By reducing cardiac fibrosis and hypertrophy, aldosterone antagonists have the potential to be beneficial in heart failure with preserved ejection fraction (HFpEF) [49]. In the Aldosterone Receptor Blockade in Diastolic Heart Failure (Aldo-DHF) trial, the effect of spironolactone on diastolic function and exercise capacity in patients with HFpEF was tested [50]. The left ventricular end-diastolic filling, left ventricular remodeling (LV mass index decreased but LA diameter not changed) and neurohumoral activation (NT pro-BNP decreased) were improved with spironolactone, demonstrating aldosterone effect on improving diastolic function and reversing cardiac remodeling. However, spironolactone had no effect on functional exercise capacity in this trial. Upon positive findings with spironolactone on diastolic function and cardiac remodeling, the Treatment of Preserved Cardiac Function Heart Failure with an Aldosterone Antagonist (TOPCAT) trial was planned to investigate whether treatment with spironolactone would reduce morbidity and mortality in patients with HFpEF [51]. The TOPCAT trial found that, compared to placebo, spironolactone did not reduce the composite of cardiovascular death, aborted cardiac arrest or heart failure hospitalization in patients with HFpEF but reduced the individual component of heart failure hospitalization. However, there was a significant interaction between treatment effect and patient recruitment strategy (natriuretic peptides vs. hospitalization with HF). In patients recruited based on previous hospitalization, spironolactone had no effect on outcome, whereas in patients recruited based on high BNP, spironolactone showed a benefit. This difference highlights the importance of patient selection criteria and recruitment of patients with true HFpEF for future trials. The efficacy of eplerenone on 6 min walking distance was evaluated in a single-center, randomized study. It was found that after 24 weeks of eplerenone treatment, there was no change in 6 min walk distance [52]. Another randomized, clinical study evaluated the effect of eplerenone on the primary outcome comprising of death from cardiovascular causes, nonfatal reinfarction, hospitalization for unstable angina, or decompensation of heart failure [53]. Eplerenone was found to have no significant effect on the primary outcome.

Phosphodiesterase-5 (PDE-5) metabolizes the nitric oxide and natriuretic peptide systems' second messenger cyclic guanosine monophosphate and thus may limit beneficial nitric oxide and natriuretic peptide actions in the heart, vasculature and kidneys. Phosphodiesterase type 5 inhibitors (PDE5I) increase cGMP levels by blocking their catabolism. PDE5I may reduce ventricular-vascular stiffening, antagonize maladaptive chamber remodeling, improve endothelial function, reduce pulmonary vascular resistance and enhance renal responsiveness to natriuretic peptides [54, 55]. Phosphodiesterase type 5 inhibitor, sildenafil, was proved to improve hemodynamic parameters in HFrEF patients [56]. The Phosphodiesterase-5

Inhibition to Improve Clinical Status and Exercise Capacity in Heart Failure with Preserved Ejection Fraction (RELAX) trial was conducted to investigate the effect of the PDE-5 inhibitor, on exercise capacity in HFpEF [57]. At the end of 24 weeks, long-term PDE-5 inhibition in HFpEF had no effect on maximal or submaximal exercise capacity, clinical status, quality of life, left ventricular remodeling, diastolic function parameters, or pulmonary artery systolic pressure.

It is known that in both the failing heart and in case of ischemia, the late sodium current is increased, leading to an Na+ accumulation in cardiac myocytes [58]. The increased Na+ concentration reverses the mode direction of the Na+/Ca2+exchanger, contributing to a Ca2+ overload in the cell. Increased diastolic Ca2+ impairs relaxation leading to diastolic dysfunction. By inhibiting the late Na+ channel, ranolazine is theoretically expected to prevent (or reduce) sodium accumulation in the myocyte. This should improve calcium extrusion through the Na+/Ca2+ exchanger and thereby improve relaxation of the myocardium. The Ranolazine for the Treatment of Diastolic Heart Failure (RALI-DHF) study was designed to evaluate the effect of ranolazine versus placebo on hemodynamics, measures of diastolic dysfunction and biomarkers in 20 patients with HFpEF [59]. After 30 min of infusion, significant decreases from baseline were observed in LVEDP and PCWP in the ranolazine group, but not in the placebo group. However, ranolazine had no effect on invasively determined relaxation parameters and the noninvasive E/E′ ratio.

In the recent PARADIGM-HF trial, the patients taking LCZ 696 showed steep reduction in the primary endpoint of CV death/heart failure hospitalization [60]. McMurray et al. noted that a subgroup of patients in the reduced EF spectrum's high end, i.e., LVEF approaching 40%, also benefits to the same extent as the overall study group [61]. Solomon et al. conducted prospective comparison of Angiotensin Receptor Neprilysin Inhibitor (ARNi) with Angiotensin Receptor Blocker (ARB) on Management of heart failure with preserved ejection fraction, PARAMOUNT trial, a double-blind randomized trial in 301 patients with heart failure with HFpEF, which compared LCZ696 with valsartan [62]. The primary endpoint, the decline in NT-proBNP, was significantly greater in the LCZ696 group than in the valsartan group. After 36 weeks, both left atrial volume and dimension, which reflect left ventricular filling pressure, also declined more with LCZ696 and there was greater improvement in the New York Heart Association (NYHA) functional class with LCZ696 than with valsartan.

These encouraging results with LCZ696 have provided the rationale for a large outcomes trial in HFpEF. Prospective Comparison of ARNI with ARB Global Outcomes in Heart Failure with Preserved Ejection Fraction (PARAGON-HF) will use a similar overall study design to that of PARAMOUNT to determine whether LCZ696 can reduce cardiovascular death or total HF hospitalizations in patients with HFpEF. PARAGON-HF will enroll 4,300 patients with HFpEF until the end of 2016.

7. Future perspectives

Diagnosis of HFpEF should only be made after complete workup and if noninvasive diagnostic data comprising of LA dilation, diastolic dysfunction and high natriuretic peptide levels, or invasively measured high LVEDP or PCWP proves indisputably the presence of high LV filling pressure. Only when more specific diagnostic criteria have emerged over time and started to be used in the clinical trials for patient recruitment, we will see improvements in outcome for this common and growing form of cardiac disease. The strategy of a tailored "precision" approach considering both the comorbidities concomitant with HFpEF and underlying pathophysiologic mechanism of reduced cardiac and vascular reserve will lead to improvement in prognosis of HFpEF.

Author details

Hakan Altay* and Seckin Pehlivanoglu

*Address all correspondence to: sakaltay@yahoo.com

Cardiology Department, Faculty of Medicine, Baskent University, Istanbul Hospital, Turkey

References

[1] Yancy CW, Jessup M, Wright RS, et al. ACCF/AHA guideline for the management of heart failure: a report of the American College of Cardiology Foundation/American Heart Association Task Force on practice guidelines. *Circulation*. 2013;128(16):e240–e327.

[2] Ponikowski P, Voors AA, Anker SD, Bueno H, Cleland JG, Coats AJ, Falk V, González-Juanatey JR, Harjola VP, Jankowska EA, Jessup M, Linde C, Nihoyannopoulos P, Parissis JT, Pieske B, Riley JP, Rosano GM, Ruilope LM, Ruschitzka F, Rutten FH, van der Meer P; Authors/Task Force Members; Document Reviewers. 2016 ESC guidelines for the diagnosis and treatment of acute and chronic heart failure: the task force for the diagnosis and treatment of acute and chronic heart failure of the European Society of Cardiology (ESC). Developed with the special contribution of the Heart Failure Association (HFA) of the ESC. *Eur J Heart Fail*. 2016;18(8):891–975.

[3] Senni M, Tribouilloy CM, Rodeheffer RJ, Jacobsen SJ, Evans JM, Bailey KR, Redfield MM. Congestive heart failure in the community: a study of all incident cases in Olmsted county, Minnesota, in 1991. *Circulation*. 1998;98:2282–2289.

[4] Owan TE, Hodge DO, Herges RM, Jacobsen SJ, Roger VL, Redfield MM. Trends in prevalence and outcome of heart failure with preserved ejection fraction. *N Engl J Med*. 2006;355:251–259.

[5] Caruana L, Petrie MC, Davie AP, McMurray JJ. Do patients with suspected heart failure and preserved left ventricular systolic function suffer from "diastolic heart failure" or from misdiagnosis? A prospective descriptive study. *BMJ*. 2000;321:215–219.

[6] Bhatia RS, Tu JV, Lee DS, Austin PC, Fang J, Haouzi A, Gong Y, Liu PP. Outcome of heart failure with preserved ejection fraction in a population- based study. *N Engl J Med*. 2006;355:260–269.

[7] Bursi F., et al. Systolic and diastolic heart failure in the community. *JAMA*. 2006; 296:2209–2216.

[8] Owan TE, Hodge DO, Davie AP, et al. Epidemiology of chronic heart failure. *Prog Cardiovasc Dis*. 2005;47:320–332.

[9] Ceia F, Fonseca C, Mota T, Morais H, Matias F, de Sousa A, et al. Prevalence of chronic heart failure in southwestern Europe: the EPICA study. *Eur J Heart Fail*. 2002;4:531–539. This study reports the prevalence of HFpEF in Portuguese reporting a higher prevalence than HFrEF.

[10] Hogg K, Swedberg K, McMurray JJ. Heart failure with preserved left ventricular systolic function; epidemiology, clinical characteristics and prognosis. *J Am Coll Cardiol*. 2004;43:317–327.

[11] Lenzen MJ, Scholte op Reimer WJ, Boersma E, et al. Differences between patients with a preserved and a depressed left ventricular function: a report from the EuroHeart Failure Survey. *Eur Heart J*. 2004;25:1214–1220.

[12] Solomon SD, Wang D, Finn P, Skali H, Zornoff L, McMurray JJV, Swedberg K, Yusuf S, Granger CB, Michelson EL, Pocock S, Pfeffer MA. Effect of candesartan on cause-specific mortality in heart failure patients: the Candesartan in Heart Failure Assessment of Reduction in Mortality and Morbidity (CHARM) program. *Circulation*. 2004;110:2180–2183.

[13] Zile MR, Gaasch WH, Anand IS, et al. Mode of death in patients with heart failure and a preserved ejection fraction: results from the Irbesartan in heart failure with preserved ejection fraction study (I-Preserve) trial. *Circulation*. 2010;121:1393–1405.

[14] Poole-Wilson PA, Uretsky BF, Thygesen K, Cleland JGF, Massie BM, Rydén L. Mode of death in heart failure: findings from the ATLAS trial. *Heart*. 2003;89:42–48.

[15] Hamaguchi S, Kinugawa S, Sobirin MA, Goto D, Tsuchihashi-Makaya M, Yamada S, et al. Mode of death in patients with heart failure and reduced versus preserved ejection fraction: report from the registry of hospitalized heart failure patients. *Circ J*. 2012;76(7):1662–1669.

[16] Campbell RT, Jhund PS, Castagno D, Hawkins NM, Petrie MC, McMurray JJ. What have we learned about patients with heart failure and preserved ejection fraction from DIG-PEF, CHARM-preserved and I-PRESERVE? *J'Coll Cardiol*. 2012;60(23):2349–2356.

[17] Yancy CW, Lopatin M, Stevenson LW, De Marco T, Fonarow GC. Clinical presentation, management and in-hospital outcomes of patients admitted with acute decompensated heart failure with pre-served systolic function: a report from the Acute Decompensated Heart Failure National Registry (ADHERE) database. *J Am Coll Cardiol*. 2006;47(1):76–84.

[18] Kass DA, Bronzwaer JG, Paulus WJ. What mechanisms underlie diastolic dysfunction in heart failure? *Circ Res*. 2004;94:1533–1542.

[19] Borlaug BA, Kass DA. Mechanisms of diastolic dysfunction in heart failure. *Trends Cardiovasc Med*. 2006;16:273–279.

[20] Oxenham HC, Young AA, Cowan BR, et al. Age related changes in myocardial relaxation using three dimensional tagged magnetic resonance imaging. *J Cardiovasc Magn Reson*. 2003;5:421–430.

[21] Paulus WJ, Tschope C. A novel paradigm for heart failure with preserved ejection fraction: comorbidities drive myocardial dysfunction and remodeling through coronary microvascular endothelial inflammation. *J Am Coll Cardiol*. 2013;62:263–271.

[22] Hogg K, McMurray J. Neurohumoral pathways in heart failure with preserved systolic function. *Prog Cardiovasc Dis*. 2005;47:357–366.

[23] Kitzman DW, Little WC, Brubaker PH, et al. Pathophysiological characterization of isolated diastolic heart failure in comparison to systolic heart failure. *JAMA*. 2002;288:2144–2150.

[24] Higginbotham MB, Morris KG, Williams RS, McHale PA, Coleman RD, Cobb FR. Regulation of stroke volume during submaximal and maximal upright exercise in normal man. *Circ Res*. 1986;58:281–291.

[25] Phan TT, Shivu GN, Abozuia K, et al. Impaired heart rate recovery and chronotropic incompetence in patients with heart failure with pre- served ejection fraction. *Circ Heart Fail*. 2010;3:29–34.

[26] Nagueh SF, Appleton CP, Gillebert TC, et al. Recommendations for the evaluation of left ventricular diastolic function by echocardiography. *J Am Soc Echocardiogr*. 2009;22(2):107–133.

[27] Murata K. Predictive significance of evaluation of left ventricular diastolic function in patients with heart failure. *Rinsho Byoki*. 2010;58:792–798.

[28] Shah AM, et al. Cardiac structure and function in heart failure with preserved ejection fraction: baseline findings from the echocardiographic study of the treatment of preserved cardiac function heart failure with an aldosterone antagonist trial. *Circ Heart Fail*. 2014;7:104–115.

[29] Borlaug BA, Nishimura RA, Sorajja P, Lam CS, Redfield MM. Exercise hemodynamics enhance diagnosis of early heart failure with preserved ejection fraction. *Circ Heart Fail*.2010;3:588–595.

[30] Maisel AS, McCord J, Nowak RM, et al. Bedside B type natriuretic peptide in the emergency diagnosis of heart failure with reduced or preserved ejection fraction. Results from the Breathing Not Properly Multinational Study. *J Am Coll Cardiol*. 2003;41:2010–2017.

[31] Anjan VY, et al. Prevalence, clinical phenotype and outcomes associated with normal B-type natriuretic peptide levels in heart failure with preserved ejection fraction. *Am J Cardiol*. 2012;110:870–876.

[32] Tschöpe C, Paulus WJ. Doppler echocardiography yields dubious estimates of left ventricular diastolic pressures. *Circulation*. 2009;120:810–820.

[33] McDonagh TA, Holmer S, Raymond I, Luchner A, Hildebrant P, Dargie HJ. NT-proBNP and the diagnosis of heart failure: a pooled analysis of three European epidemiological studies. *Eur J Heart Fail*. 2004;6:269–273.

[34] Januzzi JL, van Kimmenade R, Lainchbury J, et al. NT-proBNP testing for diagnosis and short-term prognosis in acute destabilized heart failure: an international pooled analysis of 1256 patients: The International Collaborative of NT-proBNP Study. *Eur Heart J*. 2006;27:330–337.

[35] Tsutamoto T, Wada A, Sakai H, Ishikawa C, Tanaka T, Hayashi M, Fujii M, Yamamoto T, Dohke T, Ohnishi M, Takashima H, Kinoshita M, Horie M. Relationship between renal function and plasma brain natriuretic peptide in patients with heart failure. *J Am Coll Cardiol*. 2006;47:582–586.

[36] Knudsen CW, Omland T, Clopton P, et al. Impact of atrial fibrillation on the diagnostic performance of Btype natriuretic peptide concentration in dyspneic patients: an analysis from the breathing not properly multinational study. *J Am Coll Cardiol*. 2005;46(5):838–844.

[37] Schocken DD, Benjamin EJ, Fonarow GC, Krumholz HM, Levy D, Mensah GA, Narula J, Shor ES, Young JB, Hong Y. Prevention of heart failure: a scientific statement from the American Heart Association Councils on Epidemiology and Prevention, Clinical Cardiology, Cardiovascular Nursing and High Blood Pressure Research; Quality of Care and Outcomes Research Interdisciplinary Working Group; and Functional Genomics and Translational Biology Interdisciplinary Working Group. *Circulation*. 2008;117:2544–2565.

[38] Chobanian AV, Bakris GL, Black HR, Cushman WC, Green LA, Izzo Jr JL, et al. The seventh report of the joint national committee on prevention, detection, evaluation and treatment of high blood pressure: the JNC 7 report. *JAMA*. 2003;289:2560–2572.

[39] Kitzman DW, Brubaker PH, Morgan TM, Stewart KP, Little WC. Exercise training in older patients with heart failure and preserved ejection fraction: a randomized, controlled, single-blind trial. *Circ Heart Fail*. 2010;3:659–667.

[40] Kitzman DW, Brubaker PH, Herrington DM, Morgan TM, Stewart KP, Hundley WG, et al. Effect of endurance exercise training on endothelial function and arterial stiffness in older patients with heart failure and preserved ejection fraction: a randomized, controlled, single-blind trial. *J Am Coll Cardiol*. 2013;62:584–592.

[41] Paulus WJ, van Ballegoij JJ. Treatment of heart failure with normal ejection fraction: an inconvenient truth! *J Am Coll Cardiol*. 2010;55:526–537.

[42] Yusuf S, Pfeffer MA, Swedberg K, et al. Effects of candesartan in patients with chronic heart failure and preserved left-ventricular ejection fraction: the CHARM-preserved trial. *Lancet*. 2003;362:777–781.

[43] Cleland JG, Tendera M, Adamus J, Freemantle N, Polonski L, Taylor J. The perindopril in elderly people with chronic heart failure (PEP-CHF) study. *Eur Heart J*. 2006;27:2338–2345.

[44] Massie BM, Carson PE, McMurray JJ, Komajda M, McKelvie R, Zile MR anderson S, Donovan M, Iverson E, Staiger C, Ptaszynska A; I-PRESERVE Investigators. Irbesartan in patients with heart failure and preserved ejection fraction. *N Engl J Med*. 2008;359(23):2456–2467.

[45] Flather MD, Shibata MC, Coats AJ, Van Veldhuisen DJ, Parkhomenko A, Borbola J, et al. Randomized trial to determine the effect of nebivolol on mortality and cardiovascular hospital admission in elderly patients with heart failure (SENIORS). *Eur Heart J*. 2005;26:215–225.

[46] Pitt B, Zannad F, Remme WJ, et al.; Randomized Aldactone Evaluation Study Investigators. The effect of spironolactone on morbidity and mortality in patients with severe heart failure. *N Engl J Med*. 1999;341(10):709–717.

[47] Zannad F, McMurray JJ, Krum H, et al.; EMPHASIS-HF Study Group. Eplerenone in patients with systolic heart failure and mild symptoms. *N Engl J Med*. 2011;364(1):11–21.

[48] Pitt B, Remme W, Zannad F, et al.; Eplerenone Post-Acute Myocardial Infarction Heart Failure Efficacy and Survival Study Investigators. Eplerenone, a selective aldosterone blocker, in patients with left ventricular dysfunction after myocardial infarction. *N Engl J Med*. 2003;348(14):1309–1321.

[49] Lacolley P, Safar ME, Lucet B, Ledudal K, Labat C, Benetos A. Prevention of aortic and cardiac fibrosis by spironolactone in old normotensive rats. *J Am Coll Cardiol*. 2001;37:662–667.

[50] Edelmann F, Schmidt AG, Gelbrich G, et al. Rationale and design of the "Aldosterone Receptor Blockade in Diastolic Heart Failure" trial: a double-blind, randomized, placebo-controlled, parallel group study to determine the effects of spironolactone on exercise capacity and diastolic function in patients with symptomatic diastolic heart failure (Aldo-DHF). *Eur J Heart Fail*. 2010;12(8):874–882.

[51] Pitt B, Pfeffer MA, Assmann SF, Boineau R, Anand IS, Claggett B, Clausell N, Desai AS, Diaz R, Fleg JL, Gordeev I, Harty B, Heitner JF, Kenwood CT, Lewis EF, O'Meara E, Probstfield JL, Shaburishvili T, Shah SJ, Solomon SD, Sweitzer MK, Yang S, McKinlay SM. Spironolactone for heart failure with preserved ejection fraction. *N Engl J Med*. 2014;370:1383–1392.

[52] Deswal A, Richardson P, Bozkurt B, Mann DL. Results of the randomized aldosterone antagonism in heart failure with preserved ejection fraction trial (RAAM-PEF). *J Card Fail*. 2011;17:634–642.

[53] Kampourides K, Tziakas D, Chalikias G, et al. Usefulness of matrix metalloproteinase-9 plasma levels to identify patients with preserved left ventricular systolic function after acute myocardial infarction who could benefit from eplerenone. *Am J Cardiol*. 2012;110:1085–1091.

[54] Vlachopoulos C, Hirata K, O'Rourke MF. Effect of on arterial stiffness and wave reflection. *Vasc Med*. 2003;8:243–248.

[55] Katz SD, Balidemaj K, Homma S, Wu H, Wang J, Maybaum S. Acute type 5 phosphodiesterase inhibition with enhances flow-mediated vasodilation in patients with chronic heart failure. *J Am Coll Cardiol*. 2000;36:845–851.

[56] Lewis GD, Shah R, Shahzad K, et al. improves exercise capacity and quality of life in patients with systolic heart failure and secondary pulmonary hypertension. *Circulation*. 2007;116(14):1555–1562.

[57] Redfield MM, Chen HH, Borlaug BA, Semigran MJ, Lee KL, Lewis G, LeWinter MM, Rouleau JL, Bull DA, Mann DL, Deswal A, Stevenson LW, Givertz MM, Ofili EO, O'Connor CM, Felker GM, Goldsmith SR, Bart BA, McNulty SE, Ibarra JC, Lin G, Oh JK, Patel MR, Kim RJ, Tracy RP, Velazquez EJ, Anstrom KJ, Hernandez AF, Mascette AM, Braunwald E; RELAX Trial. Effect of phosphodiesterase-5 inhibition on exercise capacity and clinical status in heart failure with preserved ejection fraction: a randomized clinical trial. *JAMA*. 2013;309(12):1268–1277

[58] Valdivia CR, Chu WW, Pu J, et al. Increased late sodium current in myocytes from a canine heart failure model and from failing human heart. *J Mol Cell Cardiol*. 2005;38:475–483.

[59] Acobshagen C, Belardinelli L, Hasenfuss G, Maier LS. Ranolazine for the treatment of heart failure with preserved ejection fraction: background, aims and design of the RALI-DHF study. *Clin Cardiol*. 2011;34:426–432.

[60] McMurray JJ, Packer M, Desai AS, Gong J, Lefkowitz MP, Rizkala AR, Rouleau JL, Shi VC, Solomon SD, Swedberg K, Zile MR; PARADIGM-HF Investigators and Committees. Angiotensin-neprilysin inhibition versus enalapril in heart failure. *N Engl J Med*. 2014;371:993–1004.

[61] Solomon S, Packer M, Zile M, et al. The angiotensin receptor neprilysin inhibitor LCZ696 is effective across the spectrum of ejection fraction in heart failure with reduced ejection fraction. *J Card Fail*. 2015;21:S45.

[62] Solomon SD, Zile M, Pieske B, et al.; for the Prospective comparison of ARNI with ARB on Management Of heart failUre with preserved ejectioN fracTion (PARAMOUNT) Investigators. The angiotensin receptor neprilysin inhibitor LCZ696 in heart failure with preserved ejection fraction: a phase 2 double-blind randomized controlled trial. *Lancet*. 2012;380:1387–1395.

4

Takotsubo Cardiomyopathy as a Neurocardiogenic Injury after Subarachnoid Hemorrhage: Hemodynamics and Fluid Management

Tatsushi Mutoh, Tomoko Mutoh, Yasuyuki Taki and Tatsuya Ishikawa

Abstract

Takotsubo cardiomyopathy (TCM) is a life-threatening systemic disorder that may occur early after aneurysmal subarachnoid hemorrhage (SAH), but precise hemodynamics and fluid management remain unclear. Although TCM is often regarded as a reversible or self-limited phenomenon, it contributes significantly to morbidity and mortality of SAH patients, especially when it is complicated with other neurogenic injuries such as severe left ventricular dysfunction, pulmonary edema, and pneumonia. The purpose of this chapter is to introduce the current practice in intensive hemodynamic monitoring and goal-directed fluid management of post-SAH TCM using advanced hemodynamic devices based on our institutional protocol and the relevant literature and to evaluate their effects on clinical outcomes.

Keywords: Takotsubo cardiomyopathy, neurogenic stress cardiomyopathy, fluid therapy, pulmonary edema, subarachnoid hemorrhage

1. Introduction

Postoperative management of aneurysmal subarachnoid hemorrhage (SAH) is sometimes complicated by systemic cardiopulmonary complications to affect a significant impact on the morbidity and mortality of the patients [1, 2]. The neuro-cardiac injury of SAH is of particular importance because of their impact on the ability to manage blood pressure and volume status, especially in the setting of cerebral vasospasm or delayed cerebral ischemia (DCI). The pattern of injury produced is commonly referred to as neurogenic stress cardiomyopathy [3]. One distinct morphological variant of stress cardiomyopathy is Takotsubo cardiomyopathy (TCM), which was first described by the Japanese physician in the early 1990s to be a reversible cardiomyopathy, the shape of which named after an octopus trap used by the native fishermen [4]. Although TCM is typically associated with acute emotional stress in postmenopausal women [5], triggers may also include physical stressors such as head trauma, intracranial bleeding, ischemic stroke, medical, and surgical procedures and catecholaminergic drugs [6]. Previous reports suggest the demographics and clinical characteristics of TCM are similar irrespective of their etiologies. However, there are notable differences in post-SAH TCM from other non-neurologic stressors in that the patients tended to be younger and more frequent in females than what is typically reported and had high in-hospital mortality (25%) [7].

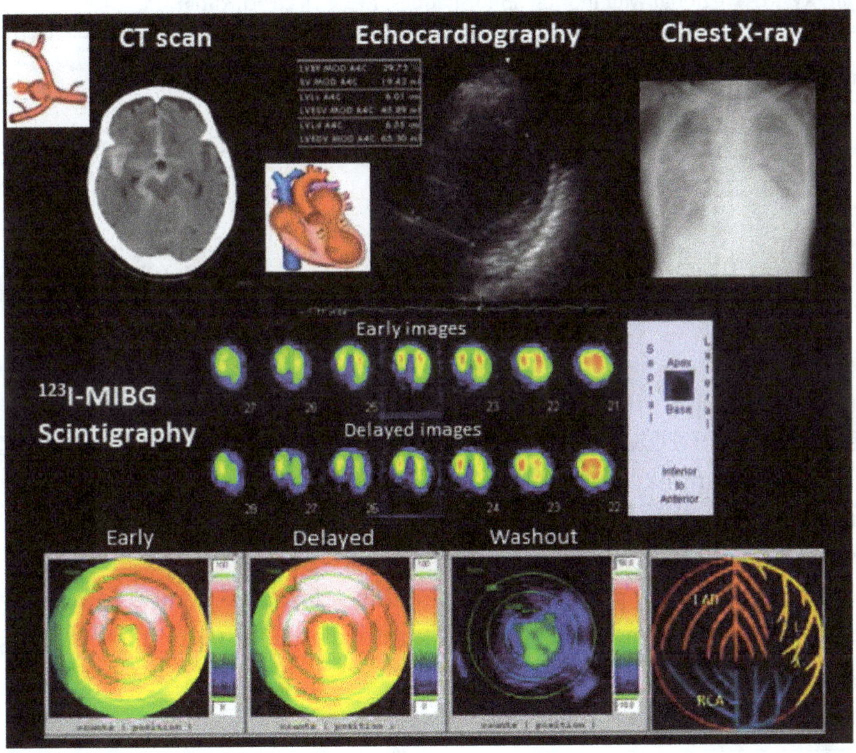

Figure 1. Subarachnoid hemorrhage-induced neurogenic injuries. Note that apical ballooning suggestive of Takotsubo cardiomyopathy (TCM) and left ventricular dysfunction detected by apical two-chamber view on initial echocardiogram. Acute pulmonary edema was also observed on chest X-ray. ^{123}I-metaiodobenzylguanidine (MIBG) SPECT depicting apical defect in the two-chamber view and the analysis of two-dimensional polar maps (bull's eyes) show decreased myocardial perfusion in apex. In 4-h delayed images, washout is increased, suggesting the presynaptic sympathetic dysfunction caused by TCM.

TCM is originally characterized by transient hypokinesis which results from apical wall motion abnormalities with sparing of the base. Although most of the TCM patients (>65%) can present such typical patterns on echocardiography (**Figure 1**), there are several different variants of regional wall motion abnormalities (RWMA) that spares the cardiac apex, as well as one that affects the right ventricle. The right ventricle involvement is noted in 26% of the patients with TCM and bilateral pleural effusions are commonly seen in these patients [8].

The diagnosis of TCM is made based on a modified version of the Mayo Clinic Criteria [9] as described in **Table 1**.

1. Transient hypokinesis, akinesis or dyskinesis of the LV mid-segments with or without apical involvement; the RWMA extend beyond a single epicardial vascular distribution; a stressful trigger is often, but not always, present.
2. Absence of obstructive coronary artery disease or angiographic evidence of acute plaque rupture.
3. New ECG abnormalities (either ST elevation and/or T wave inversion) or modest elevation in cardiac troponin.
4. Absence of other precipitants such as pheochromocytoma and myocarditis.
LV: left ventricular; RWMA: regional wall motion abnormalities; ECG: electrocardiogram.

Table 1. The Mayo Clinic published diagnostic criteria for TCM after SAH.

Patients with akinesis or hypokinesis of left ventricular (LV) apical segments with preserved contractility of the basal segments are considered to have the apical variant of TCM (apical ballooning), while those with akinesis of the basal segments with preserved contractility of the apex and mid-ventricular segments are classified as having reverse TCM (non-apical ballooning).

A massive release of catecholamines into the systemic circulation after aneurysmal rupture has been considered responsible for SAH-induced TCM. In view of the literature reviews (**Table 1**), the incidence of TCM in SAH patients ranges from 0.8 to 17% [1, 2, 7, 10–12], which makes it a relatively common postoperative complication. However, the management of TCM becomes cumbersome in the setting of volumetric and hemodynamic therapy for DCI. In this chapter, we will review the current practice in intensive hemodynamic monitoring and goal-directed fluid management of post-SAH TCM using advanced hemodynamic devices based on our institutional protocol and the relevant literature and to evaluate their effects on clinical outcomes (**Table 2**).

	Total number	**TCM [*n* (%)]**	**LVEF <40% [*n* (%)]**	**Mean age (years)**	**Female (%)**	**Poor grade (%)**	**DCI (%)**	**Poor outcome (%)**
Mutoh et al. [12]	575	46 (8)	20 (43)	64	70	87	33	48
Talahma et al. [1]	800	18 (2.2)	N/A	63	78	33	N/A	44
Kilbourn et al. [2]	63	11 (17)	N/A	61	72	82	N/A	80
Inamasu et al. [10]	391	30 (7.7)	8 (27)	62	63	83	27	57
Abd et al. [7]	2276	19 (0.8)	14 (74)	45	100	58	N/A	N/A
Lee et al. [11]	661	8 (1.2)	4 (50)	56	100	88	38	N/A

Table 2. Incidence and characteristics of TCM in patients after subarachnoid hemorrhage.

2. Pathophysiology of post-SAH TCM

The underlying mechanism of TCM is not fully understood. Several theories have been proposed to explain its pathophysiology including excessive sympathetic stimulation, microvascular dysfunction, coronary artery vasospasm, and abnormal myocardial tissue metabolism [1]. An excessive release of catecholamines (catecholamine surge or sympathetic storming) immediately after insult associated with aneurysm rupture seems to have a pivotal role in the development of TCM. In fact, patients with TCM are at risk for fatal arrhythmias particularly those with SAH combined with intra-sylvian/intracerebral hematoma that involves the right insular cortex where sympathetic hyperactivation can occur [13, 14].

The deleterious effect of such brain–heart interactions may contribute to explain the observation that the outcome of patients with SAH can be predicted by measuring the levels of circulating catecholamine or myocardial sympathetic function. Using an isotope dilution technique, Naredi et al. [15] suggest that patients with subarachnoid hemorrhage exhibited a threefold increase in plasma norepinephrine within 48 h persisted throughout 7–10 days and normalized thereafter. Indeed, nuclear imaging using ^{123}I-meta-iodobenzylguanidine (MIBG), a radioactive marker allowing mapping of the autonomic nervous system of the heart also support the existence of sympathetic dysfunction (**Figure 1**) as a result of overactivation in the area of ventricular wall dysfunction with preserved coronary blood flow [16].

Histopathological findings support this theory since patients presented with typical TCM showed extensive area of myocardial thinning and myocyte edema at the cardiac apex in which degenerative myocardium with histiocyte and lymphocyte infiltration, and contracture-like necrotic bands, but a less severe pathology at the base [17, 18]. Oxidative stress can lead to myocardial necrosis, remodelling, and contractility disturbances [8]. Neuropathological evidence of Lewy body-like cytoplasmic inclusions in both dorsal nuclei of the vagus nerve suggests that disorders of the parasympathetic nervous system may also be associated with a consequence of TCM [17].

On the other hand, the predominance of TCM in female subjects implicates possible properties of genetic predisposition and/or estrogen deficiency [8]. Goodloe et al. [19] investigated functional adrenergic polymorphisms in 28 TCM patients to suggest that TCM was enriched for variants within functional domains, although the polymorphism frequencies were similar to population controls as described previously. Kuo et al. [20] presented a case series of 18 TCM patients and concluded that the lack of estrogen replacement in the postmenopausal state may predispose women to Takotsubo cardiomyopathy. Based on the results from TCM in a mother–sister pair, it has been suggested that the segregating rare variants in four genes (ADH5, CACNG1, EPHA4, and PRKCA) [19] may synergistically confer myocardial vulnerability and risk for TCM in the setting of a postmenopausal hormonal environment and a catecholamine trigger.

The available literature provides no clear answer about the safety of general anesthesia in SAH patients complicated with TCM, and whether the treatment of the aneurysms should be surgical or endovascular. However, it appears that TCM may not be a contraindication to surgical obliteration of the aneurysms as long as the patient is hemodynamically stable [10], while multiple other reports showed that endovascular intervention is the preferred modality of treatment in these patients [21]. In fact, 37–61% of patients underwent surgical clipping for their aneurysms which elucidate the safety of anesthesia for microsurgical clipping even in the setting of TCM [1, 10, 12]. Furthermore, neither clipped nor coiled patients developed serious perioperative cardiopulmonary complications, although relatively higher incidence of fatal procedure-related complications was demonstrated in patients underwent coiling [10].

3. Hemodynamics of TCM after SAH

The hemodynamic changes of TCM that occur during the course of SAH are not fully understood, presumably because of the complicated underlying acute pathophysiological mechanisms that could merely be an innocent finding reflecting the general population.

Although the RWMA associated with TCM is transient with resolution generally within several days to weeks [22, 23], it contributes significantly to cardiopulmonary hemodynamics following SAH, especially when it is combined with other neurogenic injuries such as pulmonary edema, cardiogenic shock, and life-threatening arrhythmia [24, 25]. The RWMA diagnosed on echocardiography have been reported in up to 20% of patients after SAH [2], which is sometimes extensive enough to reduce left ventricular ejection fraction (LVEF). Therefore, in addition to pulmonary edema and hypoxia, TCM may lead to low cardiac output (CO) and hypotension to reduce cerebral perfusion pressure. The incidence of SAH-induced LV dysfunction has been estimated at around 5–10% [26], the development of which following TCM can increase the risk of DCI [11, 27] and poor outcome [12]. Moreover, TCM is associated with a 25% incidence of left ventricular outflow tract (LVOT) obstruction [28], and thus we have to be carefully monitor the cardiac functions to avoid increased intraventricular pressure gradient particularly when treating the related cardiogenic shock or post-SAH DCI.

4. Intensive fluid management for post-SAH TCM

4.1. Hemodynamic monitoring

Cardiovascular monitoring is essential for the diagnostic and therapeutic management of critically ill patients. Of particular, early hemodynamic assessment is importance for adequate cerebral circulation in patients with SAH. Echocardiography is currently the most frequently used noninvasive imaging modality for bedside assessment of LV function [29–31], but is not ideal for real-time monitoring of systolic function because of its high intra- and inter-observer variability [32].

Hemodynamic monitoring is essential for the diagnosis and therapeutic management of critically ill patients. Several different methods and techniques are used to monitor patients with cardiopulmonary complications, although none are ideal (i.e., noninvasive, safe, reproducible, assessing both preload and lung edema volumes, as well as cardiac function) [33]. Unfortunately, the use of such monitoring devices has been limited in neurocritical care, presumably due to inexperience and complexity of handling multiple hemodynamic parameters (e.g., pulmonary artery catheter) [34]. Recently, several studies examined acute hemodynamic changes following SAH using an advanced bedside transpulmonary thermodilution (TPTD) device [12, 35–38].

The single-indicator TPTD method incorporated into the PiCCO/PulsioFlex (Pulsion Medical Systems, Munich, Germany) or EV-1000 (Edwards Lifesciences, Irvine, CA, USA) system measures the change in temperature over time at a thermistor-tipped peripheral arterial catheter inserted into the femoral or brachial artery by triplicate injections of 15-mL boluses of ice-cold saline via the central venous line [39]. The TPTD algorithm calculates CO by analysis of the thermodilution curve using the Stewart–Hamilton equations, which are less-invasive but comparable with those by the established PAC technique [40].

The accuracy of continuous CO measurements, superiority of the TPTD-derived volumetric parameters for estimating cardiac preload (based on global end-diastolic volume (GEDV)) compared with measurement using fluid balance, central venous pressure or a pulmonary artery catheter [41], and the utility of EVLW to discriminate pulmonary edema [37, 42] have been validated in clinical studies in SAH. These hemodynamic data can provide to analyze the cardiac function index (CFI, normal value: 4.5–6.5 per minute), which is the ratio of CO to GEDV [39]. Previous data suggest that CFI is closely related to the LV fractional area of change measured by echocardiography [43] and that CFI can be used to accurately assess the effects of positive inotropic therapy with dobutamine in acute circulatory failure [29].

4.2. Hemodynamic parameters for monitoring TCM

We have recently demonstrated that CFI measured by TPTD provides reliable real-time estimation of LV systolic function in 46 patients with TCM [12]. This study has an advantage of including the *largest* reported number of patients with post-SAH TCM who were successfully monitored for cardiac performance and volume status for approximately 14 days. CFI behaves like an index of LV systolic function because (1) it is fairly well correlated with the echocardiographic LVEF and reliably tracks treatment-induced changes in LVEF, and (2) it is not affected by fluid loading, but increased after administration of an inotropic agent. The decrease in CFI of <4.0 per minute is valuable for detecting LV dysfunction in TCM defined by LVEF <40% (sensitivity of 82% and specificity of 84%), which is the point at which inotropic support should be considered.

At initial measurement on day 0 during the first 24 h after SAH, depression of LV systolic function (CFI 3.3 per minute) mainly attributable to low CO (2.2 L/min/m^2) was observed for patients with TCM. Hypovolemia defined by decreased GEDV (635 mL/m^2) was notable in patients with LV dysfunction (LVEF <40%). In our population, we could not detect any significant difference in HR, MAP, CVP, or SVRI between the groups with and without LV dysfunction throughout the acute period of 2 weeks after SAH. It has also been suggested that TCM combined with LV dysfunction has a longer duration of low CFI

(<4.0 per minute, corresponding to predicted LVEF <40% [29]) with a mean difference of 4 days and more frequencies of pulmonary edema defined by EVLW > 14 mL/kg after day 4 (55%) (**Figure 2**).

4.3. Choice of drugs for post-SAH TCM patients

Medical treatment of arterial vasospasm following aneurysmal subarachnoid hemorrhage (SAH) generally consists of triple H (hypertensive-hypervolemia-hemodilution) therapy [44, 45] or its modification [46–48], which frequently relies on inotropic agents in order to increase CO. Although the optimal treatment is still a matter of debate, given the relationship between catecholamine hypersecretion and subsequent development of TCM, intensivists are often

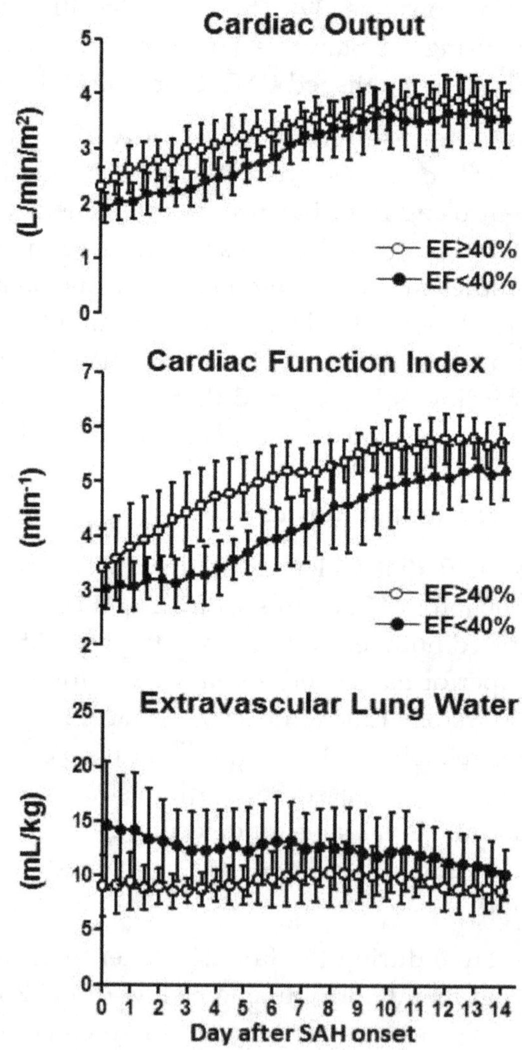

Figure 2. Changes in hemodynamic parameters over 2 weeks in 30 patients with Takotsubo cardiomyopathy following subarachnoid hemorrhage. Note that cardiac function index more clearly traces changes in cardiac function than cardiac output particularly in patients with left ventricular dysfunction [ejection fraction (EF) < 40%]. Increased extravascular lung water in this subgroup can also be detected. Modified with permission from Ref. [12].

reluctant to use inotropes and vasopressors even in patients who may benefit from cardiogenic shock or hemodynamic therapy for DCI. Although there is general agreement in the literature about avoiding vasopressors in TCM patients because of the adverse effects on catecholamine hypersensitivity, the recent data suggest that vasopressors may be used safely by careful monitoring of the hemodynamic parameters [1, 49]. In fact, most patients (61%) had already been administered vasopressors prior to the diagnosis of TCM, in which more than 60% remained on the same treatment and most of them (86%) had good outcome [1]. There is only a case of TCM reported as a direct effect of catecholamine stimulation, including an anecdotal case of de novo TCM in a patient treated with dobutamine for symptomatic SAH vasospasm [50]. In select patients, the use of intra-aortic balloon pump (IABP) may be beneficial as an adjunctive therapy of patients with comorbid DCI and TCM who become intolerant to aggressive pharmacologic hemodynamic augmentation [51].

Milrinone could be a good alternative when inotropes are required in TCM and when dobutamine infusion is associated with tachycardia [52]. The use of milrinone has been proposed to augment the cerebral perfusion in TCM giving its combined inotropic and vasodilating properties [53]. Milrinone is a phosphodiesterase-III inhibitor that increases calcium influx in the myocardium which leads to increased cardiac contractility without β-agonist action, resulting in less tachycardia [52] and myocardial oxygen consumption [54]. However, milrinone may induce hypotension as a result of peripheral vasodilatory property, which may require intensive hemodynamic monitoring during the management.

In the case of concurrent LVOT obstruction associated with post-SAH TCM that may have a paradoxical decrease in CO following administration of inotropic pressors, discontinuation of the inotropes and maintenance of hypervolemia may be required in order to optimize cerebral perfusion and prevent ischemia [27]. If a patient with TCM is deteriorating and has a low CO with LVOT, cardiogenic shock, and progressive multiorgan failure, temporary LV assist devices (LVAD) or extracorporeal membrane oxygenation (ECMO) as a bridge-to-recovery may be useful, as there is a possibility that the ventricular function will recover fully [55].

The role of β-blockers in SAH patients with TCM remains unclear. Patients who had been treated with β-blockers prior to the SAH were associated with a lower risk of developing TCM [56]. In one small study (n = 18), the use of β-blockers prior to or after the diagnosis of TCM was not associated with a significant difference in neurological outcome [1]. The role of a newer inotropic agent levosimendan is more controversial, with mixed expert opinion based on preclinical and limited clinical experience [1, 55]. Future studies on the effectiveness of these drugs in prevention or treatment of TCM may be warranted in larger population.

4.4. TPTD-guided early goal-directed fluid management

Fluid management of peri- and postoperative SAH patients is aimed primarily at maintaining CO to increase cerebral blood flow, and at preventing hypovolemia by minimizing cardiopulmonary complications [44, 57, 58]. The practical usefulness of early goal-directed fluid therapy (EGDT) with TPTD has been proposed in SAH patients including those suffered from TCM [12, 36, 37, 41, 42, 59].

Hemodynamic stability is defined as CO ≥3 L/min/m², GEDV ≥680 mL/m², and ELWI ≤14 mL/kg (the upper limits chosen were the values associated with a higher risk of mortality in patients with pulmonary edema) [60]. If CO fell below the target value due to hypovolemia, patients received 500 mL of either crystalloid fluid or 6% hydroxyethyl starch. If this fluid loading did not increase the GEDV to above the target value, and the low CO persisted for at least 8 h, 25% albumin solution was administered. If the low CO persisted even with hypervolemia (GEDV ≥ 850 mL/m²) and fluid therapy for at least 12 h, inotropic support was initiated with dobutamine [61] or milrinone [12, 37] to maintain CO above the target value. If the patient had elevated EVLW (>14 mL/kg) and any signs of congestive heart failure or pulmonary edema (such as bilateral pulmonary infiltrates or cardiomegaly with a cardiothoracic ratio >50% on chest radiography), furosemide (5 mg bolus) was administered intravenously.

According to our institutional protocol, clinical deterioration due to DCI or evidence of cerebral vasospasm on transcranial Doppler ultrasonography (mean flow velocity in the middle cerebral artery >120 cm/s) was treated with hyperdynamic therapy with incremental doses of dobutamine (3 μg/kg/min, maximum 15 μg/kg/min) or milrinone (0.125 μg/kg/min, maximum 0.75 μg/kg/min) to raise the CO above the normal limit (>5.0 L/min/m²) or to resolve the deficit [12, 62, 63]. Recovery of RWMA [64] and the absence of LVOT obstruction were confirmed by echocardiography before the initiation of hyperdynamic therapy to avoid adverse effects due to the use of inotropic agents [27].

4.5. Outcome of EGDT in post-SAH TCM

In TCM patients managed with aforementioned post-SAH EGDT, multivariate logistic regression analysis showed that persisted low CFI (<4.0 per minute) for ≥4 days was independently associated with DCI (odds ratio, 1.87) and poor functional outcome at 3 months (modified Rankin Scale of 4–6: odds ratio, 1.92). In addition, coexisting pulmonary edema (EVLW > 12 mL/kg) also increased the risk of poor functional outcome at 3 months (odds ratio, 1.85). The results may have an advantage of EGDT because neither a lower LEVF nor the presence of concomitant pulmonary edema correlated with unfavorable outcomes in 30 SAH patients with TCM managed by conventional fluid management using echocardiography and standard hemodynamic parameters [10]. Furthermore, the finding that EGDT has a lower incidence of therapy-related pulmonary edema than standard care [65] may support the value of intensive hemodynamic monitoring.

5. Conclusion

TCM is a well-recognized neurogenic stress-induced complication early after SAH. It is a self-limiting condition but often adds an additional layer of clinical morbidity to a patient particularly suffering from DCI. Our clinical data suggest that prolonged cardiac dysfunction and concurrent pulmonary edema can increase the risk of DCI, contributing to poor functional outcome in patients with SAH complicated with TCM. Serial measurements of CFI and EVLW may provide an easy bedside method of estimating changes in LVEF in TCM and predicting the outcome, as well as detecting fluid therapy-related cardiopulmonary complications.

Acknowledgements

The authors gratefully acknowledge the financial support of Grants: Grant-in-Aid for Scientific Research from the Japan Society for the Promotion of Science (15K10966) and Life Science Foundation of Japan.

Author details

Tatsushi Mutoh[1,2*], Tomoko Mutoh[2], Yasuyuki Taki[2] and Tatsuya Ishikawa[1]

*Address all correspondence to: tmutoh@tiara.ocn.ne.jp

1 Research Institute for Brain and Blood Vessels-AKITA, Akita, Japan

2 Institute of Development, Aging and Cancer, Tohoku University, Sendai, Japan

References

[1] Talahma M, Alkhachroum AM, Alyahya M, et al. Takotsubo cardiomyopathy in aneurysmal subarachnoid hemorrhage: Institutional experience and literature review. *Clin Neurol Neurosurg* 2016; 141:65–70.

[2] Kilbourn KJ, Ching G, Silverman DI, et al. Clinical outcomes after neurogenic stress induced cardiomyopathy in aneurysmal sub-arachnoid hemorrhage: A prospective cohort study. *Clin Neurol Neurosurg* 2015; 128:4–9.

[3] Lee VH, Oh JK, Mulvagh SL, et al. Mechanisms in neurogenic stress cardiomyopathy after aneurysmal subarachnoid hemorrhage. *Neurocrit Care* 2006; 5:243–249.

[4] Templin C, Ghadri JR, Diekmann J, et al. Clinical features and outcomes of Takotsubo (stress) cardiomyopathy. *N Engl J Med* 2015; 373:929–938.

[5] Dote K, Sato H, Tateishi H, et al. Myocardial stunning due to simultaneous multivessel coronary spasms: A review of 5 cases. *J Cardiol* 1991; 21:203–214.

[6] Bybee KA, Prasad A. Stress-related cardiomyopathy syndromes. *Circulation* 2008; 118:397–409.

[7] Abd TT, Hayek S, Cheng JW, et al. Incidence and clinical characteristics of Takotsubo cardiomyopathy post-aneurysmal subarachnoid hemorrhage. *Int J Cardiol* 2014; 176: 1362–1364.

[8] Roshanzamir S, Showkathali R. Takotsubo cardiomyopathy a short review. *Curr Cardiol Rev* 2013; 9:191–196.

[9] Scantlebury DC, Prasad A. Diagnosis of Takotsubo cardiomyopathy. *Circ J* 2014; 78:2129–2139.

[10] Inamasu J, Ganaha T, Nakae S, et al. Therapeutic outcomes for patients with aneurysmal subarachnoid hemorrhage complicated by Takotsubo cardiomyopathy. *Acta Neurochir (Wien)* 2016; 158:885–893.

[11] Lee VH, Connolly HM, Fulgham JR, et al. Tako-tsubo cardiomyopathy in aneurysmal subarachnoid hemorrhage: An underappreciated ventricular dysfunction. *J Neurosurg* 2006; 105:264–270.

[12] Mutoh T, Kazumata K, Terasaka S, et al. Impact of transpulmonary thermodilution-based cardiac contractility and extravascular lung water measurements on clinical outcome of patients with Takotsubo cardiomyopathy after subarachnoid hemorrhage: A retrospective observational study. *Crit Care* 2014; 18:482.

[13] Hirashima Y, Takashima S, Matsumura N, et al. Right sylvian fissure subarachnoid hemorrhage has electrocardiographic consequences. *Stroke* 2001; 32:2278–2281.

[14] Takahashi C, Hinson HE, Baguley IJ. Autonomic dysfunction syndromes after acute brain injury. *Handb Clin Neurol* 2015; 128:539–551.

[15] Naderi S, Ozguven MA, Bayhan H, et al. Evaluation of cerebral vasospasm in patients with subarachnoid hemorrhage using single photon emission computed tomography. *Neurosurg Rev* 1994; 17:261–265.

[16] Christensen TE, Bang LE, Holmvang L, et al. ^{123}I-MIBG scintigraphy in the subacute state of Takotsubo cardiomyopathy. *JACC Cardiovasc Imaging* 2016;

[17] Aoki Y, Kodera S, Watanabe T, et al. Autopsy findings in Takotsubo cardiomyopathy with special reference to the autonomic nervous system. *Int J Cardiol* 2016; 203:236–237.

[18] van der Bilt IA, Vendeville JP, van de Hoef TP, et al. Myocarditis in patients with subarachnoid hemorrhage: A histopathologic study. *J Crit Care* 2016; 32:196–200.

[19] Goodloe AH, Evans JM, Middha S, et al. Characterizing genetic variation of adrenergic signalling pathways in Takotsubo (stress) cardiomyopathy exomes. *Eur J Heart Fail* 2014; 16:942–949.

[20] Kuo BT, Choubey R, Novaro GM. Reduced estrogen in menopause may predispose women to Takotsubo cardiomyopathy. *Gend Med* 2010; 7:71–77.

[21] Manto A, De Gennaro A, Manzo G, et al. Early endovascular treatment of aneurysmal subarachnoid hemorrhage complicated by neurogenic pulmonary edema and Takotsubo-like cardiomyopathy. *Neuroradiol J* 2014; 27:356–360.

[22] Gianni M, Dentali F, Grandi AM, et al. Apical ballooning syndrome or Takotsubo cardiomyopathy: A systematic review. *Eur Heart J* 2006; 27:1523–1529.

[23] Sharkey SW, Lesser JR, Maron BJ. Cardiology patient page. Takotsubo (stress) cardiomyopathy. *Circulation* 2011; 124:e460–462.

[24] Pilgrim TM, Wyss TR. Takotsubo cardiomyopathy or transient left ventricular apical ballooning syndrome: A systematic review. *Int J Cardiol* 2008; 124:283–292.

[25] Ahmed S, Ungprasert P, Ratanapo S, et al. Clinical characteristics of Takotsubo cardiomyopathy in North America. *N Am J Med Sci* 2013; 5:77–81.

[26] Spina R, Baron D, Wong S, et al. Severe stress (Takotsubo) cardiomyopathy following subarachnoid haemorrhage. *Int J Cardiol* 2016; 210:119–121.

[27] Zada G, Terterov S, Russin J, et al. Cerebral vasospasm and concurrent left ventricular outflow tract obstruction: Requirement for modification of hyperdynamic therapy regimen. *Neurocrit Care* 2010; 12:265–268.

[28] El Mahmoud R, Mansencal N, Pilliere R, et al. Prevalence and characteristics of left ventricular outflow tract obstruction in Tako-tsubo syndrome. *Am Heart J* 2008; 156:543–548.

[29] Jabot J, Monnet X, Bouchra L, et al. Cardiac function index provided by transpulmonary thermodilution behaves as an indicator of left ventricular systolic function. *Crit Care Med* 2009; 37:2913–2918.

[30] Lee VH, Abdelmoneim SS, Daugherty WP, et al. Myocardial contrast echocardiography in subarachnoid hemorrhage-induced cardiac dysfunction: Case report. *Neurosurgery* 2008; 62:E261–E262; discussion E262.

[31] Cinotti R, Piriou N, Launey Y, et al. Speckle tracking analysis allows sensitive detection of stress cardiomyopathy in severe aneurysmal subarachnoid hemorrhage patients. *Intensive Care Med* 2016; 42:173–182.

[32] McGowan JH, Cleland JG. Reliability of reporting left ventricular systolic function by echocardiography: A systematic review of 3 methods. *Am Heart J* 2003; 146:388–397.

[33] Merenkov VV, Kovalev AN, Gorbunov VV. Bedside lung ultrasound: A case of neurogenic pulmonary edema. *Neurocrit Care* 2013; 18:391–394.

[34] Stevens RD, Naval NS, Mirski MA, et al. Intensive care of aneurysmal subarachnoid hemorrhage: An international survey. *Intensive Care Med* 2009; 35:1556–1566.

[35] Yoneda H, Nakamura T, Shirao S, et al. Multicenter prospective cohort study on volume management after subarachnoid hemorrhage: Hemodynamic changes according to

severity of subarachnoid hemorrhage and cerebral vasospasm. *Stroke* 2013; 44:2155–2161.

[36] Mutoh T, Kazumata K, Yokoyama Y, et al. Comparison of postoperative volume status and hemodynamics between surgical clipping and endovascular coiling in patients after subarachnoid hemorrhage. *J Neurosurg Anesthesiol* 2015; 27:7–15.

[37] Mutoh T, Kazumata K, Kobayashi S, et al. Serial measurement of extravascular lung water and blood volume during the course of neurogenic pulmonary edema after subarachnoid hemorrhage: Initial experience with 3 cases. *J Neurosurg Anesthesiol* 2012; 24:203–208.

[38] Tagami T, Kuwamoto K, Watanabe A, et al. Optimal range of global end-diastolic volume for fluid management after aneurysmal subarachnoid hemorrhage: A multicenter prospective cohort study. *Crit Care Med* 2014; 42:1348–1356.

[39] Sakka SG, Reuter DA, Perel A. The transpulmonary thermodilution technique. *J Clin Monit Comput* 2012; 26:347–353.

[40] Profant M, Vyska K, Eckhardt U. The stewart-hamilton equations and the indicator dilution method. *SIAM J Appl Math* 1978; 34:666–675.

[41] Mutoh T, Kazumata K, Ishikawa T, et al. Performance of bedside transpulmonary thermodilution monitoring for goal-directed hemodynamic management after subarachnoid hemorrhage. *Stroke* 2009; 40:2368–2374.

[42] Mutoh T, Kazumata K, Ueyama-Mutoh T, et al. Transpulmonary thermodilution-based management of neurogenic pulmonary edema after subarachnoid hemorrhage. *Am J Med Sci* 2015; 350:415–419.

[43] Ritter S, Rudiger A, Maggiorini M. Transpulmonary thermodilution-derived cardiac function index identifies cardiac dysfunction in acute heart failure and septic patients: An observational study. *Crit Care* 2009; 13:R133.

[44] Suarez JI, Tarr RW, Selman WR. Aneurysmal subarachnoid hemorrhage. *N Engl J Med* 2006; 354:387–396.

[45] Vergouwen MD, Vermeulen M, van Gijn J, et al. Definition of delayed cerebral ischemia after aneurysmal subarachnoid hemorrhage as an outcome event in clinical trials and observational studies: Proposal of a multidisciplinary research group. *Stroke* 2010; 41:2391–2395.

[46] Muench E, Horn P, Bauhuf C, et al. Effects of hypervolemia and hypertension on regional cerebral blood flow, intracranial pressure, and brain tissue oxygenation after subarachnoid hemorrhage. *Crit Care Med* 2007; 35:1844–1851.

[47] Mutoh T, Ishikawa T, Yasui N. Application of the FloTrac™ arterial pressure-based continuous cardiac output monitor to dobuta-induced hyperdynamic therapy for

cerebral vasospasm after subarachnoid hemorrhage. *No Shinkei Geka* 2009; 37:1085–1093.

[48] Mori K, Arai H, Nakajima K, et al. Hemorheological and hemodynamic analysis of hypervolemic hemodilution therapy for cerebral vasospasm after aneurysmal subarachnoid hemorrhage. *Stroke* 1995; 26:1620–1626.

[49] Mittal M, Radhakrishnan M, UmamaheswaraRao GS. Management of catecholamine-induced stunned myocardium – a case report. *J Clin Anesth* 2015; 27:527–530.

[50] Saito R, Takahashi T, Noshita N, et al. Takotsubo cardiomyopathy induced by dobutamine infusion during hypertensive therapy for symptomatic vasospasm after subarachnoid hemorrhage – case report. *Neurol Med Chir (Tokyo)* 2010; 50:393–395.

[51] Al-Mufti F, Morris N, Lahiri S, et al. Use of intra-aortic-balloon pump counterpulsation in patients with symptomatic vasospasm following subarachnoid hemorrhage and neurogenic stress cardiomyopathy. *J Vasc Interv Neurol* 2016; 9:28–34.

[52] Mrozek S, Srairi M, Marhar F, et al. Successful treatment of inverted Takotsubo cardiomyopathy after severe traumatic brain injury with milrinone after dobutamine failure. *Heart Lung* 2016;

[53] Naidech A, Du Y, Kreiter KT, et al. Dobutamine versus milrinone after subarachnoid hemorrhage. *Neurosurgery* 2005; 56:21–27.

[54] Mager G, Klocke RK, Kux A, et al. Phosphodiesterase III inhibition or adrenoreceptor stimulation: Milrinone as an alternative to dobutamine in the treatment of severe heart failure. *Am Heart J* 1991; 121:1974–1983.

[55] Lyon AR, Bossone E, Schneider B, et al. Current state of knowledge on Takotsubo syndrome: A position statement from the taskforce on Takotsubo syndrome of the heart failure association of the european society of cardiology. *Eur J Heart Fail* 2016; 18:8–27.

[56] Liang CW, Chen R, Macri E, et al. Preadmission beta-blockers are associated with decreased incidence of neurogenic stunned myocardium in aneurysmal subarachnoid hemorrhage. *J Stroke Cerebrovasc Dis* 2013; 22:601–607.

[57] Rabinstein AA, Lanzino G, Wijdicks EF. Multidisciplinary management and emerging therapeutic strategies in aneurysmal subarachnoid haemorrhage. *Lancet Neurol* 2010; 9:504–519.

[58] Sen J, Belli A, Albon H, et al. Triple-H therapy in the management of aneurysmal subarachnoid haemorrhage. *Lancet Neurol* 2003; 2:614–621.

[59] Mutoh T, Kazumata K, Ajiki M, et al. Goal-directed fluid management by bedside transpulmonary hemodynamic monitoring after subarachnoid hemorrhage. *Stroke* 2007; 38:3218–3224.

[60] Kirov MY, Kuzkov VV, Bjertnaes LJ: Extravascular lung water in sepsis. In: Vincent JL, ed. Yearbook of intensive care and emergency medicine, Berlin: Springer; 2005: pp.449–461.

[61] Hadeishi H, Mizuno M, Suzuki A, et al. Hyperdynamic therapy for cerebral vasospasm. *Neurol Med Chir (Tokyo)* 1990; 30:317–323.

[62] Mutoh T, Ishikawa T, Kobayashi S, et al. Performance of third-generation FloTrac/Vigileo system during hyperdynamic therapy for delayed cerebral ischemia after subarachnoid hemorrhage. *Surg Neurol Int* 2012; 3:99.

[63] Mutoh T, Ishikawa T, Suzuki A, et al. Continuous cardiac output and near-infrared spectroscopy monitoring to assist in management of symptomatic cerebral vasospasm after subarachnoid hemorrhage. *Neurocrit Care* 2010; 13:331–338.

[64] Banki N, Kopelnik A, Tung P, et al. Prospective analysis of prevalence, distribution, and rate of recovery of left ventricular systolic dysfunction in patients with subarachnoid hemorrhage. *J Neurosurg* 2006; 105:15–20.

[65] Mutoh T, Kazumata K, Terasaka S, et al. Early intensive versus minimally invasive approach to postoperative hemodynamic management after subarachnoid hemorrhage. *Stroke* 2014; 45:1280–1284.

5

Complexity of Sarcomere Protein Gene Mutations in Restrictive Cardiomyopathy

Shuai Wang and Daoquan Peng

Abstract

Restrictive cardiomyopathy (RCM) is characterized by impaired filling of the ventricles in the presence of normal wall thickness and systolic function. Although idiopathic RCM is rare compared to other types of cardiomyopathy, the effects are severe. Until recently, many sarcomere genes previously described to be causative mutations in hypertrophic cardiomyopathy and dilated cardiomyopathy have been reported in RCM. Nowadays, it is accepted that primary RCM is also within the spectrum of sarcomere disease. However, the relationship between the identified mutations in sarcomere genes and clinical manifestation are complex, and the possible pathogenic mechanisms are not fully understood. Besides, many RCM-related sarcomere mutations were reported to cause variable clinical phenotype. Occasionally, "phenotype transition" may also be seen in an individual who was previously diagnosed with RCM.

Keywords: restrictive cardiomyopathy, sarcomere, gene mutation

1. Introduction

Restrictive cardiomyopathy (RCM) is characterized by impaired filling of the ventricles in the presence of normal wall thickness and systolic function. While RCM is rare compared to other primary cardiomyopathies, most affected individuals have severe signs and symptoms of heart failure and majority die shortly after diagnosis unless they receive a cardiac transplant [1]. According to the etiology, RCM has been classified as primary or secondary. Secondary RCM refers to the conditions in association with local inflammation (Loeffler cardiomyopathy, endomyocardial fibrosis, and eosinophilic endomyocardial disease) or infiltrative (amyloidosis and sarcoidosis) or storage disease (hemochromatosis, glycogen storage disease, and Fabry disease, etc.) [2]. Primary RCM includes RCM ascribed to inherited or sporadically acquired mutations or in many cases due to unknown etiology. So far, through mutation screening of different individuals and families presenting the RCM phenotype, mutations in multiple sarcomere genes have been identified to be linked with RCM, which has greatly expanded our understanding about "idiopathic RCM." However, the relationship between the identified sarcomeric mutations and clinical manifestation are complex and many puzzles still exist. The mechanism behind the genotype-phenotype correlation is not clearly understood. Most of these RCM-associated sarcomeric mutations, when mutated at specific sites, are also known to induce HCM or DCM. Even people carrying the same mutation of the same sarcomeric gene may exhibit heterogenetic manifestations. "Phenotype transition" may even been seen at a late stage of RCM resulting in atypical RCM.

2. Multiple sarcomeric gene mutations in human RCM

The sarcomere contains different protein involved in muscle contraction. Two major components are actin, which constitutes the backbone of the thin filament, and myosin, which makes up the thick filament. The interaction of myosin and actin causing the sliding of the thin filaments along the thick filaments results in muscle contraction and force development. Association and disassociation of myosin and actin are regulated in a Ca^{2+}-dependent manner by the troponin-alphatropomysin (Tm) complex. The actin-myosin contractile apparatus, which consists of five thin filament proteins (actin, tropomyosin, and troponin T, I, and C) and three thick filament proteins (myosin heavy chain, essential light chain, and regulatory light chain), plays a key role in regulating the sarcomere function. So far, except for troponin C, mutations in the other thin filament and thick filament proteins have all been identified in RCM. Besides, a series of mutations in other regulatory sarcomere proteins such as myosin-binding protein C, titin, and Z-disc proteins also have been recognized to induce diastolic dysfunction resulting in a restrictive phenotype.

2.1. Cardiac troponin mutation

Cardiac troponin is located at regular intervals along the thin filament and consists of three subunits: cardiac troponin C (cTnC), troponin I (cTnI), and troponin T (cTnT). cTnC acts as a Ca^{2+} sensor, which confers Ca^{2+} sensitivity to muscle contraction [3]. Cardiac TnI is the inhibitory subunit, primarily functioning to prevent actin and myosin from interacting in the absence of Ca^{2+}. The cTnT subunit binds to tropomyosin (Tm) and is responsible for transmitting the Ca^{2+}-binding signal from cTn to Tm [4]. Electrical depolarization of the cell membrane opens the L-type calcium channels and allows Ca^{2+} influx, which incites release of Ca^{2+} from sarcoplasmic reticulum due to opening of the ryanodine receptors. The released Ca^{2+} binds to cardiac troponin C and induces conformational changes in the troponin T-tropomyosin complex, resulting in displacement of cTnI from actin and subsequent association of actin with myosin. Currently, nine mutations in genes encoding cTnI and three dominant mutations in genes encoding cTnT have been reported in human RCM and no mutations have been identified in cTnC yet.

2.1.1. Troponin I mutation

The gene of cardiac TnI (*TNNI3*) is situated on the 19th chromosome (19q13.4) and consists of eight exons and seven introns. The mature molecule of cTnI is 209 a.a long and consists of five domains: (1) N-terminal domains, (2) IT-arm, (3) inhibitory domain, (4) regulatory domain, and (5) C-terminal mobile domains [5]. Until now, RCM-related cTnI mutations are found located in the inhibitory domain and the C-terminal domain.

2.1.1.1. *Missense mutations located at the inhibitory domain*

The inhibitory domain of hcTnI spans residues 137–148 [6, 7], some also reported a different border of this region (residues 129–148) [6, 8]. In the absence of Ca^{2+}, residues 138–148 of the inhibitory domain interact with actin [9] and shift the tropomyosin molecule, impeding the antomyosin-complex formation [10]. Two of the RCM mutations are localized within this important region. The first one is 797T→A nucleotide substitution of exon 7, which led to a Leu144Gln (L144Q) amino acid substitution [11]. The second mutation is 799C→T nucleotide substitution of exon 7 that leads to an Arg145Trp (R145W) amino acid substitution [11].

Data from *in vitro* experiment showed that both L144Q and R145W alter myofilament sensitivity to Ca^{2+}. Skinned cardiac fiber experiment, which measures the Ca^{2+}-buffering capacity of the myofilament while measuring the development of tension and maximal force, revealed that these two mutations resulted in increase of Ca^{2+} sensitivity of force development in skinned fibers from transgenic mice. In addition, a significant increase in the basal force was shown compared to WT cardiac fiber [12]. Measurement of myofilament ATPase activity revealed that L144Q and R145W mutant showed an increase in the basal ATPase at low Ca^{2+} concentrations. Besides, fibers from these two mutants exhibited markedly increased Ca^{2+} sensitivity of ATPase activity [13].

2.1.1.2. *Missense mutations located at the mobile C-terminal domain*

The mobile C-terminal domain of hcTnI is further divided into the H4 α-helix (residues 164–188) and the C-terminal part (residues 199–210) [5]. 865G→A nucleotide substitution of exon 7 that led to an Ala171Thr amino acid substitution and an 886A→G nucleotide substitution of exon 7, which resulted in a Lys178Glu (K178E) amino acid substitution both occurred within the H4 α-helix region and have been identified in RCM patients. Since these two mutations are known to be located within the actin-binding sites (residues 173–181) [14, 15], K178E and Ala171Thr mutations may influence the inhibitory function through actin binding.

Although the structure of the C-terminal part of hcTnI which consists of residues 190–210 is not fully understood, it is critical for a full inhibitory activity and Ca^{2+} sensitivity of force development because it binds to actin and helps to maintain the thin filament in a blocked state [16]. Mutations occurred at the C-terminal domain may destabilize or decrease its interactions with actin in the absence of Ca^{2+}, consequently relieving cTnI inhibition [17]. Up to now, RCM-related mutant Asp190His (D190H), Arg192His (R192H), and Arg204His (R204H) have been localized within the conserved C-terminal region of the protein [11, 18]. *In vitro* experiments revealed that two of these mutants D190H and R192H markedly increased the filament sensitivity to Ca^{2+}, while another mutation R204H has been reported to result in a disruption of the normal interaction between cTnI-cTnC and cTnI-cTnT. It remains to be further determined what conformational changes happened in these mutant that lead to disrupted interaction between cTnI-actin and cTnI-cTnC.

2.1.1.3. Two deletion mutations

Deletion of nucleotides usually causes frame shift and the introduction of a premature stop codon. Two deletion mutations of *TNNI3* which impaired relaxation of myocardium and resulted in a restrictive filling pattern were reported to be located in exon 7 and cause truncation of C-terminal portion of cTnI. The truncated cTnI which lost its C-terminal portion is susceptible to degradation and has reduced inhibitory capacity on the thin filament since C-terminal contains the second binding domain for actin and cTnC [19, 20].

2.1.2. Troponin T mutation

cTnT anchors the troponin complex to Tm and plays a critical role in modulating ATPase activation when Ca^{2+} concentrations achieve threshold levels. Until now, three different mutations in the cTnT gene (*TNNT2*) linked to RCM have been identified. However, the molecular pathogenesis of these cTnT mutations is not clear [20–22].

3. α-Cardiac actin (*ACTC*)

Actin is a major constituent of the thin filament and spans the length of thin filament. Together with myosin, actin generates force and transmits this force from the sarcomere to the surrounding syncytium via the thin filament [23]. RCM mutations in the ACTC gene are extremely rare and only one ACTC mutation has been reported in RCM (nucleotide substitution in exon 5 g. 4642G→C which lead to an Asp313His amino acid substitution). However, the significance of this variant is uncertain.

4. α-Tropomyosin (*TPM1*)

In cardiac muscles, tropomyosin together with troponin forms the principal mechanism by which contractility is regulated in response to the Ca^{2+} concentration. In the absence of Ca^{2+}, tropomyosin prevents productive myosin head binding. In systole, tropomyosin moves in response to Ca^{2+} binding to allow partial myosin attachment, which resulted in further shift of tropomyosin to expose fully the interaction site on actin [24]. Recently, a novel missense mutation in α-tropomyosin, c.835A>C p.Asn279His has been identified in a patient with primary RCM [25]. However, the significance of this variant is not clear since family evaluation did not show cosegregation.

5. β-Myosin heavy chain (*MYH7*)

Myosin is a dimeric protein consisting of two heavy chains and two associated pairs of light chains. The ~23-kb long human *MYH7* gene, located on chromosome 14, contains 40 exons that direct the synthesis of the 1935 amino acid β-myosin heavy chain [26]. Although over

500 disease-causing point mutations have been found in human *MYH7* gene, most of them are reported in HCM, only four of these variants are identified in patients with primary RCM [27–32]. The understanding about the genotype-phenotype correlation between the reported MYH7 mutation and RCM are very limited. MYH7 contains different functional domains, including the globular head domain (S1), the neck or hinge region (S2), and the tail (light meromyosin) [33, 34]. Although many mutations have been identified to cluster in functional hotspots due to the development of high throughput sequencing, all the above mentioned RCM-related *MYH7* mutations located at regions where no definite function has been assigned to so far [28]. Besides, whether haploinsufficiency may contribute to the consequence of the variants is not clear.

6. Ventricular myosin essential light chain (*MYL3*) and ventricular myosin regulatory light chain (*MYL2*)

Myosin assembles into hexamers comprising two heavy chains and two pairs of each light chain isoform. The light chain forms a stabilizing collar around the α-helical neck of the heavy chain, a region of the myosin multimer thought to function as the level arm. Mutation in the gene encoding the essential light chain of myosin (*MYL3* Met149Val) and the regulatory light chain of myosin (MYL2 Glu22Lys) was previously reported to correlate with marked diastolic dysfunction and restrictive physiology both in human and transgenic mice [35]. Interestingly, carriers with simultaneous mutation in both *MYL3* and MYL2 showed different phenotypes. While patients with heterozygous mutation in MYL2 (p.Gly57Glu) and homozygous mutation in *MYL3* (p.Glu143Lys) had severe, early onset RCM, double heterozygote for these variants have no evidence of cardiomyopathy [25, 36]. It is speculated that Glu143Lys substitution may be responsible for this heterogeneity through a loss of function mechanism. This specula tion is based on (1) carriers with one mutant allele were clinically silent [36], while homozygotes for the mutation have severe, early-onset cardiomyopathy [25]. If the cardiomyopathy was caused by a dominant-negative mechanism, an intermediate phenotype in heterozygotes would be expected. (2) The substitution occurs in a surface-exposed loop of the essential light chain [37], which makes it less likely to disrupt protein conformation or stability. The site-directed mutagenesis of the corresponding loop domain was confirmed to have no effect on binding between light and heavy chains [38]. Further study using transgenic animal models may help to answer this question.

7. Myosin-binding protein C (*MYBPC3*)

Cardiac myosin-binding protein C is a modular polypeptide located at the C-zone in the striated muscles and binds myosin heavy chain in thick filament and titin in elastic filaments [39]. More than 150 mutations identified in MYBPC3 have been reported, which is the most common genetic cause of HCM [40, 41]. Recently, variants of MYBPC3 have also been reported to be RCM-causing mutation [42, 43].

8. Titin (*TTN*)

The giant protein titin acts as the third filament system of the sarcomere, in addition to the actin and myosin filament. It physically connects myosin fibers to actin polymers and is attached to the Z-line. Titin consists of four structurally and functionally distinct regions. (1) The N-terminal titin binds to various Z-disk proteins and acts as an anchor, which is composed of Z-repeats and multiple immunoglobulin (Ig) domains. (2) Elastic I-band region contains the important PEVK portion (proline, glutamate, valine, and lysine) and acts as the molecular spring. (3) Stabilizing A-band region binds to the thick muscle filaments and contains Ig-like, fibronectin type III (fibronection3) domain. (4) M-band region contains the unique serine-threonine kinase domain modulating titin expression and turnover, with C-terminus of titin embedding in the M-line [44–46]. When the sarcomere is stretched during diastole, the I-band segments gradually lengthen and develop passive tension and therefore, titin is a major determinant of the stiffness of myocardium [47].

Currently, two mechanisms are known to modulate titin's passive stiffness. (1) Titin-based passive tension is critically defined by the ratio of the two major adult cardiac isoforms (N2BA and N2B). As a general rule, longer titin isoforms with longer PEVK repeats in the I-band have more elasticity, whereas shorter isoforms provide more passive stiffness [48]. In adult cardiac muscle, two major isoforms are present: the long compliant N2BA and the shorter stiff N2B. In healthy adult, the ratio of N2BA to N2B in human left ventricle is 40:60 [49]. Moreover, the right ventricle expresses more N2BA than does the left ventricle [50]. In conditions with concentric remodeling such as hypertension or aortic stenosis with diastolic function, a decreased N2BA:N2B ratio was shown [51, 52]. (2) Another more short-term mechanism modulating titin's passive stiffness is caused by post-translational modification influencing phosphorylation states. Titin could be phosphorylated at the PEVK domain and the cardiac-specific N2B domain, and phosphorylated titin exhibited decreased titin-based passive tension [53].

Titin, known to be the major disease-causing gene for DCM, is encoded by a single gene *TTN* on chromosome 2q31 [54]. Interestingly, recent clinical and genetic studies have established the role of titin defects in the pathophysiology of diastolic dysfunction and RCM. A de novo missense mutation of Titin c.22862A > G replacing adenine by guanine at position 109 of exon 226, resulting in the substitution of an evolutionally conserved tyrosine by cysteine (p.Y7621C) has been reported to result in early-onset family RCM with severe heart failure [55]. Structural analysis revealed that p.Y7621C mutation is likely to disrupt the hydrophobic core within fibronectin3 domain, which locates in the A/I junction region [55]. However, how this *TTN* mutation might affect cardiac function and lead to the consecutive development of RCM is unknown.

9. Myopalladin (*MYPN*)

Myopalladin (MYPN) is an Ig-domain family member protein that has been reported to be a key intermediate molecule at the Z-disc involved in sarcomere/Z-disc assembly and regulation of gene expression in cardiac cells [56]. Through genetic screening for *MYPN* mutations in large cohorts of patients with cardiomyopathy, 15 *MYPN* variants were identified, of which a nonsense mutation (p.Q529X) was identified in an RCM family with variable penetrance [57]. Q529X was found to disturb different functional domains of MYNP. MYNP contains five Ig domains (two N-terminal and three C-terminal). Central and C-terminal domains of MYPN bind at the Z-disc to α-actinin and nebulette (NEBL), respectively. This actinin-MYPN-NEBL complex tethers actin and titin to the Z-disc and may play roles in the signaling and regulation of gene expression in response to muscle stress. The N-terminal domain of MYNP binds cardiac ankyrin repeat protein (CARP), which is involved in the control of muscle gene expression [58]. Q529X mutation truncates the C-terminus of MYNP, including the NEBL- and α-actinin-binding domains. Comparative immunohistochemistry of human heart tissue was performed on specimens from the siblings with RCM and from normal control subjects without *MYPN* mutation as well as in neonatal rat cardiomyocytes (NRCs) expressing green fluorescent protein (GFP) chimeras of WT- and Q529X-MYPN. Disrupted sarcomeric Z-discs with abnormally diffuse MYPN codistributed focally with abnormal sarcomeric α-actin, localization were seen in the specimen from siblings with RCM and NRCs expressing Q529X-MYPN [57]. Therefore, losing the NEBL and α-actinin-binding domain results in severe disturbance of sarcomere/Z-disc assembly, which may have impact on early myofibrillogenesis and resulted in RCM. Besides, since MYPN localizes both at sarcoplasm and nucleus, mutant MPPN-Q529X protein in the nucleus was reported to result in downregulation of CARP expression and upregulation of MLP and desmin, augmenting fibrotic restrictive remodeling [59]. In addition, truncated proteins are usually unstable due to decay of mRNA and/or protein degradation through the lysosome or ubiquitin-proteasome system. Although *MYPN* mRNA was not affected by the Q529X-MYPN mutation in the myocardium, mutant MYPN was relatively unstable compared with WT protein [57]. Therefore, insufficient quantities of the protein (haploinsufficiency) may be partly involved in dysfunction of the protein.

10. Mutations cause variable phenotypes

The molecular mechanisms by which gene mutation cause cardiomyopathy can usually be explained by two alternative ways. One is mutation may cause structural and functional change in the protein, which should be analyzed in four different levels: (1) change in the deoxyribonucleic acid sequence, (2) the actual amino acid change, (3) the changes in Ca^{2+} sensitivity of force development and ATPase activity, and (4) the change in protein-protein interaction. The other mechanism may involve insufficient quantities of the protein due to instability of the mutant protein leading to haploinsufficiency [23].

However, it is now evident that different mutations in one gene could cause multiple phenotypes. It is also intriguing that even for a given single mutation and even within a single family disparate phenotypes can be seen. For example, the cTnT lle79Asn mutation has been shown to be associated with HCM, DCM, and RCM within a single pedigree [60]. This implies that factors just beyond the pathogenic sarcomere mutation influence the phenotype. Therefore, the model of sarcomeric cardiomyopathy as monogenic disease following simple Mendelian pattern of inheritance is an oversimplification. Theoretically, a discrete number of reasons can account for phenotypic diversity. (1) First of all, patients may carry more than one disease-associated mutations, which is underestimated in most cases. Recent genotyping suggests that multiple cardiomyopathy patients have more than one mutation in the same gene or mutations in different genes. For example, in a study carried out in 292 HCM patients, 13 were found to carry at least 2 mutations [61, 62]. However, the number of patients carrying at least two mutations is likely to be significantly underestimated since many genetic studies typically investigate less than 15 genes for mutations associated with cardiomyopathy [63]. (2) Secondly, different expression and the incorporation rate of the mutant sarcomeric proteins in the heart may also contribute to the heterogeneity of the disease. A few examples in HCM have been published. Heterozygous individuals carrying the βMHC Lys207Gln mutation developed an HCM phenotype, but a homozygous individual developed a DCM-like phenotype [61]. In another case, homozygous carriers of cTnT Ser179Phe mutation exhibited profound left and right ventricular hypertrophy [64] while heterozygous carriers had little or no hypertrophy [65]. (3) Third, mutant proteins are usually unstable due to decay of mRNA and/or degradation through the lysosome or ubiquitin-proteasome system, especially in the case of nonsense mutation [66]. Because of genetic polymorphisms, individuals with RCM are likely to have substantial difference in their genome sequence including disease-modifier genes which are involved in post-translational or translational regulation, resulting in different amounts of mutant protein. This mechanism may interfere with the development of the phenotype and explain different penetrance of a specific mutation. (4) Lastly, sarcomere gene mutation induces serials of maladaptive features, ranging from the prolongation of cardiomyocyte action potential to microvascular dysfunction, from intracellular calcium abnormality to dysregulation of collagen turn-over, and from energetic derangement to abnormal sympathetic activation [67]. The extent and the rate at which each of these features occur and evolve are quite variable within individual patients. Therefore, the clinical heterogeneity of a specific sarcomere gene mutation may partly be ascribed to different stages of disease progression [68]. Although epigenetics and environmental factors are likely to be relevant in sarcomeric cardiomyopathies, there have been no studies yet describing how epigenetic modification and environmental factors may affect phenotype in sarcomeric RCM.

11. Phenotype transition

Occasionally, with the progression of disease, "phenotype transition" may be seen in a given individual who was initially diagnosed with a specific type of cardiomyopathy. This situation could often be seen in patients who was initially diagnosed with HCM and gradually developed into end-stage of the disease. The morpho-functional manifestation in this advanced stage usually exhibits two extremes: hypokinetic-dilated from or hypokinetic-restrictive form which could be hard to distinguish from primary DCM and RCM [68]. The "HCM to RCM" transition has been discussed above. There is another situation that patients initially diagnosed with primary RCM could undergo persistent cardiac remodeling resulting atypical phenotype at a later stage of the disease. Although the main impairment of RCM is diastolic dysfunction, deterioration of systolic function has been observed in some patients. In a retrospective study, it was reported that 16% of 94 primary RCM patients was observed to have systolic dysfunction [69]. Another study carried out in pediatric RCM reveals that although all the 18 children had preserved ventricular systolic function at diagnosis, 6 of them later presented a deteriorated ventricular systolic function and eventually required inotropic support [70]. In the RCM model using transgenic mice noticeable impaired systolic was observed over a time of 10 months. By the time, those RCM mice presented with signs of severely aggravated congestive heart failure and some of them died [71]. This disease progression is consistent with some of the clinical observation, suggesting that systolic dysfunction may be responsible for the end-stage lethal heart failure. As for the mechanism, some proposed that ischemia may be a bridge between the progression of diastolic dysfunction and the development of systolic function, based on evidence of ischemia observed in hearts for autopsy from RCM patients and transgenic RCM mice [71–73]. Besides, it is presumed that reduced capillary density due to interstitial fibrosis and increased extravascular compressive force in the restrictive heart may also induce ischemia [74]. Of note, although an RCM patient may appear to have systolic dysfunction and low cardiac output, enlargement of ventricle is seldom seen, probably because the molecular mechanism and sarcomeric mechanics of RCM and DCM are opposite [75].

12. Summary

In the past decades, clinical and genetic studies suggest that primary RCM is part of a spectrum of sarcomeric disease. Since RCM is associated with severe prognosis, ongoing and future basic science will continue to dissect the precise pathways driving how these mutations remodel the heart, and identify rational therapies targeting pathophysiological aspects to interrupt the emergency of pathology. On the other hand, it is also important to realize that genes contain information that is essential for the development of the phenotype but not necessarily complete. The final phenotype is determined not only by the causal mutation but also by the modifier genes, each exerting a modest effect, epigenetic factors, which link the gene to the phenotype, and the environmental factors, as in the case of complex phenotypes observed in single-gene disorders with Mendelian pattern of inheritance. Thus, while advances in molecular genetics of cardiovascular diseases are gradually changing our classical understanding of the disease and the phenotype-based approach to the practice of medicine, currently they are unlikely to be sufficient to trigger a full switch from a phenotype-based to genotyped-based medicines. A comprehensive understanding of molecular mechanism of the pathogenesis integrating the genetic, epigenetic, transcriptomic, and proteomic profiles is necessary.

Author details

Shuai Wang and Daoquan Peng*

*Address all correspondence to: pengdq@hotmail.com

1 Department of Cardiovascular Medicine, The Second Xiangya Hospital of Central South University, Changsha, Hunan, China

References

[1] Mogensen J, Arbustini E. Restrictive cardiomyopathy. *Curr Opin Cardiol.* 2009;24:214–220.

[2] Kushwaha SS, Fallon JT, Fuster V. Restrictive cardiomyopathy. *N Engl J Med.* 1997;336:267–276.

[3] Gordon AM, Homsher E, Regnier M. Regulation of contraction in striated muscle. *Physiol Rev.* 2000;80:853–924.

[4] Gordon AM, Regnier M, Homsher E. Skeletal and cardiac muscle contractile activation: tropomyosin "rocks and rolls". *News Physiol Sci.* 2001;16:49–55.

[5] Katrukha IA. Human cardiac troponin complex. Structure and functions. *Biochemistry (Mosc).* 2013;78:1447–1465.

[6] Takeda S, Yamashita A, Maeda K, Maeda Y. Structure of the core domain of human cardiac troponin in the Ca^{2+}-saturated form. *Nature.* 2003;424:35–41.

[7] Kobayashi T, Patrick SE, Kobayashi M. Ala scanning of the inhibitory region of cardiac troponin i. *J Biol Chem.* 2009;284:20052–20060.

[8] Brown LJ, Sale KL, Hills R, Rouviere C, Song L, Zhang X, Fajer PG. Structure of the inhibitory region of troponin by site directed spin labeling electron paramagnetic resonance. *Proc Natl Acad Sci U S A.* 2002;99:12765–12770.

[9] Lindhout DA, Sykes BD. Structure and dynamics of the c-domain of human cardiac troponin c in complex with the inhibitory region of human cardiac troponin i. *J Biol Chem.* 2003;278:27024–27034.

[10] Farah CS, Miyamoto CA, Ramos CH, da Silva AC, Quaggio RB, Fujimori K, Smillie LB, Reinach FC. Structural and regulatory functions of the NH_2- and COOH-terminal regions of skeletal muscle troponin i. *J Biol Chem.* 1994;269:5230–5240.

[11] Mogensen J, Kubo T, Duque M, Uribe W, Shaw A, Murphy R, Gimeno JR, Elliott P, McKenna WJ. Idiopathic restrictive cardiomyopathy is part of the clinical expression of cardiac troponin i mutations. *J Clin Invest.* 2003;111:209–216.

[12] Gomes AV, Liang J, Potter JD. Mutations in human cardiac troponin i that are associated with restrictive cardiomyopathy affect basal atpase activity and the calcium sensitivity of force development. *J Biol Chem.* 2005;280:30909–30915.

[13] Kobayashi T, Solaro RJ. Increased Ca^{2+} affinity of cardiac thin filaments reconstituted with cardiomyopathy-related mutant cardiac troponin i. *J Biol Chem.* 2006;281:13471–13477.

[14] Gomes AV, Potter JD. Cellular and molecular aspects of familial hypertrophic cardiomyopathy caused by mutations in the cardiac troponin i gene. *Mol Cell Biochem.* 2004;263:99–114.

[15] Tripet B, Van Eyk JE, Hodges RS. Mapping of a second actin-tropomyosin and a second troponin c binding site within the c terminus of troponin i, and their importance in the Ca^{2+}-dependent regulation of muscle contraction. *J Mol Biol.* 1997;271:728–750.

[16] Galinska A, Hatch V, Craig R, Murphy AM, Van Eyk JE, Wang CL, Lehman W, Foster DB. The c terminus of cardiac troponin i stabilizes the Ca^{2+}-activated state of tropomyosin on actin filaments. *Circ Res*. 2010;106:705–711.

[17] Rarick HM, Tu XH, Solaro RJ, Martin AF. The c terminus of cardiac troponin i is essential for full inhibitory activity and Ca^{2+} sensitivity of rat myofibrils. *J Biol Chem*. 1997;272:26887–26892.

[18] Gambarin FI, Tagliani M, Arbustini E. Pure restrictive cardiomyopathy associated with cardiac troponin i gene mutation: mismatch between the lack of hypertrophy and the presence of disarray. *Heart*. 2008;94:1257.

[19] Kostareva A, Gudkova A, Sjoberg G, Morner S, Semernin E, Krutikov A, Shlyakhto E, Sejersen T. Deletion in tnni3 gene is associated with restrictive cardiomyopathy. *Int J Cardiol*. 2009;131:410–412.

[20] Kaski JP, Syrris P, Burch M, Tome-Esteban MT, Fenton M, Christiansen M, Andersen PS, Sebire N, Ashworth M, Deanfield JE, McKenna WJ, Elliott PM. Idiopathic restrictive cardiomyopathy in children is caused by mutations in cardiac sarcomere protein genes. *Heart*. 2008;94:1478–1484.

[21] Peddy SB, Vricella LA, Crosson JE, Oswald GL, Cohn RD, Cameron DE, Valle D, Loeys BL. Infantile restrictive cardiomyopathy resulting from a mutation in the cardiac troponin t gene. *Pediatrics*. 2006;117:1830–1833.

[22] Miller T, Szczesna D, Housmans PR, Zhao J, de Freitas F, Gomes AV, Culbreath L, McCue J, Wang Y, Xu Y, Kerrick WG, Potter JD. Abnormal contractile function in transgenic mice expressing a familial hypertrophic cardiomyopathy-linked troponin t (i79n) mutation. *J Biol Chem*. 2001;276:3743–3755.

[23] Xu Q, Dewey S, Nguyen S, Gomes AV. Malignant and benign mutations in familial cardiomyopathies: insights into mutations linked to complex cardiovascular phenotypes. *J Mol Cell Cardiol*. 2010;48:899–909.

[24] McKillop DF, Geeves MA. Regulation of the interaction between actin and myosin subfragment 1: evidence for three states of the thin filament. *Biophys J*. 1993;65:693–701.

[25] Caleshu C, Sakhuja R, Nussbaum RL, Schiller NB, Ursell PC, Eng C, De Marco T, McGlothlin D, Burchard EG, Rame JE. Furthering the link between the sarcomere and primary cardiomyopathies: restrictive cardiomyopathy associated with multiple mutations in genes previously associated with hypertrophic or dilated cardiomyopathy. *Am J Med Genet A*. 2011;155A:2229–2235.

[26] Buvoli M, Hamady M, Leinwand LA, Knight R. Bioinformatics assessment of beta-myosin mutations reveals myosin's high sensitivity to mutations. *Trends Cardiovasc Med*. 2008;18:141–149.

[27] Greenway SC, Wilson GJ, Wilson J, George K, Kantor PF. Sudden death in an infant with angina, restrictive cardiomyopathy, and coronary artery bridging: an unusual

phenotype for a beta-myosin heavy chain (myh7) sarcomeric protein mutation. *Circ Heart Fail*. 2012;5:e92–e93.

[28] Colegrave M, Peckham M. Structural implications of beta-cardiac myosin heavy chain mutations in human disease. *Anat Rec (Hoboken)*. 2014;297:1670–1680.

[29] Karam S, Raboisson MJ, Ducreux C, Chalabreysse L, Millat G, Bozio A, Bouvagnet P. A de novo mutation of the beta cardiac myosin heavy chain gene in an infantile restrictive cardiomyopathy. *Congenit Heart Dis*. 2008;3:138–143.

[30] Rai TS, Ahmad S, Ahluwalia TS, Ahuja M, Bahl A, Saikia UN, Singh B, Talwar KK, Khullar M. Genetic and clinical profile of Indian patients of idiopathic restrictive cardiomyopathy with and without hypertrophy. *Mol Cell Biochem*. 2009;331:187–192.

[31] Koppole S, Smith JC, Fischer S. Simulations of the myosin ii motor reveal a nucleotide-state sensing element that controls the recovery stroke. *J Mol Biol*. 2006;361:604–616.

[32] Yu BL, Xiang R, Hu D, Peng DQ. A novel myh7 mutation in a family with cardiomyopathy presenting with restrictive physiology and varying degrees of left ventricle hypertrophy. *Eur Heart J*. 2015;36:178.

[33] Miroshnichenko NS, Balanuk IV, Nozdrenko DN. Packing of myosin molecules in muscle thick filaments. *Cell Biol Int*. 2000;24:327–333.

[34] Walsh R, Rutland C, Thomas R, Loughna S. Cardiomyopathy: a systematic review of disease-causing mutations in myosin heavy chain 7 and their phenotypic manifestations. *Cardiology*. 2010;115:49–60.

[35] Sanbe A, Nelson D, Gulick J, Setser E, Osinska H, Wang X, Hewett TE, Klevitsky R, Hayes E, Warshaw DM, Robbins J. In vivo analysis of an essential myosin light chain mutation linked to familial hypertrophic cardiomyopathy. *Circ Res*. 2000;87:296–302.

[36] Olson TM, Karst ML, Whitby FG, Driscoll DJ. Myosin light chain mutation causes autosomal recessive cardiomyopathy with mid-cavitary hypertrophy and restrictive physiology. *Circulation*. 2002;105:2337–2340.

[37] Rayment I, Holden HM, Whittaker M, Yohn CB, Lorenz M, Holmes KC, Milligan RA. Structure of the actin-myosin complex and its implications for muscle contraction. *Science*. 1993;261:58–65.

[38] Ho G, Chisholm RL. Substitution mutations in the myosin essential light chain lead to reduced actin-activated atpase activity despite stoichiometric binding to the heavy chain. *J Biol Chem*. 1997;272:4522–4527.

[39] Oakley CE, Hambly BD, Curmi PM, Brown LJ. Myosin binding protein c: structural abnormalities in familial hypertrophic cardiomyopathy. *Cell Res*. 2004;14:95–110.

[40] Bahrudin U, Morisaki H, Morisaki T, Ninomiya H, Higaki K, Nanba E, Igawa O, Takashima S, Mizuta E, Miake J, Yamamoto Y, Shirayoshi Y, Kitakaze M, Carrier L, Hisatome I. Ubiquitin-proteasome system impairment caused by a missense cardiac myosin-binding protein c mutation and associated with cardiac dysfunction in hypertrophic cardiomyopathy. *J Mol Biol*. 2008;384:896–907.

[41] Olivotto I, d'Amati G, Basso C, Van Rossum A, Patten M, Emdin M, Pinto Y, Tomberli B, Camici PG, Michels M. Defining phenotypes and disease progression in sarcomeric cardiomyopathies: contemporary role of clinical investigations. *Cardiovasc Res*. 2015;105:409–423.

[42] Wu W, Lu CX, Wang YN, Liu F, Chen W, Liu YT, Han YC, Cao J, Zhang SY, Zhang X. Novel phenotype-genotype correlations of restrictive cardiomyopathy with myosin-binding protein c (mybpc3) gene mutations tested by next-generation sequencing. *J Am Heart Assoc*. 2015; Jul 10;4(7)

[43] Zou Y, Wang J, Liu X, Wang Y, Chen Y, Sun K, Gao S, Zhang C, Wang Z, Zhang Y, Feng X, Song Y, Wu Y, Zhang H, Jia L, Wang H, Wang D, Yan C, Lu M, Zhou X, Song L, Hui R. Multiple gene mutations, not the type of mutation, are the modifier of left ventricle hypertrophy in patients with hypertrophic cardiomyopathy. *Mol Biol Rep*. 2013;40:3969–3976.

[44] Bang ML, Centner T, Fornoff F, Geach AJ, Gotthardt M, McNabb M, Witt CC, Labeit D, Gregorio CC, Granzier H, Labeit S. The complete gene sequence of titin, expression of an unusual approximately 700-kDa titin isoform, and its interaction with obscurin identify a novel z-line to i-band linking system. *Circ Res*. 2001;89:1065–1072.

[45] Lange S, Xiang F, Yakovenko A, Vihola A, Hackman P, Rostkova E, Kristensen J, Brandmeier B, Franzen G, Hedberg B, Gunnarsson LG, Hughes SM, Marchand S, Sejersen T, Richard I, Edstrom L, Ehler E, Udd B, Gautel M. The kinase domain of titin controls muscle gene expression and protein turnover. *Science*. 2005;308:1599–1603.

[46] Labeit S, Kolmerer B. Titins: giant proteins in charge of muscle ultrastructure and elasticity. *Science*. 1995;270:293–296.

[47] Gerull B. The rapidly evolving role of titin in cardiac physiology and cardiomyopathy. *Can J Cardiol*. 2015;31:1351–1359.

[48] Freiburg A, Trombitas K, Hell W, Cazorla O, Fougerousse F, Centner T, Kolmerer B, Witt C, Beckmann JS, Gregorio CC, Granzier H, Labeit S. Series of exon-skipping events in the elastic spring region of titin as the structural basis for myofibrillar elastic diversity. *Circ Res*. 2000;86:1114–1121.

[49] Cazorla O, Freiburg A, Helmes M, Centner T, McNabb M, Wu Y, Trombitas K, Labeit S, Granzier H. Differential expression of cardiac titin isoforms and modulation of cellular stiffness. *Circ Res*. 2000;86:59–67.

[50] Neagoe C, Opitz CA, Makarenko I, Linke WA. Gigantic variety: expression patterns of titin isoforms in striated muscles and consequences for myofibrillar passive stiffness. *J Muscle Res Cell Motil*. 2003;24:175–189.

[51] Williams L, Howell N, Pagano D, Andreka P, Vertesaljai M, Pecor T, Frenneaux M, Granzier H. Titin isoform expression in aortic stenosis. *Clin Sci (Lond)*. 2009;117:237–242.

[52] Warren CM, Jordan MC, Roos KP, Krzesinski PR, Greaser ML. Titin isoform expression in normal and hypertensive myocardium. *Cardiovasc Res*. 2003;59:86–94.

[53] Hidalgo C, Granzier H. Tuning the molecular giant titin through phosphorylation: role in health and disease. *Trends Cardiovasc Med*. 2013;23:165–171.

[54] Hinson JT, Chopra A, Nafissi N, Polacheck WJ, Benson CC, Swist S, Gorham J, Yang L, Schafer S, Sheng CC, Haghighi A, Homsy J, Hubner N, Church G, Cook SA, Linke WA, Chen CS, Seidman JG, Seidman CE. Heart disease. Titin mutations in ips cells define sarcomere insufficiency as a cause of dilated cardiomyopathy. *Science*. 2015;349:982–986.

[55] Peled Y, Gramlich M, Yoskovitz G, Feinberg MS, Afek A, Polak-Charcon S, Pras E, Sela BA, Konen E, Weissbrod O, Geiger D, Gordon PM, Thierfelder L, Freimark D, Gerull B, Arad M. Titin mutation in familial restrictive cardiomyopathy. *Int J Cardiol*. 2014;171:24–30.

[56] Bang ML, Mudry RE, McElhinny AS, Trombitas K, Geach AJ, Yamasaki R, Sorimachi H, Granzier H, Gregorio CC, Labeit S. Myopalladin, a novel 145-kilodalton sarcomeric protein with multiple roles in z-disc and i-band protein assemblies. *J Cell Biol*. 2001;153:413–427.

[57] Purevjav E, Arimura T, Augustin S, Huby AC, Takagi K, Nunoda S, Kearney DL, Taylor MD, Terasaki F, Bos JM, Ommen SR, Shibata H, Takahashi M, Itoh-Satoh M, McKenna WJ, Murphy RT, Labeit S, Yamanaka Y, Machida N, Park JE, Alexander PM, Weintraub RG, Kitaura Y, Ackerman MJ, Kimura A, Towbin JA. Molecular basis for clinical heterogeneity in inherited cardiomyopathies due to myopalladin mutations. *Hum Mol Genet*. 2012;21:2039–2053.

[58] Otey CA, Dixon R, Stack C, Goicoechea SM. Cytoplasmic ig-domain proteins: cytoskeletal regulators with a role in human disease. *Cell Motil Cytoskeleton*. 2009;66:618–634.

[59] Huby AC, Mendsaikhan U, Takagi K, Martherus R, Wansapura J, Gong N, Osinska H, James JF, Kramer K, Saito K, Robbins J, Khuchua Z, Towbin JA, Purevjav E. Disturbance in z-disk mechanosensitive proteins induced by a persistent mutant myopalladin causes familial restrictive cardiomyopathy. *J Am Coll Cardiol*. 2014;64:2765–2776.

[60] Menon SC, Michels VV, Pellikka PA, Ballew JD, Karst ML, Herron KJ, Nelson SM, Rodeheffer RJ, Olson TM. Cardiac troponin t mutation in familial cardiomyopathy with variable remodeling and restrictive physiology. *Clin Genet*. 2008;74:445–454.

[61] Alpert NR, Mohiddin SA, Tripodi D, Jacobson-Hatzell J, Vaughn-Whitley K, Brosseau C, Warshaw DM, Fananapazir L. Molecular and phenotypic effects of heterozygous, homozygous, and compound heterozygote myosin heavy-chain mutations. *Am J Physiol Heart Circ Physiol*. 2005;288:H1097–H1102.

[62] Friedrich FW, Bausero P, Sun Y, Treszl A, Kramer E, Juhr D, Richard P, Wegscheider K, Schwartz K, Brito D, Arbustini E, Waldenstrom A, Isnard R, Komajda M, Eschenhagen T, Carrier L, Project EHF. A new polymorphism in human calmodulin iii gene promoter is a potential modifier gene for familial hypertrophic cardiomyopathy. *Eur Heart J*. 2009;30:1648–1655.

[63] Frisso G, Limongelli G, Pacileo G, Del Giudice A, Forgione L, Calabro P, Iacomino M, Detta N, Di Fonzo LM, Maddaloni V, Calabro R, Salvatore F. A child cohort study from

southern Italy enlarges the genetic spectrum of hypertrophic cardiomyopathy. *Clin Genet*. 2009;76:91–101.

[64] Maron BJ, Thompson PD, Puffer JC, McGrew CA, Strong WB, Douglas PS, Clark LT, Mitten MJ, Crawford MH, Atkins DL, Driscoll DJ, Epstein AE. Cardiovascular preparticipation screening of competitive athletes. A statement for health professionals from the sudden death committee (clinical cardiology) and congenital cardiac defects committee (cardiovascular disease in the young), American Heart Association. *Circulation*. 1996;94:850–856.

[65] Ho CY, Lever HM, DeSanctis R, Farver CF, Seidman JG, Seidman CE. Homozygous mutation in cardiac troponin t: implications for hypertrophic cardiomyopathy. *Circulation*. 2000;102:1950–1955.

[66] Vosberg HP. The ubiquitin-proteasome system may be involved in the pathogenesis of hypertrophic cardiomyopathy. *Cardiovasc Res*. 2005;66:1–3.

[67] Ferrantini C, Belus A, Piroddi N, Scellini B, Tesi C, Poggesi C. Mechanical and energetic consequences of hcm-causing mutations. *J Cardiovasc Transl Res*. 2009;2:441–451.

[68] Olivotto I, Cecchi F, Poggesi C, Yacoub MH. Patterns of disease progression in hypertrophic cardiomyopathy: an individualized approach to clinical staging. *Circ Heart Fail*. 2012;5:535–546.

[69] Ammash NM, Seward JB, Bailey KR, Edwards WD, Tajik AJ. Clinical profile and outcome of idiopathic restrictive cardiomyopathy. *Circulation*. 2000;101:2490–2496.

[70] Weller RJ, Weintraub R, Addonizio LJ, Chrisant MR, Gersony WM, Hsu DT. Outcome of idiopathic restrictive cardiomyopathy in children. *Am J Cardiol*. 2002;90:501–506.

[71] Du J, Liu J, Feng HZ, Hossain MM, Gobara N, Zhang C, Li Y, Jean-Charles PY, Jin JP, Huang XP. Impaired relaxation is the main manifestation in transgenic mice expressing a restrictive cardiomyopathy mutation, r193h, in cardiac tni. *Am J Physiol Heart Circ Physiol*. 2008;294:H2604–H2613.

[72] Jean-Charles PY, Li YJ, Nan CL, Huang XP. Insights into restrictive cardiomyopathy from clinical and animal studies. *J Geriatr Cardiol*. 2011;8:168–183.

[73] Palka P, Lange A, Ward C. A fatal case of idiopathic restrictive cardiomyopathy. *Cardiol Young*. 2003;13:469–471.

[74] Maron MS, Olivotto I, Maron BJ, Prasad SK, Cecchi F, Udelson JE, Camici PG. The case for myocardial ischemia in hypertrophic cardiomyopathy. *J Am Coll Cardiol*. 2009;54:866–875.

[75] Robinson P, Mirza M, Knott A, Abdulrazzak H, Willott R, Marston S, Watkins H, Redwood C. Alterations in thin filament regulation induced by a human cardiac troponin t mutant that causes dilated cardiomyopathy are distinct from those induced by troponin t mutants that cause hypertrophic cardiomyopathy. *J Biol Chem*. 2002;277:40710–40716.

6

Hypertrophic Cardiomyopathy: Treatment, Risk Stratification, and Implantable Defibrillators

Peter Magnusson

Abstract

Hypertrophic cardiomyopathy (HCM) affects 1:500 individuals, and in majority of cases, a mutation in sarcomere proteins can explain the disease. Phenotype is heterogeneous and thus the prognosis. Many patients suffer from dyspnoea, especially at exercise. Unfortunately, sudden cardiac death (SCD) does occur at all ages and is a major cause of death in young adults. There is no proven pharmacological treatment to reduce hypertrophy or fibrosis, but beta-blockers are first-line treatment. In patients with obstruction, myectomy is preferred in the young, but in older patients, alcohol septal ablation is tried to reduce symptoms and possibly prognosis. Risk stratification of sudden cardiac death is challenging. The major established risk factors are extreme myocardial thickness, non-sustained ventricular tachycardia, unexplained syncope, abnormal exercise blood pressure response, and family history of sudden cardiac death. In 2014, a novel risk calculator was developed that also takes age, outflow gradient, and left atrial seize into account. Implantable defibrillator treatment is effective in HCM, but complications requiring surgery and inappropriate shocks remain a problem.

Keywords: complications, hypertrophic cardiomyopathy, implantable defibrillator, inappropriate shock, risk stratification, risk markers, sudden cardiac death

1. Diagnosis

Hypertrophic cardiomyopathy (HCM) implies increased ventricular thickness that is not only a response to hypertension, aortic stenosis, or any other loading condition with abnormal loading of the ventricle [1]. In adults, a wall thickness of ≥15 mm is typically required for diagnosis. In borderline cases (≥13 mm), a thorough evaluation including family history is needed [1, 2]. In siblings, parents or children of a HCM patient, 13-mm thickness is enough for diagnosis [1, 2]. In children and adolescents, a wall thickness more than two standard deviations in the corresponding age group should raise suspicion of the diagnosis of HCM [3]. An ultrasound of the heart, echocardiography, typically reveals the diagnosis of HCM. Echocardiography is usually readily available, but occasionally other imaging techniques are needed. Cardiac magnetic resonance (CMR), computed tomography (CT) or rarely positron emission tomography (PET) is sometimes used for diagnostic purposes or to gain additional information for optimal disease management [4]. The hypertrophied segment is almost always affecting the left ventricle even though right wall involvement does occur [1, 2]. Typically, the septal part is enlarged, either the basal part or the middle part, but could affect lateral, posterior and apical part, or a combination thereof [1]. A concentric hypertrophic is often associated with secondary causes of hypertrophy but does occur as HCM entity. If an isolated hypertrophy solely involves the basal part of the septal wall in an elderly and no other signs or family history of HCM is found, often an explanation such as hypertension is the major cause [1, 2]. Even though the diagnosis of most cases of HCM is straight forward, careful attention to other causes and robust imaging techniques, including a cardiologist with expertise in the field, is warranted. Because HCM is a life-long disease with consequences not only for the patient but also for relatives, a correct diagnosis is indeed important.

2. Symptoms and signs

Dyspnoea is the predominant symptom of HCM that leads to evaluation with an echocardiogram. Shortness of breath is pronounced at exertion due to relaxation disturbance of the left ventricle during diastole and/or outflow tract obstruction. This latter form is called hypertrophic obstructive cardiomyopathy, and the obstruction is often dynamic with regard to filling pressure, heart rate and body position and affected by medications with effect on the cardiovascular system. Often the patient has an adopted life style to decreased physical stamina, and often the diagnostic presentation is rather vague including tiredness. The HCM diagnosis is often delayed or sometimes misclassified from the initial diagnostic work-up.

A progressive HCM may sometimes lead to deterioration of the systolic function of the left ventricle. The ventricle dilates and hypertrophic segments remodel into dilatation, which sometimes can make it difficult to discern from other cardiomyopathies with dilated morphology. This condition is called end stage and indicates a worse prognosis [5–8].

Chest pain without coronary disease may also lead the physician to evaluate alternative diagnosis, and sometimes HCM is revealed. Microvascular dysfunction and fibrosis are part of the disease progression; biopsies show myocardial disarray, and modern PET imaging techniques confirm structural and functional abnormalities, which explain symptoms. However, biopsies are not indicated as part of routine evaluation as the same information would be gained non-invasively [2, 4]. Syncope evaluation is sometimes the initial work-up that leads to the diagnosis of HCM. The mechanisms could be either hemodynamic or cardiac arrhythmias [9]. Less specific symptoms such as pre-syncope, near-syncope or vertigo will often include ECG and that in turn will lead to suspicion of morphological disease.

Atrial fibrillation is common among HCM, and thus, the risk of embolization stroke warrants effective anticoagulants even without other risk factors [10, 11]. The CHADSVASC score is not validated for HCM patients, and current guidelines recommend warfarin/dual oral anticoagulants if no contraindication is present [2].

Unfortunately, the first manifestation of HCM could be sudden cardiac death (SCD). In such cases, the autopsy confirms or at least suspects HCM even though the microscopy and post-mortem genetic evaluation will aid. A conclusive diagnosis of HCM is of uttermost importance because of the inheritance pattern and relatives need to be evaluated.

3. Inheritance

In more than half of the HCM cases, modern genetic panels can explain the cause of HCM and partly predict the outcome [12–14]. Of all mutations associated with HCM, the vast majority affects myosin proteins: beta-myosin heavy chain (MYH7) and myosin-binding protein (MYBPC3). Other components of the actin-myosin filaments, such as troponins or tropomyosin, rarely explain disease [2]. However, there is a steady increase in disease causing mutations due to increased research activities and widened genetic panels in everyday practise.

The mutations of HCM are autosomal dominant with the exception of the X-linked Danon disease due to lysosome-associated membrane protein 2 [15]. The most common metabolic disease causing hypertrophy of the heart is Anderson-Fabry, which is a storage dysfunction of the lysosomes. In children, hypertrophy of the heart is part of a syndrome, and constellations of malformations may lead suspicion towards Noonans disease, LEOPARD or even more rare diseases. In adults, amyloidosis should be part of the differential diagnosis. A correct molecular diagnosis can sometimes provide clinicians with specific treatment options and thus improve prognosis for the individual.

Family-history taking is a compulsory part of the initial evaluation of a patient with a suspected or conformed hypertrophy. The clinician should systematically document the patients' report on family members who died suddenly or suffered from unexplained syncope or other symptoms suggesting an inheritance. This history taking may include not only first or secondary degree relatives and but also often tedious and administrative efforts to search for older documents, medical records, military service tests like ECG and autopsy protocols. In families who have members who moved to other regions or emigrated from the country, this can be especially challenging. A portion of detective abilities and a critical approach to information from historical medical records or a patients' explanation to a sudden death may be unmasked by a pedigree of suspected HCM. In these efforts, a specialized health care provider trained in history taking, administrative paths and updated knowledge of genetic counselling including bioinformatics will be valuable in conjunction with the cardiologist.

4. Epidemiology

Since the first descriptions of hypertrophy of the heart, numerous labels have been used [2, 16]. Still hypertrophic *obstructive* cardiomyopathy is frequently used, sometimes to stress that an individual patient is symptomatic due to obstructive. While this can be illustrative in a case eligible for septal reductive procedures such as myectomy or alcohol ablation, it can often confuse health care providers, patients and relatives. Furthermore, since the dynamic state of the disease, it can be difficult to assess even though guidelines provide support for establishing degree of obstruction using pharmacological and physiological provocations of obstructiveness. Nowadays, guidelines recommend the usage of HCM and avoid former nomenclature [2].

In echocardiographic studies of populations in the USA, the prevalence of HCM is 1:500, which has been confirmed in other geographical parts of the world with highly available resources of diagnostic tools [17, 18]. Interestingly, also if patients without hypertrophy (phenotype) but who have mutations associated with HCM (genotype), the prevalence is 1:350 [19]. This makes HCM the most prevalent inherited myocardial disease. Because of the high prevalence, a basic knowledge about the disease is needed among a broad spectrum of heath care providers and managers.

The public awareness of HCM has been increased. This is probably due the journalistic attention to sudden death among young people especially during sport activities. In fact, in some countries and certain sport associations, screening of members of athletes is established. However, the approach to screening has been a matter of controversies and the benefits questioned and criticism of the resources it takes and the number of borderline cases that has to be evaluated and managed [20–23].

Nevertheless, HCM or at least unexplained post-mortem left ventricular hypertrophy is considered the most common cause of sudden cardiac death among sport persons younger than 35 years of age; HCM accounts for a half of the cases [24]. A historical perspective on this topic found HCM as a major cause of sudden death in the young [25]. A recent study in Denmark of all cases of SCD in the country reported a lower number [26]. From this Danish cohort, the cases of HCM were further analysed with regard to medical attention before death and about half of the cases had been evaluated for symptoms associated with HCM [26]. This stresses the importance of a qualified disease management including risk stratification of sudden cardiac death.

5. Pharmacological treatment

Recommendations of pharmacological treatment are based on smaller trials or empirical findings on HCM patients or evidence from other patient groups. No drug has been proven to reverse disease progression, but reduction in symptoms can often be achieved. Treatment strategies are based on whether the patient suffers from left ventricular outflow tract obstruction or not. A peak gradient of ≥30 mmHg is considered as obstruction, but one should bear in mind that this varies over time due to the hemodynamic situation [2].

The principle behind treatment options in patients with obstruction is to avoid severe dehydration with risk of low filling pressures, which could be deleterious for certain patients. Therefore, dehydration, drugs with vessel dilatation actions, or increase in heart rate is disadvantageous. Atrial arrhythmias are frequently encountered in HCM, and often a trigger of unbearable symptoms leads the patient to hospitalization. If the patient is admitted within 48 hours or properly anticoagulated, direct electrical conversion is preferred. However, this is often not the case. In such circumstances, beta-blockers are the drug of choice and digoxin should be avoided due to inotropic increase in myocardium [2].

The first-line treatment option is beta-blocking agents [2]. Notably, the beta-blocker carvedilol exerts vaso-dilating effects and should be avoided. Historically, propranolol was used, but nowadays metoprolol is often the drug of choice. Unfortunately, beta-blockers commonly imply side effects like cognitive impairment and exercise intolerance. This limit dosage titration and compliance to the drug may be questioned. It is important to recognize side effects and discuss alternatives rather than prompt withdrawal, which could possibly provoke worsening of symptoms and cause arrhythmias due to rebound effects on beta-receptors.

The calcium channel antagonist verapamil is often the drug of choice when beta-blockers are not reducing symptoms enough or not tolerated due to side effects. Diltiazem is an alternative choice but not dihydropyridine calcium antagonists because of their vascular effects. Contraindications of verapamil are systolic heart failure and conduction disturbances, i.e., bundle branch block.

The class 1A drug disopyramide has been studied in HCM cohorts and may relieve obstructive symptoms and are considered safe with regard to risk of ventricular arrhythmias. It can be prescribed in addition to beta-blockers. In practise, intolerance is frequent due to anticholinergic side effects (dry mucous membrane, urinary retention, and obstipation), and in some countries, it is not available.

In patients without obstructive component of HCM, the same principle to diminish relaxation disturbance of the left ventricle holds true. Loop diuretics and thiazides can be used without the same precautions as in HCM with obstruction. If disease progression reaches the crossroad with decreased systolic function with ejection fraction below 50%, treatment options include the same drugs as in heart failure due to other causes: beta-blockers, ACE/ARB-inhibitors, aldosterone receptor blockers, and diuretics.

6. Septal reduction therapy

In patients with symptoms due to pronounced obstruction (≥50 mmHg) despite pharmacological treatment, invasive options remain. Myectomy requires open-heart surgery and can be performed concomitant mitral plasty or replacement [27]. The incision is typically up to 70 mm and provides long-term success even though complications, i.e., atrioventricular block, aortic valve insufficiency, septal shunts occur. Perioperative death is 1–4% and increase with age, left atrial size, and female sex [28].

Alcohol septal ablation implies injection in an arterial branch with resulting necrosis and decreased obstruction. It is less invasive but requires careful judgement of the targeted vessel and still AV-block complications in up to 20% of patients in some series and overall mortality comparable to myectomy. Typically, alcohol ablation is the preferred method for older patients and can be performed multiple times in the same patient. It is important to stress that the decision to performed either alcohol septal ablation or myectomy should be done in centres with expertise in the field and adequate volumes.

There has been a preference of myectomy over alcohol ablation in the USA compared to Europe. The low number of myectomies in Europe has been criticized by experts [29].

Moreover, both myectomy and alcohol septal ablation result in scarring tissue, which have been reported to be a substrate for ventricular arrhythmias have been a matter of debate. However, in larger series, both methods seem to be safe at middle or long-term follow-ups even if individual risk stratification is important even after successful septum reduction procedure [30].

7. Pacemaker therapy

A pacemaker protects from bradycardia and is indicated in high degree AV-block, tachy-brady, and occasionally to reduce outflow gradients in patient where options are not suitable [2, 31]. Ventricular pacing from the right apical part may relieve obstruction by an electrical dyssynchrony between septal and lateral segments of the left ventricle. Earlier studies showed promising results, but current guidelines have constrained indications to include selected patients described above [2, 31, 32]. In the case of indication of an implantable cardioverter defibrillator (ICD) in patients with obstruction, patients should be considered for a dual chamber system for this reason.

Cardiac resynchronization therapy (CRT) has evaluated in smaller observational trial of HCM patients [33]. The experience is that it provides improved exercise capacity, functional class and ejection fraction, and biomarker levels. The vast experience and solid scientific ground of CRT treatment in patients with functional class II–IV, EF ≤ 35% despite optimal pharmacological treatment in left bundle branch block gives a rationale for usage in HCM patients with end-stage heart failure [31, 34, 35].

8. End-stage heart failure

Lowering EF is a predictor of worse outcome and is sometimes called 'burned-out HCM.' It is important to recognize the beginning of this stage and take prompt action including optimal pharmacologic treatments and device therapy. Notably, many patients have supernormal EF for several years, and when EF is below 50%, this is a turning point. An EF < 50% also predicts risk of life threatening ventricular arrhythmias. This marks a risk for appropriate ICD therapy and should thus imply consideration for preventing sudden cardiac death [34, 35].

If not CRT is enough in end-stage heart failure due to HCM, the same approach as in life threatening heart failure should apply. Rarely, very small left ventricular chamber cavity or intractable ventricular arrhythmia situation without systolic dysfunction may be an indication. Totally, 1–7% of all transplants have HCM as the indication [36]. Left ventricular assist devices may be an option, and continuous axial flow assist therapy has shown promising results in a small series [37].

9. Risk assessment

HCM is heterogeneous disease in many aspects including the risk of sudden cardiac death. The combined risk of cardiovascular mortality is estimated to 6% per year [2]. The cardiovascular mortality constitutes heart failure, sudden cardiac death, and stroke. Many HCM cohorts from highly specialized centres do not necessarily reflect the mortality of the whole HCM population. In fact, a report with less selection bias reported a mortality of 2% [2]. In elderly patients, above 65 years old, the mortality is similar to age- and sex-matched population according to US data [2]. However, sudden cardiac death does occur at all ages and is notably high in early adulthood when sudden cardiac death otherwise is rare.

Survivors of cardiac arrest due to spontaneous ventricular fibrillation or sustained ventricular tachycardia with hemodynamic compromise have 33% mortality at seven years or 41% appropriate ICD therapy at five years [2, 38]. The survival after a cardiac arrest is approximately 10% in the general population. Because of the low chance of survival of cardiac arrest, these patients need an ICD. Thus, these patients are eligible for ICDs as secondary prevention of SCD, and the decision to implant is usually straight forward.

In patients who had not experienced a life threatening ventricular arrhythmia (primary prevention), the decision to implant an ICD requires careful judgement of clinical risk markers and consideration of comorbidities and risk of complications.

There have been three guidelines covering the complex task of ICD as primary prevention of SCD; a joint guideline between the American College of Cardiology/American Heart Association and European Society of Cardiology from 2003, an updated guideline 2011 from ACC/AHA and an ESC guideline launched in August 2014 [2, 39, 40]. The 2003 and 2011 guidelines provide readily evaluated risk factors from history taking, echocardiography and exercise test. Often, one risk factor is considered enough for offering an ICD, but there are differences between countries and centres. It has also not been conclusive if more than risk factor actually correlates with increased risk of appropriate ICD therapy even though more recent studies point in that direction. In addition, possible risk markers have been suggested based on observational studies on ICD cohorts or case reports or expert opinions.

According to guidelines from 2003 and 2011, five major risk factors are established: nonsustained ventricular tachycardia (NSVT), family history of sudden cardiac death (FHSCD), abnormal blood pressure response (ABPRE), unexplained syncope, and MWT 30 mm. A meta-analysis from 2010 based on 30 articles confirmed these risk factors [41]. From this meta-analysis, the presence of left ventricular outflow tract obstruction showed convincing evidence to support in association with SCD. There also seemed to be higher risk for younger patients even though there is no age above which could be safe, but SCD occurs at all ages in HCM [2]. Atrial dilatation and subsequent atrial fibrillation also correlated with SCD in some studies [2]. In patients with concomitant coronary ischemic disease, there was possibly an additional risk as well as in the small subset of patients with left ventricular apical aneurysms [2]. Genetic factors are indirectly included because of the risk factor FHSCD but guideline stress phenotype on an individual level; however, the presence of certain mutations, especially in the cases of double or multiple mutations, there seemed to be an increased risk. ECG is abnormal in 90% of HCM patients, and efforts have been made to correlate abnormalities to risk of SCD suggesting QRS amplitudes and/or fragmentation as risk markers [2]. However, ECG pattern has not been part of guidelines. SCD in athletes due to HCM is well known, and 2003 guideline considered intense (competitive) physical exertion a possible risk factor [39]. Fibrosis assessed on CMR has been studied is advocated as risk factor but is not yet part of guidelines [42, 43].

The evolving criticism on guidelines resulted in a completely new algorithm to assess 5-year risk of SCD in HCM [44]. The article preceding the guidelines change in August 2014 argued that previous guideline considered the clinical parameters left ventricular hypertrophy as binary (30 mm), and in the new guideline, it is treated as continuous [2]. They also included age as the validation work was based on cohorts where risk was higher in the young. Atrial enlargement was again considered a risk factor and included in the algorithm are treated as a continuous variable. The new European algorithm is based on 3,675 patients from six centres and follow-up time of more than 24,000 patient years. One of the centres constituted an external validation. Since the introduction of the 2014 ESC guidelines, external validation work has been published [45]. These two reports support for using the new guidelines. The sophisticated statistics behind the new guideline resulting in a formula with a prognostic index as an exponential function have been overcome by an open access link where a clinician within a few minutes can calculate 5-year risk in an individual patient [2, 46]. However, one should consider the aim of the new guidelines carefully and recognize its limitations. The authors of the new algorithm considered the rationale for the new approach because previous guideline would lead to overuse of ICD; many patients would experience harm of the ICD and never have benefit of the device. One should bear in mind that the underlying patient cohorts were adults and risk stratification in children and adolescent should be used with caution. Hypertrophic as part of metabolic disease or syndromes were not part of study base. Paradoxically, extreme left myocardial thickness 35 mm had low SCD risk, but this subset of patient was few and the model does not seem to cover all ranges. Furthermore, the model does not take into account the obstruction only at exercise but at rest.

Even though the new model has been widely recognized, it is still unclear to what degree it is actually used globally. Recently, an independent assessment of the ESC risk model concluded that the model was unreliable because many patients with SCD or appropriate ICD therapy had a low risk score. The implementation of new guidelines may take time or require further refinement. Probably it will not replace previous strategies completely but serve as important tool. Risk stratification is and will always be a complex task.

10. Age and gender

Most studies found no significant association with age and sudden death in HCM cohorts, but these studies are typically ICD populations selected from tertiary centres [47]. Furthermore, usually these studies do not take age- and sex-matched comparison with general population into account. Many studies on ICD cohorts lack statistical power to detect differences at different age strata. In two studies, there was an inverse relationship between age and sudden cardiac death, but in the majority of studies, no association was demonstrated [2]. In a recently published nationwide Swedish study without selection, bias age was not significantly associated with appropriate ICD therapy [34, 35]. In American guidelines, age is not part of risk stratification, whereas in the European guidelines, age is part of the equation based on validation of cohorts, which showed an increased risk in younger patients [2]. The association between age and other risk factors is quite complicated, but there seems to be data supporting the rationale for offering ICDs with NSVT, severe left ventricular hypertrophy (LVH) and unexplained syncope in younger patients [2]. Age is further complicated by the individual comorbidities and the discrepancy between biological and calendric age. From other guidelines on general ICD candidates, guidelines state at least 2 years of life expectancy to be eligible for an ICD. An experienced clinician may reflect about age in the individual case but cannot neglect local resources and risk of complications in addition to effective patient communication on prognosis.

Most HCM cohorts have a majority of males. In the six cohorts in the ESC risk algorithm, the proportion of males ranged from 59 to 72% (mean 64%) [2]. This pattern is also seen in several ICD cohorts [34, 35, 47]. However, there does not seem to be a significant difference with regard to risk of appropriate ICD therapy in these cohorts. It is important to recognize the individual risk factor profile rather than gender itself. Neither previous nor current guidelines use gender as part of risk stratification. Notably, females may have a higher risk for complications related to the ICD system [47].

11. Nonsustained ventricular tachycardia (NSVT)

The presence of NSVT has been part on guidelines since it first appeared in 2003 after several reports on the association to sudden cardiac death in HCM. This is in contrast to general ICD population with ischemic or dilated CM with low EF in which NSVT is not part of guidelines The definition of NSVT is at least three beats in a row of ventricular origin but varies with regard to cycle length; the formal cut-off of 100 bpm is seldom used, and 120 or 150 bpm is typically used [2]. The association of life threatening arrhythmias does not seem to vary with length or cycle length. The maximal duration of NSVT is 30 seconds while longer duration is called sustained ventricular tachycardia. The diagnosis of NSVT could be from an ambulatory monitor such as Holter for 24–48 hours as prescribed in the evaluation of HCM patients. However, sometimes NSVT is detected from telemetry in the ward or from a cardiac device, i.e., a pacemaker EGM or implantable loop recorder. Interestingly, NSVT seems to be quite common in ICD recipients. Thus, the more often a HCM patient is monitored for NSVT, the higher the likelihood for detecting the risk factor NSVT. Prolonged monitoring with implantable devices or non-invasive ECG patches is currently not indicated without a history of syncope but remains to be evaluated in the future.

12. Syncope

Syncope deserves special attention when it comes to interviewing the patient about the actual episode. This includes observations from witness about duration (which often may be overestimated) and signs before or after the loss of consciousness. Certain situations may be typical for vaso-vagal syncope (i.e., defection, micturition), situational or orthostatic hypotension. Carotid sinus mechanism for syncope can sometimes be reproduced. The body position and activity may aid important clues. If exercise-induced syncope is experienced, this should imply prompt evaluation because a malignant cause is likely. Notably, tiredness and seizure may indicate epilepsy but do not rule out cardiac causes as severe cerebral hypoxia mimics the clinical scenario. In some studies, unexplained syncope within six months seems to predict worse outcome to higher extent [2]. Nevertheless, a syncopal episode suggestive or arrhythmic cause independent of when it happened should warrant careful evaluation.

13. Family history

A family history of SCD is a dramatic event. Relatives of the victim have to deal with their own attitude and subsequent risk assessment beside emotional impact of the lost relative. Unfortunately, not every physician is aware of the inheritance component in family of SCD or the family does not seek medical advice due to this. Documentation from possibly related HCM is often lacking, misinterpreted or unavailable. Current European guidelines state SCD in the first-degree relative before the age of 40, but no age cut-off when SCD can be attributed to HCM [2]. The underlying studies are quite heterogeneous using different age limit. This risk factor is further complicated as it does not take into account second- or third-degree relatives nor the number of siblings in a family. It is understandable that the motivation for patient and clinicians is usually high when there is case of SCD in the family. However, the scientific basis is less strong than for NSVT, unexplained syncope, or MWT, based on three studies, whereas several other studies could not prove an association [2, 48]. If this inability is due to power problems of studies because of the limited number of patients included and/or few outcome of events, is difficult to judge. The heterogeneity of definitions and relative short follow-up time may also influence the results. Statistical methods often account for uni- and multi-variable influence of risk factors but have difficulties to prove interaction between risk factors in smaller samples with few events.

14. Wall thickness

In patients with a ≥30 mm maximal wall thickness, there was a three-fold increased risk, which makes it a comparatively strong risk factor. Later analyses suggest a U-shaped correlation to sudden cardiac death [49]. As mentioned above, this risk factor has been treated as binary risk factor previously, at least theoretically, but in practise, it is likely that number patients have been offered an ICD even if they did not fulfil this criterion formally. For example, in a 25-year-old patient with otherwise long-life expectancy, a 29 mm thickness would probably be enough for most clinicians. Another limit is the fact that hypertrophy can be more or less unevenly distributed, and it is not known if this influences risk. Moreover, echocardiography does not always provide accurate estimations and certain parts, i.e., apical parts may be difficult to trace. Other imaging techniques may resolve this problem in individuals. The progression of disease is difficult to predict, but in a young patient, it is more likely and effect of hypertensive disease is more easy to rule out. Future validation work on this risk factor will hopefully elucidate this factor better. Here, CMR and PET may add important knowledge of not only structural findings but also functional and metabolic disturbances associated with risk of arrhythmia.

15. Exercise blood pressure response

The assessment of this risk factor requires referral for ergometer bicycle test or any other exercise test. In series of HCM patients, one third of patients show abnormal blood pressure response [2, 50]. The definition of abnormal blood pressure response varies, but with regard to risk stratification, a failure to increase systolic pressure at least 20 mmHg or a fall of 20 mmHg from peak pressure is considered relevant [2]. This risk factor seems to be more pronounced in patients younger than 40 years old. In some studies, this risk factor has not been analysed because not all patients were systematically assessed. This is understandable as if a clinician already has data enough to support the decision to implant an ICD, there is a rationale for omitting this test as is does not add clinical insight for further management of the individual patient. In the new guidelines, the authors took the decision to abandon exercise test as part of risk stratification, and it remains to be seen if upcoming guidelines will stick to this policy.

16. Atrial fibrillation and left atrial diameter

The increased filling pressures of the left ventricle will result in wall stress of left atrium and risk of dilatation. There is a well-known risk of atrial fibrillation and a dilated left atrium, and this in turn increases risk of embolic events. In a recent study, AF was a stronger risk factor than the established five major risk factors in both univariable and multivariable analyses in HCM-ICD cohort [34, 35]. AF should be considered as a sole factor for risk stratification and lead to an ICD, but in patients implanted based on the five major risk factors, AF predicted high probability of appropriate ICD therapy [2, 34, 35].

Left atrial diameter is assessed by echocardiography using a parasternal projection and is now part of the risk model algorithm [46]. It is handled as a continuous variable, but it does not take into account the different shapes of the atrium as some patients have elongated atrium mostly visualized in an apical four-chamber view. Neither is the volume calculated, but a simple diameter in one projection sometimes allows inter-user variability and anatomical variation difficult to standardize.

17. LVOT obstruction

The outflow gradient of the left chamber may vary and change with exercise or can be provoked by drugs. In the meta-analysis, they concluded that LVOT gradient should be reassessed as a risk factor based on evidence from numerous observational studies [41, 51, 52]. This also holds true when developing the new algorithm and was then included and treated as a continuous variable.

18. CMR, CT and PET

Cardiac magnetic resonance using a contrast-enhanced technique has demonstrated association with arrhythmias, and substantial amount of fibrosis may be suggestive increased risk for SCD [53]. The accurate delineation and spatial resolution of CMR may aid in cases where echocardiography is inadequate. However, to assess association between CMR-derived baseline data and outcome such as SCD or appropriate ICD therapy will follow-up time and large cohorts with enough events to prove association. Therefore, CMR has been included in the first prospective registry on HCM patients, and this will hopefully provide gain of insight in this matter. CMR uses magnetic fields instead of ionizing radiation, but contraindication needs to be considered. Notably, ICD patients should be assessed before a device is implanted even though newer ICD model may allow CMR at least 1.5 Tesla investigations but gives rise to artefacts. PET can be used in conjunction within either CT or CMR and is a promising field for research with functional, structural and metabolic assessment, which is available.

19. Driving

While most HCM patients have no driving restrictions, patients with ICD devices need special considerations. This advice needs to be in harmony with national laws besides checking international guidelines that provide update recommendation on this topic. A survivor of cardiac arrest should not drive for the first six months after the event, and careful assessment of cognitive function is then advised. The same considerations should be made after stroke, epilepsy, diabetes and other medical conditions. The risk after an arrhythmic event is highest in the first few months, which makes six-month restriction reasonably. In primary prevention of ICD patients, there is no restriction except for unexplained syncope with a typical restriction in the first 6 months. Professional driving (buss, truck, taxi) is not accepted for ICD carriers, independent of indication (primary or secondary) in most countries. Other vehicles, including trains and aeroplanes, need to be considered and legal actions taken.

20. Pregnancy

Pregnancy implies increased loading pressures, and in last semester, a cardiovascular demand may increase risk. HCM is a heterogeneous disease, and risk of SCD during pregnancy needs to be addressed based on individual factors. Few women need to give up a wish to become a biological mother; however, there are fatal cases reported, but these have been in patients with a known high risk. Because of the non-negligible risk, females are advised to plan pregnancy and counselling should be offered during the pregnancy and delivery by a multidisciplinary team. In the rare case of need for ICD implant during pregnancy, efforts need to be taken to provide protection from radiation or using echocardiography to assess position of leads.

21. Combinations of risk markers and modifiers

The new algorithm takes several risk factors into account and weights them using a formula [46]. But even this method has the same lack of accurate estimation of mediating or possibly protective interaction between markers. All markers are somewhat surrogates and life-time risk can never be exactly assessed in the individual. Long-term follow-up in all studies is actually typically less than 10 years for the majority of the patient, and risk is not linear. Besides, risk markers are assessed at the time for decision to implant and may change during the course and should therefore be re-assessed every 1–3 years. Again, a multicentre, international, prospective registry will provide more insights in the challenge to stratify risk in HCM.

22. Children

Risk stratification in children equals adult strategy in many ways, but primary prevention is typically based on two or more risk factors rather than one. Historically, epicardial lead has been used in a growing child, but nowadays subcutaneous ICD may be a more attractive option. A single device (ICD-VVI) is usually sufficient as pacing indication is rare in the young, and this approach seems to limit complications.

23. ICD therapy

ICD is an effective way to prevent sudden cardiac death in HCM. The landmark trial by Maron et al. demonstrated 11% annual rate in secondary and 5% annual rate in primary prevention [54]. Several studies have confirmed the usefulness on ICD in HCM [47]. Schinkel et al. performed a meta-analysis of 2,190 patients from 16 cohorts (mean age 42 years, 62% males) with 83% primary prevention indication [47]. The summary estimate for appropriate ICD therapy was 3.3% per year (95% confidence interval 2.2–4.4%). A later nationwide ICD cohort of unselected patients reported 4.5% appropriate ICD therapy in primary prevention and 7.0% in secondary prevention [34, 35].

It should be noted that *not* every appropriate ICD therapy is indeed lifesaving. A ventricular arrhythmia can self-terminate, which can lead to an overestimation of benefit of ICD. Therefore, it is important to programme a number of intervals to at least 30 before therapy. The detection zones should be carefully considered, and antitachycardia pacing (ATP) should be used to avoid unnecessary shocks. However, the risk of a sustained ventricular below detection zone could lead to fatal hemodynamic collapse including pulseless electrical tachycardia or recurrent ventricular fibrillation when ventricles are finally exhausted. Patients on amiodarone are known to have a slower rate than otherwise [2]. Earlier there have been worries about the efficacy in hypertrophic heart due to increased myocardial mass to discharge, but large series of a patient show efficacy of ICD discharges with very few exceptions. The discussion on DFT testing preoperatively could be extended to HCM populations, but the trend to induce patients more rarely, if at all, will continue for HCM patients. One may argue that induction is not without risk; devices have high voltage and sufficient margin, and the clinical situation is not exactly the same as during implant. Moreover, it may be advisable to choose a type and brand of ICD device capable of wave form optimization and to deliver high voltage discharges. Different devices offer different solutions to avoid T-wave oversense, which should be reflected upon. A T-wave oversense leads to double counting and will deliver inappropriate shocks. Technical failure of lead, fracture and insulation defects, or external noise could lead inappropriate shocks. The overall annual risk of inappropriate shocks is 4.8% in a meta-analysis [47] and confirmed in later analyses of unselected populations [55]. Hopefully, with programming optimization, this could likely be reduced. The most common cause of inappropriate shocks is atrial arrhythmias, predominantly. In addition to programming longer duration, longer cycle length, discrimination algorithm should be considered such as interval stability, but one should neglect the risk of misdiagnosis simultaneous ventricular arrhythmias that need appropriate therapy. Furthermore, other actions to avoid atrial tachycardia and to reduce rapid atrioventricular conduction are needed: beta-blockers, antiarrhythmics, and occasionally His-ablation.

Compared to other ICD populations where ATP is effective in a vast majority of cases, the proportion of ATP success was less in HCM-ICD cohorts. This has been seen in other HCM trials, and HCM possibly carries an increased risk of rapid ventricular tachycardia or ventricular fibrillation to a larger extent than other ICD groups.

ICD systems offer an alert function for the patient if technical failure or essential clinical episode takes place. Remote monitoring of ICD devices is standard, and this increases safety as it detects technical problems between follow-ups in clinic or detects atrial fibrillation, which implies decision to anticoagulated.

24. Death despite ICD

The efficacy of ICDs to prevent sudden cardiac death leads to a swift in cases of death. The vast majority of death in the ICD population dies because of progressive heart failure. The standardized mortality was 3.4 (95% confidence interval 2.4–4.5) compared to general population [56]. This implies that heart failure care needs to be addressed if improved survival should be achieved. Importantly, a holistic approach to device patient is warranted, and one should not just focus on the prevention of arrhythmia death.

25. Implant procedure

The procedure to implant an ICD in a HCM patient is essentially the same as in other indication. The vascular access is typically from the left side either through cephalic cut-down or punctures of the axillary or subclavian vein. The ventricular lead is implanted in the apical region of the right ventricle if R-waves and thresholds are acceptable in this position. It is important to check for T-wave oversensing before deciding the final position of the lead. In obstructive HCM, it is of special importance to implant the lead in apex as this could facilitate reduction in outflow gradient if AV-pacing is tried. For the same reason, an atrial lead (ICD-DR) is often preferred. Furthermore, many HCM patients have high beta-blocking dosage, conduction defects or paroxysmal atrial fibrillation with the help of AV synchronous pacing. The ventricle lead could be either single or dual coil. There is a tendency to increased use of single-coil system as possible defibrillation threshold difference is negligible, easier to implant and extract. The device could be implanted subcutaneously or intramuscular. As described above, less number of patients is induced nowadays. The typical procedure time is less than 1 hour, and the patient can often be discharged the same day. The battery of an ICD in a modern system lasts for 8–10 years, depending on amount pacing and, in few cases, the demand of therapies. CRT system in end-stage HCM has been tried with preliminary promising results.

26. Health-related quality of life

In a British study from 1995 on HCM patients, health-related quality of life was decreased [57]. Since then, improvement of health care has been made, and there may be different outcomes in a HCM population that is not selected from a specialized centre. Recently, a study on HCM patients with ICDs confirmed poor quality of life, regardless of sex, age, or primary/secondary indication [58]. Instead, atrial fibrillation and systolic heart failure are determinants of poor quality of life, especially physical aspects. Notably, inappropriate, but appropriate therapies are associated with poorer mental health. To further address quality of life issues, qualitative studies may provide valuable insights.

27. S-ICD

An subcutaneous-ICD (S-ICD) system contains a subcutaneously implanted lead (in an L-configuration) connected to a device inserted subcutaneously, or preferably intramuscular. It effectively terminates ventricular arrhythmias and can offer supportive post-chock pacing. Current devices cannot be used in patients who need permanent pacing, but technical solutions are developed to combine a leadless pacemaker system communicating with an S-ICD system. This is beneficial in patients with abnormal vascular anatomy, i.e., malformations or vessel occlusions. But, in young patient, there is an increasing interest in S-ICD to save vessels for future interventions and avoid short-term and long-term vessel-related complications. S-ICD has been used in HCM, but careful pre-operative assessment of possibly risk of T-wave oversense is of importance in this group. The cost of S-ICD device is currently much larger than for transvenous device, but this probably diminishes. Studies so far have shown a promising short-term use of S-ICD among HCM patients [59].

28. Future perspectives

There remain many challenges in the field of HCM. A detailed understanding of pathophysiologic mechanism of disease progression, arrhythmia substrate and triggers and molecular-genetic base of the heterogeneous disease is crucial. This could lead to improvement in the therapeutic arsenal, but this development relies on scientific progress in the field of cardiology and basic sciences. Multicentre, prospective registries and other international collaborations to evaluate outcome and refine risk stratification are promising [60, 61].

Author details

Peter Magnusson

Address all correspondence to: peter.magnusson@regiongavleborg.se

1 Cardiology Research Unit, Department of Medicine, Karolinska Institute, Karolinska University Hospital, Solna, Stockholm, Sweden

2 Centre for Research and Development, Uppsala University/Region Gävleborg, Gävle, Sweden

References

[1] Elliott P, Andersson B, Arbustini E, Bilinska Z, Cecchi F, Charron P, Dubourg O, Kühl U, Maisch B, McKenna WJ, Monserrat L, Pankuweit S, Rapezzi C, Seferovic P, Tavazzi L, Keren A. Classification of the cardiomyopathies: a position statement from the European Society of Cardiology Working Group on Myocardial and Pericardial Diseases. Eur Heart J. 2008;29(2):270-6. DOI: 10.1093/eurheartj/ehm342

[2] Elliott PM, Anastasakis A, Borger MA, Borggrefe M, Cecchi F, Charron P, Hagege AA, Lafont A, Limongelli G, Mahrholdt H, McKenna WJ, Mogensen J, Nihoyannopoulos P, Nistri S, Pieper PG, Pieske B, Rapezzi C, Rutten FH, Tillmanns C, Watkins H. 2014 ESC Guidelines on diagnosis and management of hypertrophic cardiomyopathy: the Task Force for the Diagnosis and Management of Hypertrophic Cardiomyopathy of the European Society of Cardiology (ESC). Eur Heart J. 2014;35(39):2733-79. DOI: 10.1093/eurheartj/ehu284

[3] Kampmann C, Wiethoff CM, Wenzel A, Stolz G, Betancor M, Wippermann CF, Huth RG, Habermehl P, Knuf M, Emschermann T, Stopfkuchen H. Normal values of M mode echocardiographic measurements of more than 2000 healthy infants and children in central Europe. Heart. 2000;83(6):667-72. DOI: 10.1136/heart.83.6.667

[4] Cardim N, Galderisi M, Edvardsen T, Plein S, Popescu BA, D'Andrea A, Bruder O, Cosyns B, Davin L, Donal E, Freitas A, Habib G, Kitsiou A, Petersen SE, Schroeder S, Lancellotti P, Camici P, Dulgheru R, Hagendorff A, Lombardi M, Muraru D, Sicari R. Role of multimodality cardiac imaging in the management of patients with hypertrophic cardiomyopathy: an expert consensus of the European Association of Cardiovascular Imaging Endorsed by the Saudi Heart Association. Eur Heart J Cardiovasc Imaging. 2015;16(3):280. DOI: 10.1093/ehjci/jeu291

[5] Kawarai H, Kajimoto K, Minami Y, et al. Risk of sudden death in end-stage hypertrophic cardiomyopathy. J Card Fail. 2011;17:459-64.

[6] Biagini E, Coccolo F, Ferlito M, et al. Dilated-hypokinetic evolution of hypertrophic cardiomyopathy: prevalence, incidence, risk factors, and prognostic implications in pediatric and adult patients. J Am Coll Cardiol. 2005;46:1543-50.

[7] Harris KM, Spirito P, Maron MS, et al. Prevalence, clinical profile, and significance of left ventricular remodeling in the end-stage phase of hypertrophic cardiomyopathy. Circulation. 2006;114:216-25.

[8] Melacini P, Basso C, Angelini A, et al. Clinicopathological profiles of progressive heart failure in hypertrophic cardiomyopathy. Eur Heart J. 2010;31:2111-23.

[9] Williams L, Frenneaux M. Syncope in hypertrophic cardiomyopathy: mechanisms and consequences for treatment. Europace. 2007;9(9):817-22. DOI: 10.1093/europace/eum093

[10] Guttmann OP, Rahman MS, O'Mahony C, Anastasakis A, Elliott PM. Atrial fibrillation and thromboembolism in patients with hypertrophic cardiomyopathy: systematic review. Heart. 2014;100(6):465-72. DOI: 10.1136/heartjnl-2013-304276

[11] Guttmann OP, Pavlou M, O'Mahony C, Monserrat L, Anastasakis A, Rapezzi C, Biagini E, Gimeno JR, Limongelli G, Garcia-Pavia P, McKenna WJ, Omar RZ, Elliott PM, Hypertrophic Cardiomyopathy Outcomes Investigators. Prediction of thromboembolic risk in patients with hypertrophic cardiomyopathy (HCM Risk-CVA). Eur J Heart Fail. 2015;17(8):837-45. DOI: 10.1002/ejhf.316.

[12] Lopes LR, Rahman MS, Elliott PM. A systematic review and meta-analysis of genotype-phenotype associations in patients with hypertrophic cardiomyopathy caused by sarcomeric protein mutations. Heart. 2013;99(24):1800-11. DOI: 10.1136/heartjnl-2013-303939.

[13] Morita H, Nagai R, Seidman JG, et al. The impact of genetic testing on hypertrophic cardiomyopathy and heart failure. J Cardiovasc Transl Res. 2010;3:297-303.

[14] Bos JM, Towbin JA, Ackerman MJ, et al. Diagnostic, prognostic, and therapeutic implications of genetic testing for hypertrophic cardiomyopathy. J Am Coll Cardiol. 2009;54:201-11.

[15] Sébillon P, Bouchier C, Bidot LD, Bonne G, Ahamed K, Charron P, Drouin-Garraud V, Millaire A, Desrumeaux G, Benaïche A, Charniot JC, Schwartz K, Villard E, Komajda M. Expanding the phenotype of LMNA mutations in dilated cardiomyopathy and functional consequences of these mutations. J Med Genet. 2003;40(8):560-7.

[16] Teare D. Asymmetrical hypertrophy of the heart in young adults. Br Heart J. 1958;20:1-18.

[17] Maron BJ, Gardin JM, Flack JM, Gidding SS, Kurosaki TT, Bild DE. Prevalence of hypertrophic cardiomyopathy in a general population of young adults. Echocardiographic analysis of 4111 subjects in the CARDIA study. Coronary artery risk development in (Young) adults. Circulation. 1995;92(4):785-9.

[18] Corrado D, Basso C, Schiavon M, Thiene G. Screening for hypertrophic cardiomyopathy in young athletes. N Engl J Med. 1998;339(6):364-9.

[19] Semsarian C, Ingles J, Maron MS, Maron BJ. New perspectives on the prevalence of hypertrophic cardiomyopathy. J Am Coll Cardiol. 2015;65(12):1249-54. DOI: 10.1016/j.jacc.2015.01.019.

[20] Caselli S, Maron MS, Urbano-Moral JA, Pandian NG, Maron BJ, Pelliccia A. Differentiating left ventricular hypertrophy in athletes from that in patients with hypertrophic cardiomyopathy. Am J Cardiol. 2014;114(9):1383-9. DOI: 10.1016/j.amjcard.2014.07.070

[21] Ostman-Smith I. Sudden cardiac death in young athletes. Open Access J Sports Med. 2011;2:85-97. DOI: 10.2147/OAJSM.S10675.

[22] Maron BJ, Haas TS, Doerer JJ, Thompson PD, Hodges JS. Comparison of U.S. and Italian experiences with sudden cardiac deaths in young competitive athletes and implications for preparticipation screening strategies. Am J Cardiol. 2009;104(2):276-80. DOI: 10.1016/j.amjcard.2009.03.037

[23] Pelliccia A, Zipes DP, Maron BJ. Bethesda Conference #36 and the European Society of Cardiology Consensus Recommendations revisited a comparison of U.S. and European criteria for eligibility and disqualification of competitive athletes with cardiovascular abnormalities. J Am Coll Cardiol. 2008;52(24):1990-6. DOI: 10.1016/j.jacc.2008.08.055

[24] Maron BJ, Epstein SE, Roberts WC. Hypertrophic cardiomyopathy: a common cause of sudden death in the young competitive athlete. Eur Heart J. 1983;4 (Suppl F):135-44.

[25] Maron BJ. Historical perspectives on sudden deaths in young athletes with evolution over 35 years. Am J Cardiol. 2015;116(9):1461-8. DOI: 10.1016/j.amjcard.2015.07.072.

[26] Lynge TH, Risgaard B, Jabbari R, Glinge C, Bundgaard H, Maron B, Haunsø S, Winkel BG, Tfelt-Hansen J. Cardiac symptoms before sudden cardiac death caused by hypertrophic cardiomyopathy: a nationwide study among the young in Denmark. Europace. 2016 Jan 27. pii: euv403. [Epub ahead of print]

[27] Yu EH, Omran AS, Wigle ED, Williams WG, Siu SC, Rakowski H. Mitral regurgitation in hypertrophic obstructive cardiomyopathy: relationship to obstruction and relief with myectomy. J Am Coll Cardiol. 2000;36(7):2219-25

[28] Desai MY, Bhonsale A, Smedira NG, Naji P, Thamilarasan M, Lytle BW, Lever HM. Predictors of long-term outcomes in symptomatic hypertrophic obstructive cardiomyopathy patients undergoing surgical relief of left ventricular outflow tract obstruction. Circulation. 2013;128(3):209-16. DOI: 10.1161/CIRCULATIONAHA

[29] Maron BJ, Yacoub M, Dearani JA. Controversies in cardiovascular medicine. Benefits of surgery in obstructive hypertrophic cardiomyopathy: bring septal myectomy back for European patients. Eur Heart J. 2011;32(9):1055-8. DOI: 10.1093/eurheartj/ehr006.

[30] Jensen MK, Prinz C, Horstkotte D, van Buuren F, Bitter T, Faber L, Bundgaard H. Alcohol septal ablation in patients with hypertrophic obstructive cardiomyopathy: low incidence of sudden cardiac death and reduced risk profile. Heart. 2013;99(14):1012-7. DOI: 10.1136/heartjnl-2012-303339.

[31] Brignole M, Auricchio A, Baron-Esquivias G, Bordachar P, Boriani G, Breithardt OA, Cleland J, Deharo JC, Delgado V, Elliott PM, Gorenek B, Israel CW, Leclercq C, Linde C, Mont L, Padeletti L, Sutton R, Vardas PE. 2013 ESC guidelines on cardiac pacing and cardiac resynchronization therapy: the task force on cardiac pacing and resynchronization therapy of the European Society of Cardiology (ESC). Developed in collaboration with the European Heart Rhythm Association (EHRA). Europace. 2013;15(8):1070-118. DOI: 10.1093/europace/eut206.

[32] Jurado Román A, Montero Cabezas JM, Rubio Alonso B, García Tejada J, Hernández Hernández F, Albarrán González-Trevilla A, Velázquez Martín MT, Coma Samartín R,

Rodríguez García J, Tascón Pérez JC. Sequential atrioventricular pacing in patients with hypertrophic cardiomyopathy: an 18-year experience. Rev Esp Cardiol (Engl Ed). 2016;69(4):377-83. DOI: 10.1016/j.rec.2015.08.023.

[33] Rogers DP, Marazia S, Chow AW, Lambiase PD, Lowe MD, Frenneaux M, et al. Effect of biventricular pacing on symptoms and cardiac remodelling in patients with end-stage hypertrophic cardiomyopathy. Eur J Heart Fail. 2008;10:507-13.

[34] Ponikowski P, Voors AA, Anker SD, Bueno H, Cleland JG, Coats AJ, Falk V, González-Juanatey JR, Harjola VP, Jankowska EA, Jessup M, Linde C, Nihoyannopoulos P, Parissis JT, Pieske B, Riley JP, Rosano GM, Ruilope LM, Ruschitzka F, Rutten FH, van der Meer P; Authors/Task Force Members; Document Reviewers. 2016 ESC Guidelines for the diagnosis and treatment of acute and chronic heart failure: the Task Force for the diagnosis and treatment of acute and chronic heart failure of the European Society of Cardiology (ESC). Developed with the special contribution of the Heart Failure Association (HFA) of the ESC. Eur J Heart Fail. 2016;18(8):891-975. DOI: 10.1002/ejhf. 592.

[35] Magnusson P, Gadler F, Liv P, Mörner S. Risk markers and appropriate implantable defibrillator therapy in hypertrophic cardiomyopathy. Pacing Clin Electrophysiol. 2016;39(3):291-301. DOI: 10.1111/pace.12801

[36] Kato TS, Takayama H, Yoshizawa S, Marboe C, Schulze PC, Farr M, Naka Y, Mancini D, Maurer MS. Cardiac transplantation in patients with hypertrophic cardiomyopathy. Am J Cardiol. 2012;110(4):568-74. DOI: 10.1016/j.amjcard.2012.04.030. Epub 15 May 2012.

[37] Wynne E, Bergin JD, Ailawadi G, Kern JA, Kennedy JL. Use of a left ventricular assist device in hypertrophic cardiomyopathy. J Card Surg. 2011;26(6):663-5. DOI: 10.1111/j. 1540-8191.2011.01331.x.

[38] Maron BJ, Spirito P, Shen WK, Haas TS, Formisano F, Link MS, Epstein AE, Almquist AK, Daubert JP, Lawrenz T, Boriani G, Estes NA 3rd, Favale S, Piccininno M, Winters SL, Santini M, Betocchi S, Arribas F, Sherrid MV, Buja G, Semsarian C, Bruzzi P. Implantable cardioverter-defibrillators and prevention of sudden cardiac death in hypertrophic cardiomyopathy. JAMA. 2007;298(4):405-12

[39] Maron BJ, McKenna WJ, Danielson GK, et al. American College of Cardiology/ European Society of Cardiology clinical expert consensus document on hypertrophic cardiomyopathy. A report of the American College of Cardiology Foundation Task Force on clinical expert consensus documents and the European Society of Cardiology Committee for practice guidelines. J Am Coll Cardiol. 2003;42:1687-713.

[40] Gersh BJ, Maron BJ, Bonow RO, et al. 2011 ACCF/AHA Guideline for the diagnosis and treatment of hypertrophic cardiomyopathy: a report of the American College of Cardiology Foundation/American Heart Association Task Force on Practice Guidelines developed in collaboration with the American Association for Thoracic Surgery, American Society of Echocardiography, American

Society of Nuclear Cardiology, Heart Failure Society of America, Heart Rhythm Society, Society for Cardiovascular Angiography and Interventions, and Society of Thoracic Surgeons. J Am Coll Cardiol. 2011;58:e212-60.

[41] Christiaans I, van Engelen K, van Langen IM, et al. Risk stratification for sudden cardiac death in hypertrophic cardiomyopathy: systematic review of clinical risk markers. Europace. 2010;12:313-21.

[42] Bruder O, Wagner A, Jensen CJ, et al. Myocardial scar visualized by cardiovascular magnetic resonance imaging predicts major adverse events in patients with hypertrophic cardiomyopathy. J Am Coll Cardiol. 2010;56:875-87.

[43] Chan RH, Maron BJ, Olivotto I, Pencina MJ, Assenza GE, Haas T, et al. Prognostic value of quantitative contrast-enhanced cardiovascular magnetic resonance for the evaluation of sudden death risk in patients with hypertrophic cardiomyopathy. Circulation. 2014;130:484-95.

[44] O'Mahony C, Jichi F, Pavlou M, Monserrat L, Anastasakis A, Rapezzi C, Biagini E, Gimeno JR, Limongelli G, McKenna WJ, Omar RZ, Elliott PM, Hypertrophic Cardiomyopathy Outcomes Investigators. A novel clinical risk prediction model for sudden cardiac death in hypertrophic cardiomyopathy (HCM risk-SCD). Eur Heart J. 2014;35(30):2010-20. DOI: 10.1093/eurheartj/eht439.

[45] Vriesendorp PA, Schinkel AFL, Liebregts M, Willems R, Ten Cate FJ, Van Cleemput J, et al. Independent validation of the novel clinical risk prediction model for sudden cardiac death in hypertrophic cardiomyopathy (HCM Risk-SCD). Eur Heart J. 2014;35(Suppl 1):210.

[46] European Society of Cardiology. HCM Risk-SCD Calculator. 2014. Available at: www.doc2do.com/hcm/webHCM.html

[47] Schinkel AF, Vriesendorp PA, Sijbrands EJ, Jordaens LJ, ten Cate FJ, Michels M. Outcome and complications after implantable cardioverter defibrillator therapy in hypertrophic cardiomyopathy: systematic review and meta-analysis. Circ Heart Fail. 2012;5(5):552-9

[48] Watkinson OT, Elliott PM. A family history of sudden death should not be a primary indication for an implantable cardioverter defibrillator in hypertrophic cardiomyopathy. Can J Cardiol. 2015;31(11):1407-9. DOI: 10.1016/j.cjca.2015.07.724

[49] O'Mahony C, Jichi F, Monserrat L, Ortiz-Genga M, Anastasakis A, Rapezzi C, Biagini E, Gimeno JR, Limongelli G, McKenna WJ, Omar RZ, Elliott PM, Hypertrophic Cardiomyopathy Outcomes Investigators. Inverted U-shaped relation between the risk of sudden cardiac death and maximal left ventricular wall thickness in hypertrophic cardiomyopathy. Circ Arrhythm Electrophysiol. 2016 Jun;9(6). pii: e003818. doi: 10.1161/CIRCEP.115.003818.

[50] Coats CJ, Rantell K, Bartnik A, Patel A, Mist B, McKenna WJ, Elliott PM. Cardiopulmonary exercise testing and prognosis in hypertrophic cardiomyopathy. Circ Heart Fail. 2015;8(6):1022-31. DOI: 10.1161/CIRCHEARTFAILURE.

[51] Elliott PM, Gimeno JR, Tomé MT, Shah J, Ward D, Thaman R, et al. Left ventricular outflow tract obstruction and sudden death risk in patients with hypertrophic cardiomyopathy. Eur Heart J. 2006;27:1933-41.

[52] Autore C, Bernabò P, Barillà CS, et al. The prognostic importance of left ventricular outflow obstruction in hypertrophic cardiomyopathy varies in relation to the severity of symptoms. J Am Coll Cardiol. 2005;45:1078-80.

[53] Ismail TF, Jabbour A, Gulati A, Mallorie A, Raza S, Cowling TE, Das B, Khwaja J, Alpendurada FD, Wage R, Roughton M, McKenna WJ, Moon JC, Varnava A, Shakespeare C, Cowie MR, Cook SA, Elliott P, O'Hanlon R, Pennell DJ, Prasad SK. Role of late gadolinium enhancement cardiovascular magnetic resonance in the risk stratification of hypertrophic cardiomyopathy. Heart. 2014;100(23):1851-8. DOI: 10.1136/heartjnl-2013-305471.

[54] Maron BJ, Shen WK, Link MS, Epstein AE, Almquist AK, Daubert JP, Bardy GH, Favale S, Rea RF, Boriani G, Estes NA 3rd, Spirito P. Efficacy of implantable cardioverter-defibrillators for the prevention of sudden death in patients with hypertrophic cardiomyopathy. N Engl J Med. 2000;342(6):365-73.

[55] Magnusson P, Gadler F, Liv P, Mörner S. Hypertrophic cardiomyopathy and implantable defibrillators in Sweden: inappropriate shocks and complications requiring surgery. J Cardiovasc Electrophysiol. 2015;26(10):1088-94. DOI: 10.1111/jce.12750.

[56] Magnusson P, Gadler F, Liv P, Mörner S. Causes of death and mortality in hypertrophic cardiomyopathy patients with implantable defibrillators in Sweden. J Cardiovasc Med (Hagerstown). 2016;17(7):478-84. DOI: 10.2459/JCM.0000000000000359.

[57] Cox S, O'Donoghue AC, McKenna WJ, Steptoe A. Health related quality of life and psychological wellbeing in patients with hypertrophic cardiomyopathy. Heart. 1997;78(2):182-7.

[58] Magnusson P, Mörner S, Gadler F, Karlsson J. Health-related quality of life in hypertrophic cardiomyopathy patients with implantable defibrillators. Health Qual Life Outcomes. 2016;14:62. DOI: 10.1186/s12955-016-0467-x.

[59] Weinstock J, Bader YH, Maron MS, Rowin EJ, Link MS. Subcutaneous implantable cardioverter defibrillator in patients with hypertrophic cardiomyopathy: an initial experience. J Am Heart Assoc. 2016 Feb 12;5(2). pii: e002488. doi: 10.1161/JAHA.115.002488.

[60] Kramer CM, Appelbaum E, Desai MY, Desvigne-Nickens P, DiMarco JP, Friedrich MG, Geller N, Heckler S, Ho CY, Jerosch-Herold M, Ivey EA, Keleti J, Kim DY, Kolm P, Kwong RY, Maron MS, Schulz-Menger J, Piechnik S, Watkins H, Weintraub WS, Wu P, Neubauer S.Hypertrophic cardiomyopathy registry: the rationale and design of an

international, observational study of hypertrophic cardiomyopathy. Am Heart J. 2015;170(2):223-30. DOI: 10.1016/j.ahj.2015.05.013.

[61] Elliott P, Charron P, Blanes JR, Tavazzi L, Tendera M, Konté M, Laroche C, Maggioni AP; EORP Cardiomyopathy Registry Pilot Investigators. European cardiomyopathy pilot registry: EURObservational Research Programme of the European Society of Cardiology. Eur Heart J. 2016;37(2):164-73. DOI: 10.1093/eurheartj/ehv497

7

Cardiac Magnetic Resonance T1 Mapping in Cardiomyopathies

Christian R. Hamilton-Craig, Mark W. Strudwick and Graham J. Galloway

Abstract

Cardiac magnetic resonance (CMR) imaging has been widely used to assess myocardial perfusion and scar and is the noninvasive reference standard for identification of focal myocardial fibrosis. However, the late gadolinium enhancement (LGE) technique is limited in its accuracy for absolute quantification and assessment of diffuse myocardial fibrosis by technical and pathophysiological features. CMR relaxometry, incorporating T1 mapping, has emerged as an accurate, reproducible, highly sensitive, and quantitative technique for the assessment of diffuse myocardial fibrosis in a number of disease states. We comprehensively review the physics behind CMR relaxometry, the evidence base, and the clinical applications of this emerging technique.

Keywords: cardiac magnetic resonance, T1 mapping, myocardial fibrosis, cardiomyopathy

1. Introduction

Cardiac Magnetic Resonance (CMR) imaging has been used widely to assess myocardial perfusion and scar [1–5]. It is the noninvasive reference standard for left and right ventricular quantitation, as well as the assessment and quantitation of focal myocardial fibrosis (after infarction or due to other causes of cellular injury). Myocardial necrosis causes high signal on late gadolinium enhancement (LGE) inversion recovery T1-weighted images with excellent signal-noise ratios, and this has become the reference standard for noninvasive scar imaging in cardiomyopathies of various causes [1–4]. However, LGE is limited in its ability to assess and quantitate diffuse (nonfocal) myocardial injury and fibrosis. LGE is affected by inconsistencies in acquisition parameters, such as choice inversion time, and in postprocessing when signal intensity thresholds may be arbitrarily applied to distinguish normal myocardium from fibrotic tissue [6, 7]. Moreover, the critical issue with LGE is that signal intensity is expressed on an arbitrary scale (*relative* signal intensity compared with "nulled" normal myocardium). Detection of myocardial fibrosis using *relative* differences between scar and normal myocardium tissue is therefore *qualitative*. Thus, in nonischemic cardiomyopathies, such as hypertension or diabetes, LGE CMR is unable to detect signal differential where the collagen deposition is diffuse and widespread throughout the myocardium [8].

2. CMR relaxometry

CMR is an evolving technique, providing valuable and comprehensive data on the anatomy and functional integrity of both the heart and coronary blood vessels. Currently, CMR is performed at magnetic field strengths of 1.5 or 3 T.

3. T1 mapping with Look–Locker

The initial technique to measure spin–lattice T1 relaxation time values was the eponymously named "Look–Locker" sequence (also known as "TI scout"). It has been widely used to estimate the optimal inversion time for assessment of myocardial LGE [9, 10]. It was originally proposed by Look and Locker in 1968 and analyzed more fully in 1970 [11] and consists of an initial inversion pulse, followed by a train of pulses with a constant, limited flip angle (7–15°).

The development of LL technique is summarized in **Table 1**.

The LL sequence has been widely applied in CMR due to its fast acquisition with minimal breath-hold requirements. The LL sequence has been used to measure T1 values in patients with myocardial fibrosis [9]. However, it suffers from significant limitations: low flip angle RF pulse exciting the magnetization and the two RR intervals in the LL sequence are not sufficient for the magnetization to return to equilibrium. This causes *underestimation* of true T1 values using LL. Furthermore, the LL T1 images with different TIs are acquired at different cardiac phases. Therefore, images are "cine" with cardiac motion effect, which requires tedious manual tracking of the myocardial borders for each phase, a labour-intensive and error-prone process, which is challenging in clinical practice. The drawing of regions of interest "ROI" in myocardial segments requires adjusting for cardiac motion, which results in including blood pool (partial volume averaging) and artificially increasing the measured T1 [12].

To address these shortcomings, several myocardial T1 mapping sequences have been created, including modified Look-Locker inversion (MOLLI) recovery.

Author	Year	Summary of research findings
Look & Locker	1968	Initial proposition of Look–Locker technique
Look & Locker	1970	Fully analyzed NMR pulse sequence to measure a spin–lattice T1 relaxation time
Kaptein et al.	1976	LL was co-opted to quickly sample the recovery after a preparation pulse during the recovery period
Gerumann	1987	T1 by Multiple Readout Pulses (TOMROP) was proposed through which the multiple samples of a particular recovery after RF preparation each correspond to a separate image
Hinson and Sobol	1988	LL method was applied without preparation pulse
Crawley and Henkelman	1988	Compared (LL, saturation recovery, inversion recovery, and stimulated echo) and concluded that LL was almost as efficient
Brix et al.	1990	TMPROP was used with 32 gradient echoes in a total acquisition time of 4 min
Kay	1991	LL single-shot IR method has been optimized and refined
Gowland	1992	LL single-shot IR method has been optimized and refined
Been et al.	1988	Improved RF preparation pulses
Gowland et al.	1989	Improved RF preparation pulses
Ordidge et al.	1990	Echo-planar imaging (EPI) was incorporated into the inversion recovery LL-based method
Gowland and Mansfield	1993	EPI was applied in vivo in less than 3 s
Freeman et al.	1998	An entire image was acquired at each point on a single recovery of longitudinal magnetization after a saturation pulse
Karlsson and Nordell	1999	EPI- with LL method has found application in pharmacokinetic modeling in the head
Daniel et al.	2004	Modified Look–Locker inversion recovery is proposed to overcome the limitations of the conventional LL approach for cardiac applications
Daniel et al.	2006	Studied the single breath-hold myocardial MR T1 mapping with MOLLI technique with high spatial resolution at 1.5 T MR-reproducibility study
Daniel et al.	2007	Investigated optimization and validation of a fully integrated pulse sequence for (MOLLI) T1 mapping of the heart
Iles et al.	2008	Evaluation of diffuse myocardial fibrosis in heart failure with cardiac magnetic resonance contrast-enhanced T1 mapping

Table 1. Summary of development of Look–Locker technique.

4. T1 mapping with Modified Look-Locker Inversion "MOLLI" recovery

Currently, the most evaluated sequence for myocardium T1 mapping is a modified Look-Locker inversion recovery (MOLLI) sequence [13, 14]. The T1 mapping identifies a significant variation between normal and abnormal myocardium. It demonstrates the myocardial fibrosis among different myocardial disorders include ischemia [15], acute/chronic infraction [16], amyloidosis [17], diabetic [18], dilated and hypertrophic cardiomyopathy [19], and heart failure [8].

MOLLI is a CMR pulse sequence that is used for accurate T1 mapping of myocardium with high spatial resolution. MOLLI is an ECG-gated pulse sequence scheme and uses three prepared Look–Locker experiments consecutively within one breath-hold over 17 heartbeats to reconstruct 11 images with different inversion times. Three successive ECG-triggered LL experiments (LL**1**, LL**2**, and LL**3**) are carried out with three, three, and five single-shot readouts, respectively, at end diastole of consecutive heartbeats to sample the recovery of longitudinal magnetization after the inversion pulse. MOLLI pulse sequence scheme is illustrated in **Figure 1**. T1 maps can be generated any time before or after contrast agent (e.g., gadolinium) administration [12].

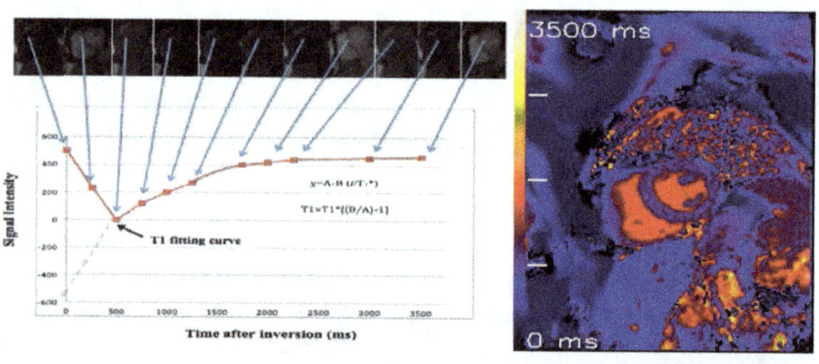

Figure 1. T1 map of a healthy volunteer: Using 17 heartbeats to reconstruct 11 images with different inversion times at end of diastole phase. By merging these images into one data set, T1 values are computed for every pixel with three parameters curve fitting. A reconstructed T1 map with parametric color scale is produced for these pixel values and the segmental and global T1 times can be estimated.

The MOLLI sequence has been described, optimized, tested, and retested in phantoms and in large cohorts of healthy volunteers [12, 14] as well as being applied in cardiomyopathies [8, 15, 17, 19, 20]. In addition, the T1 mapping with MOLLI has been validated against histopathology for assessment of myocardial fibrosis. It demonstrated that the precontrast "native T1" has a linear correlation with the percentage of myocardial fibrosis as measured histologically on invasive myocardial biopsy. T1 times postcontrast administration (10–15 min) had an inverse linear relationship with collagen content in myocardial fibrosis subjects [8, 21, 22].

- Precontrast "Native" T1 = predominant signal from *myocytes* (replacement fibrosis or intracellular accumulation, e.g., Fabry disease)

- Postcontrast T1 = predominant signal from *interstitial* space (interstitial fibrosis)

T1 mapping can be generated for different segments of the myocardium (base, mid-cavity, and apex) within a single breath-hold of about 15–20 s. However, the apex T1 values with MOLLI are slightly higher than basal and mid-cavity. The increasing in T1 values may be caused by partial volume effect and some degree of overestimation effect in apical level of left ventricle [23–25].

T1 mapping with MOLLI has a greater reproducibility, accuracy, and an excellent overall inter- and intra-observer agreement over a wide range of TIs as compared with the traditional LL sequence [13, 14].

However, the T1 mapping with MOLLI sequence is sensitive to extremes of heart rate (bradycardia or tachycardia) [14] leading to a slight underestimation of T1 values. This may be corrected though *heart rate correction* by changing the timing of the readouts with respect to the inversion pulses at different heart rates.

Moreover, MOLLI is also limited by long breath-hold for about 15–20 s (17 heartbeats to acquire the final T1 maps). This may be difficult for elderly and pulmonary compromised patients and generates respiratory and motion artifacts [26]. Modern in-line processing provides registration tools to reduce motion artifacts before the computation of final T1 maps (motion-corrected or "MoCo MOLLI") [27]. A shortened Modified Look-Locker inversion recovery (*shMOLLI*) with shorter breath-holds has been validated and recently applied for cardiomyopathies [28, 29].

5. MRI field strength

At 1.5 T, the pre- and postcontrast (10 mins) T1 times of normal myocardium are 980 ± 53 ms and 470 ± 26 ms, respectively [14]. Precontrast T1 values of myocardial fibrosis (Infarction scar) are significantly longer than those of normal myocardium (1060 ± 61 ms vs. 987 ± 34 ms) [20]. The postcontrast T1 times (10 mins) were significantly shorter in chronic infarct scar compared with normal myocardium at 0.15 mmol/kg (390 ± 20 ms vs. 483 ± 23 ms, respectively) [20].

3 T: T1 mapping at higher magnetic field (3 T) has been reported in a few studies of interstitial myocardial fibrosis, but minimal data exist for ultra-high field at 7 T. 3 T data are similar to 1.5 T, the precontrast T1 was longer, and postcontrast T1 was shorter in myocardial fibrosis patients compared with normal myocardium. Puntmann et al. [30] reported higher precontrast T1 values for hypertrophic and nonischemic dilated cardiomyopathies at 3 T compared with controls (Hypertrophic 1.254 ± 43 ms, and nonischemic dilated cardiomyopathy 1.239 ± 57 ms vs. healthy 1.070 ± 55 ms). Also, the postcontrast T1 values (10 mins) at 3 T were shorter in hypertrophic and dilated cardiomyopathies compared with healthy (hypertrophic: 307 ± 47 ms, dilated cardiomyopathies: 296 ± 43 ms vs. controls: 402 ± 58 ms) [30].

There are studies published for normal and diffuse myocardial fibrosis of myocardium T1 values, as described comprehensively in **Tables 2** and **3**:

First author (Ref.#)	Sample size	T1/T2* mapping sequence	Result of T1 or T2* mapping (ms)
Wacker et al. [31]	5	srTFL, segmented T2* gradient echo pulse	T1 = 1219 ± 72 ms T2* = 35 ± 3 ms
Sebastian et al. [32]	12	LL	T1 = 1033 ± 126 ms T2* = NA
Messroghli et al, [33]	15	MOLLI	T1 = 980 ± 53 ms T2* = NA
Messroghli et al. [34]	20	MOLLI	T1 = 939 ± 63 ms T2* = NA
Sparrow et al, [35]	15	MOLLI	T1 = 980 ± 53 ms T2* = NA
Iles et al. [8]	20	VAST	T1 = 975 ± 62 ms T2* = NA
Li et al. [36]	13	2 echo times GRE	T1 = NA T2* = 33 ± 6.5 ms
Reeder et al. [37]	5	Multi echo GRE	T1 = NA T2*= 38 ± 6 ms
Anderson et al. [38]	15	Multi echo GRE	T1 = NA T2*= 52 ± 16 ms
Positano et al. [39]	15	Multi echo GRE	T1 = NA T2* = 38 ± 9.2 ms in endocardial sectors, and 33.1 ± 8.4 ms in epicardial sectors
Messroghli et al. [40]	20	Multi echo GRE	T1 = NA T2* = 27.9 ± 3.4 ms in anteroseptal and 23.1 ± 5.2 ms in inferolateral
Piechnik et al. [28]	342	shMOLLI	T1 = 962 ± 25 ms T2* = NA Heart rate only physiologic factors effect on myocardial T1 values

Note: NA, not applicable; srTFL, saturation recovery turboFLASH; LL, Look-Locker; MOLLI, modified Look–Locker inversion recovery sequence; VAST, inversion recovery gradient echo sequence with Variable Sampling of the k-space in Time; GRE, gradient pulse sequence; shMOLLI, short modified Look-Locker sequence.

Table 2. Healthy clinical studies using T1 and T2*.

First author (Ref. #)	Cardiac disease category	Patient sample size	T1 mapping method	Summary of findings
Franck Thuny	Systemic sclerosis	37	MOLLI	LV diastolic dysfunction had a shorter 15 min postcontrast T1 time (ms) than those with a normal diastolic function (431 ± 7 vs. 464 ± 8, p = 0.01).
Helene Thibault	Type II diabetic patient	24	MOLLI	Mean myocardial T1 relaxation time was significantly shorter in diabetic patients than in volunteers both at 5 (312 ± 5 vs. 361 ± 6 milliseconds, respectively, p < 0.001) and 15 min (405 ± 6 vs. 456 ± 5 milliseconds, respectively, p < 0.001) after gadolinium injection.
Andris H Ellims	Hypertrophy cardiomyopathy	51	VAST	Postcontrast myocardial T1 time was significantly shorter in patients with HCM compared with controls, consistent with diffuse myocardial fibrosis (498 ± 80 ms vs. 561 ± 47 ms, p < 0.001).
Beatrice A Marzluf	Patients with NH_2-terminal portion of the precursor of brain natriuretic peptide (NT-proBNP)	37	N/A	In patients with NT-proBNP levels >400 pg/ml mean T1 was significantly shorter than in patients with NT-proBNP <400 pg/ml (374.6 ± 51.1 vs. 404.6 ± 34.4 ms, p = 0.042) and controls (509.4 ± 46.5 ms, p < 0.001).
Christopher T Sibley	Nonischemic cardiomyopathy	73	LL	47 patients had a focal myocardial scar and 26 without scar tissue. The midwall circumferential strain (Ecc) was reduced (−13.0 +/− 5.4%) and mean T1 time was 478 +/ − 70 ms in patients with no scar tissue.
Jellis et al. [18]	Type II diabetic patients	67	VAST	Subjects has a shorter post contrast T1 = 434 ± 20 ms. Postcontrast T1 was associated with Echocardiography diastolic dysfunction (Em r = 0.28, p = 0.020; E/Em r =−0.24, p = 0.049).
Messroghli et al. [13]	Acute myocardial infarction	8	Inversion recovery (IR)-prepared fast gradient echo sequence	T1 precontrast value of the infarcted myocardium was significantly prolonged compared with noninfarcted normal myocardium (+18 ± 7%). T1 10-min postcontrast value of the infarct was significantly reduced compared with normal myocardium (−27 ± 4%).
Messroghli et al. [20]	Acute and chronic myocardial infarction	24	MOLLI	In chronic MI, the precontrast T1 relaxation time of hyper-enhanced areas was higher than T1 of remote areas (1060 ± 61 vs. 987 ± 34 ms, p < 0.0001). In acute MI, the precontrast T1 value of hyper-enhanced areas was higher

First author (Ref. #)	Cardiac disease category	Patient sample size	T1 mapping method	Summary of findings
				than remote areas (1197 ± 76 vs. 1011 ± 66). The hyper-enhanced in acute is higher than chronic infarction.
Flacke and Sebastian [32]	Acute and chronic myocardial infarction	10	LL	Mean T1 values of the normal myocardium postcontrast was 536 ± 66 ms, chronically infracted precontrast and postcontrast was 1000 ± 67 ms and 408 ± 43 ms, respectively.
Sparrow et al. [35]	Myocardial Fibrosis in Chronic Aortic Regurgitation	8	Molli	There is a significant difference in segmental averaged T1 relaxation between in abnormal wall motion vs. Normal control segments in 10, 15, and 20 min after administration Gd: (510 vs. 476 ms, 532 vs 501 ms, and 560 vs. 516 ms, respectively).
Iles et al. [8]	Chronic heart failure	25	VAST	Postcontrast myocardial T1 times were shorter in heart failure subjects than in controls (383 ± 17 ms vs. 564 ± 23 ms) even when excluding areas of regional fibrosis. T1 15-min postcontrast values correlated significantly with collagen volume fraction on myocardial biopsies ($R = -0.7$).
Maceira 2005	Cardiac amyloidosis	22	Segmented inversion recovery sequence	Subendocardial T1 in amyloid patients was shorter than in controls (at 4 min: 427 ± 73 vs. 579 ± 75 ms; $p < 0.01$).

Table 3. Clinical studies using T1 mapping for myocardial diffuse fibrosis in clinical patients.

6. Limitations of T1 mapping

Challenges remain with myocardial relaxometry for T1 mapping. These include technical challenges such as variations of T1 times at different field strength and across different vendors, and the rapidity in growth of pulse sequences being released as product and as works-in-progress (WIP), calling into question both the inherent accuracy and the level agreement between these techniques. Furthermore, the variations in T1 relaxometry values with different contrast doses and image timing require further investigation to establish the test–retest and intersite reproducibility of this technique. Next, the challenges to application of T1 mapping to clinical practice include establishment of robust normal ranges in large cohorts across multiple ethnic groups and the observation that T1 mapping appears to be a highly sensitive technique, with the ability to discriminate healthy normal myocardium and identify very early changes in substrate. However, this technique lacks specificity; a wide variety of conditions prolong native T1 and/or shorten postcontrast myocardial T1. Therefore, further clinical data are required in order to establish the use of these parameters in relation to disease (e.g., early detection of target organ damage in systemic conditions such as hypertension or diabetes), to inform treatment decisions, and their ability to predict or alter clinical outcomes.

7. Conclusions

Myocardial T1 mapping using quantitative relaxometry is an emerging and important tool in the assessment of global myocardial fibrosis. It is a highly sensitive marker of disease, but is not specific, with changes in myocardial T1 occurring in many different conditions. Nevertheless, the high sensitivity and excellent reproducibility of the technique offer a tool for the early detection of myocardial damage, over-and-above techniques such as the CMR LGE technique and other modalities such as speckle tracking echocardiography, pulse wave velocity, and tissue tagging. Native T1 mapping is proving to be a robust indicator of early myocardial disease in many conditions, and normal ranges and guidelines for postprocessing have been published by the Society of Cardiovascular Magnetic Resonance [41]. Myocardial T1 mapping is a rapidly evolving technique, now with longitudinal prognostic data emerging, and normal ranges established at 1.5 and 3.0 T in healthy humans and in aging persons. Further questions remain as to the standardization of pulse sequences across field strengths and between vendors, the affect of contrast type, dose and timing, the postprocessing software, and the interpretation of T1 mapping results to inform clinical practice.

Acknowledgements

The author acknowledges the contribution of Dr Qurain Alshammari's to the background work.

Abbreviations

CMR	cardiac magnetic resonance
LL	Look- Locker
LGE	late gadolinium enhancement
LV	left ventricle
MOLLI	modified Look-Locker inversion recovery
MRI	magnetic resonance imaging
ROI	regions of interest
RV	right ventricle
*sh*MOLLI	shortened modified Look-Locker inversion recovery

Author details

Christian R. Hamilton-Craig[1,2*], Mark W. Strudwick[3] and Graham J. Galloway[1,4]

*Address all correspondence to: c.hamiltoncraig@uq.edu.au

1 Centre for Advanced Imaging, University of Queensland, Brisbane, Australia

2 Department of Radiology, University of Washington, Seattle, WA, USA

3 Medical Imaging and Radiation Science, Monash University, Australia

4 Translational Research Institute, Brisbane, Australia

References

[1] Croisille P, Revel D, Saeed M. Contrast agents and cardiac MR imaging of myocardial ischemia: from bench to bedside. European Radiology 2006;16:1951–1963.

[2] Judd RM, Atalay MK, Rottman GA, Zerhouni EA. Effects of myocardial water exchange on T1 enhancement during Bolus administration of MR contrast agents. Magnetic Resonance in Medicine 1995;33:215–223.

[3] Lima JAC. Myocardial viability assessment by contrast-enhanced magnetic resonance imaging. Journal of the American College of Cardiology 2003;42:902–904.

[4] Kim RJ, Chen E-L, Lima JoAC, Judd RM. Myocardial Gd-DTPA kinetics determine MRI contrast enhancement and reflect the extent and severity of myocardial injury after acute reperfused infarction. Circulation 1996;94:3318–3326.

[5] Mahrholdt H, Wagner A, Judd RM, Sechtem U, Kim RJ. Delayed enhancement cardiovascular magnetic resonance assessment of non-ischaemic cardiomyopathies. European Heart Journal 2005;26:1461–1474.

[6] Simonetti OP, Kim RJ, Fieno DS et al. An improved MR imaging technique for the visualization of myocardial infarction. Radiology 2001;218:215–223.

[7] Spiewak M, Malek LA, Misko J et al. Comparison of different quantification methods of late gadolinium enhancement in patients with hypertrophic cardiomyopathy. European Journal of Radiology 2010;74:e149–e153.

[8] Iles L, Pfluger H, Phrommintikul A et al. Evaluation of diffuse myocardial fibrosis in heart failure with cardiac magnetic resonance contrast-enhanced T1 mapping. Journal of the American College of Cardiology 2008;52:1574–1580.

[9] Amano Y, Takayama M, Kumita S. Contrast-enhanced myocardial T1-weighted scout (Look–Locker) imaging for the detection of myocardial damages in hypertrophic cardiomyopathy. Journal of Magnetic Resonance Imaging 2009;30:778–784.

[10] Karlsson M, Nordell B. Analysis of the Look-Locker T1 mapping sequence in dynamic contrast uptake studies: simulation and in vivo validation. Magnetic Resonance Imaging 2000;18:947–954.

[11] Look DC, Locker DR. Time saving in measurement of NMR and EPR relaxation times. The Review of scientific Instruments 1970;41:250–251.

[12] Messroghli DR, Radjenovic A, Kozerke S, Higgins DM, Sivananthan MU, Ridgway JP. Modified Look-Locker inversion recovery (MOLLI) for high-resolution T1 mapping of the heart. Magnetic Resonance in Medicine 2004;52:141–146.

[13] Messroghli DR, Niendorf T, Schulz-Menger J, Dietz R, G. FM. T1 Mapping in patients with acute myocardial infarction. Journal of Cardiovascular Magnetic Resonance 2003;5:353–359.

[14] Messroghli DR, Plein S, Higgins DM et al. Human myocardium: single-breath-hold MR T1 mapping with high spatial resolution—reproducibility study. Radiology 2006;238:1004–1012.

[15] Goldfarb JW, Arnold S, Han J. Recent Myocardial infarction: assessment with unenhanced T1-weighted MR imaging1. Radiology 2007;245:245–250.

[16] Messroghli DR, Greiser A, Fröhlich M, Dietz R, Schulz-Menger J. Optimization and validation of a fully-integrated pulse sequence for modified look-locker inversion-recovery (MOLLI) T1 mapping of the heart. Journal of Magnetic Resonance Imaging 2007;26:1081–1086.

[17] Karamitsos TD, Piechnik SK, Banypersad SM et al. Noncontrast T1 mapping for the diagnosis of cardiac amyloidosis. Journal of American College of Cardiology: Cardiovascular Imaging 2013;6:488–497.

[18] Jellis C, Wright J, Kennedy D et al. Association of imaging markers of myocardial fibrosis with metabolic and functional disturbances in early diabetic cardiomyopathy. Circulation: Cardiovascular Imaging 2011;4:693–702.

[19] Dass S, Suttie JJ, Piechnik SK et al. Myocardial tissue characterization using magnetic resonance non-contrast T1 mapping in hypertrophic and dilated cardiomyopathy. Circulation: Cardiovascular Imaging 2012.

[20] Messroghli DR, Walters K, Plein S et al. Myocardial T1 mapping: application to patients with acute and chronic myocardial infarction. Magnetic Resonance in Medicine 2007;58:34–40.

[21] Sibley CT, Noureldin RA, Gai N et al. T1 mapping in cardiomyopathy at cardiac MR: comparison with endomyocardial biopsy. Radiology 2012;256:724–732.

[22] Bull S, White SK, Piechnik SK et al. Human non-contrast T1 values and correlation with histology in diffuse fibrosis. Heart 2013;99:923–927.

[23] Lima JAC, Jeremy R, Guier W et al. Accurate systolic wall thickening by nuclear magnetic resonance imaging with tissue tagging: correlation with sonomicrometers in normal and ischemic myocardium. Journal of the American College of Cardiology 1993;21:1741–1751.

[24] Forbat SM, Karwatowski SP, Gatehouse PD, Firmin DN, Longmore DB, Underwood SR. Rapid measurement of left ventricular mass by spin echo magnetic resonance imaging. British Journal of Radiology 1994;67:86–90.

[25] Aurigemma G, Davidoff A, Silver K, Boehmer J, Pattison N. Left ventricular mass quantitaton using single-phase cardiac magnetic resonance imaging. The American Journal of Cardiology 1992;70:259–262.

[26] Solano JP, Gomes B, Higginson IJ. A comparison of symptom prevalence in far advanced cancer, AIDS, heart disease, chronic obstructive pulmonary disease and renal disease. Journal of Pain and Symptom Management 2006;31:58–69.

[27] Messroghli DR, Rudolph A, Abdel-Aty H et al. An open-source software tool for the generation of relaxation time maps in magnetic resonance imaging. BMC Medical Imaging 2010:10–16.

[28] Piechnik S, Ferreira V, Lewandowski A et al. Normal variation of magnetic resonance T1 relaxation times in the human population at 1.5 T using ShMOLLI. Journal of Cardiovascular Magnetic Resonance 2013;15:13.

[29] Piechnik S, Ferreira V, Dall'Armellina E et al. Shortened Modified Look-Locker Inversion recovery (ShMOLLI) for clinical myocardial T1-mapping at 1.5 and 3 T within a 9 heartbeat breathhold. Journal of Cardiovascular Magnetic Resonance 2010;12:69.

[30] Puntmann VO, Voigt T, Chen Z et al. Native T1 mapping in differentiation of normal myocardium from diffuse disease in hypertrophic and dilated cardiomyopathy. JACC: Cardiovascular Imaging 2013;6:475–484.

[31] Wacker CM, Bock M, Hartlep AW et al. Changes in myocardial oxygenation and perfusion under pharmacological stress with dipyridamole: assessment using T*2 and T1 measurements. Magnetic Resonance in Medicine 1999;41:686–695.

[32] Sebastian J. Flacke SEF, and Christine H. Lorenz measurement of the Gadopentetate Dimeglumine partition coefficient in human myocardium in vivo: normal distribution and elevation in acute and chronic infarction. Radiology 2001;218:703–710.

[33] Messroghli DR, Plein S, Higgins DM et al. Human myocardium: single-breath-hold MR T1 mapping with high spatial resolution-reproducibility study. Radiology 2006;238:1004–1012.

[34] Messroghli DR, Greiser A, Frohlich M, Dietz R, Schulz-Menger J. Optimization and validation of a fully-integrated pulse sequence for modified look-locker inversion-

recovery (MOLLI) T1 mapping of the heart. Journal of Magnetic Resonance Imaging 2007;26:1081–1086.

[35] Sparrow P, Messroghli DR, Ridgway SP, Bainbridge G, Sivanthan MU. Myocardial T1 mapping for detection of left ventricular myocardial fibrosis in chronic aortic regurgitation: pilot study. American Journal of Roentgenology 2006;187:630–635.

[36] Li D, Dhawale P, Rubin PJ, Haacke EM, Gropler RJ. Myocardial signal response to dipyridamole and dobutamine: Demonstration of the BOLD effect using a double-echo gradient-echo sequence. Magnetic Resonance in Medicine 1996;36:16–20.

[37] Reeder SB, Faranesh AZ, Boxerman JL, McVeigh ER. In vivo measurement of T2 star and field inhomogeneity maps in the human heart at 1.5 T. Magnetic Resonance in Medicine 1998;39:988–998.

[38] Anderson LJ, Holden S, Davis B et al. Cardiovascular T2-star (T2*) magnetic resonance for the early diagnosis of myocardial iron overload. European Heart Journal 2001;22:2171–2179.

[39] Positano V, Pepe A, Santarelli MF, Scattini B, De Marchi D, et al. Standardized T2* map of normal human heart in vivo to correct T2* segmental artefacts. NMR in Biomedicine 2007;20:578–590.

[40] Messroghli DR, Wassmuth R, Zagrosek A, Rudolph A, Schulz-Menger J. Assessment of myocardial T2* from pixel-by-pixel maps on a clinical MR system. Journal of Cardiovascular Magnetic Resonance 2008;10(Suppl 1):A240.

[41] Moon JC, Messroghli DR, Kellman P et al. Myocardial T1 mapping and extracellular volume quantification: a Society for Cardiovascular Magnetic Resonance (SCMR) and CMR Working Group of the European Society of Cardiology consensus statement. Journal of Cardiovascular Magnetic Resonance 2013;15.

8

Invasive Treatment in Advanced (Stage-D) Heart Failure

Kaan Kırali, Özge Altaş Yerlikhan and Hakan Hançer

Abstract

Heart failure is a complex, true pandemic clinical syndrome and is responsible for 5% of hospitalizations globally. Severe heart failure can manifest as two lethal clinical entities: (1) acute cardiac decompensation with cardiogenic shock after large acute myocardial infarction with mortality rates approaching 50% or after cardiac surgery with mortality rates higher than 65% and (2) chronic destructive cardiac remodeling or acute decompensative exacerbations of cardiomyopathies with one-year mortality of approximately 80% (worse than most types of cancer). Interventional therapies aim first to improve symptoms and life expectancy in patients with severe heart failure syndrome, second to prevent left ventricular remodeling, and third to bridge patients to long-term mechanical circulatory support or transplantation. Several treatment options can be used to stabilize patients. In particular, new percutaneous mitral valve interventions and short-term circulatory support devices open up a new temporary treatment area in symptomatic Stage-D heart failure. The durable or curable surgical destination treatment will be only permanent ventricular assist devices or heart transplantation. This chapter focuses on the treatment steps and new approaches in hospitalized Stage-D heart failure patients.

Keywords: heart failure, heart transplantation, ventricular assist device, ECMO, ECLS

At end-stage, any type of cardiomyopathy (CMP) causes a complex clinical heart failure (HF) syndrome, which results from structural and/or functional impairment of ventricular filling or ejection. This dire clinical situation can cause an adverse vicious cycle that is ultimately fatal if not treated by pharmacological or invasive mechanical support or heart transplantation (HTx). Left ventricular functional abnormalities range from normal-sized left ventricle (LV) with preserved left ventricular ejection fraction (LVEF) to severe left ventricular dilatation (LVD) with markedly reduced LVEF. Reduced LVEF is defined as the clinical diagnosis of HF and LVEF ≤40%, which means a clinic and functional association of systolic and/or diastolic LVD.

Abnormal systolic and/or diastolic functions impair left ventricular contractile and relaxation functions that result in increasing left ventricular end-diastolic volume (LVEDV) and left ventricular end-systolic volume (LVESV), as well as left ventricular end-diastolic diameter (LVEDD) and left ventricular end-systolic diameter (LVESD), with the alteration of the left ventricular shape from conical form to spherical form. Adverse elevation of preload and afterload results in increasing left ventricular end-diastolic pressure (LVEDP) and left ventricular end-systolic pressure (LVESP). Inadequate unloading is the primary cause of diastolic LVD due to left ventricular overloading, and ineffectual ejection is the primary cause of systolic LVD due to left ventricular overstretching. This LVD induces overpressure behind the LV, which is initially transient but becomes permanent over time. Increasing left atrial pressure (LAP) in acute decompensation of LVD results in pulmonary congestion and pulmonary edema; however, chronic overload causes increasing pulmonary vascular resistance (PVR) and pulmonary hypertension (PHT). Decompensation of the LV and increased right ventricular afterload also impairs the right ventricle (RV) over time. Both preload pressures defined as pulmonary capillary wedge pressure (PCWP) and central venous pressure (CVP) increase during cardiac failure and cause pulmonary and systemic symptoms. Sympathetic stimulation causes a rise of systemic vascular resistance (SVR) that worsens cardiac decompensation due to increased left ventricular afterload. The goals of HF therapy are decreasing both preloads to prevent tissue-congestion, increasing cardiac output (CO) via lowering both afterloads, and improving contractility of both ventricles to increase blood oxygenation and tissue perfusion.

Clinical appearance depends on systolic and/or diastolic ventricular dysfunction, and all treatment strategies are designed according to the HF-classification from Stage-A to Stage-D (**Table 1**). In the twenty-first century, new treatment options have facilitated delay or interruption of this cardiac deterioration and even enabled functional recovery and structural regeneration through corrective anatomic, functional, hemodynamic, and mechanical interventions and clinical medical improvement (**Figure 1**) [1]. Therapeutic and curative percutaneous or surgical treatments should be performed to rescue the damaged heart, and in this way, to recovery the deterioration of the heart and to prevent the development of HF. So, by definition, of left ventricular recovery presupposes that the patient can tolerate a moderate myocardial dysfunction and remain clinically and hemodynamically stable thereafter. Preinvasive therapy is usually implemented in Stage-C HF and consists of medical treatment, home rest, physical activity restriction, and closer medical follow-up.

Stage-D, advanced, end-stage, or refractory HF are various terms used to describe very sick patients (**Table 2**) [2]. Patients with decompensated Stage-D HF should be hospitalized for invasive, aggressive, effective, and interventive treatment combinations [3]. There are clinical clues that may assist clinicians in identifying patients who are progressing toward advanced HF (**Table 3**) [4]. Stage-D patients are those with truly refractory HF who might be eligible for specialized, advanced treatment strategies including mechanical circulatory support (MCS), procedures to facilitate fluid removal, continuous inotropic infusions, other innovative or experimental surgical procedures, or for end-of-life care, such as hospice [5]. After patients' clinical status improves, they will be bridged to destination treatment or HTx. The Interagency Registry for Mechanically Assisted Circulatory Support (INTERMACS) has developed seven

AHA/ACC	Stage-A	Stage-B	Stage-C			Stage-D (end-stage)		
	NYHA class	I	II	III-A	III-B		IV	
		INTERMACS		7		6 5 4	3 2	1
			STATUS			2	1-B	1-A

Stage-A: At high risk for developing HF without structural heart disease

Stage-B: Asymptomatic HF with structural heart disease, but without signs or symptoms of HF

Stage-C: Symptomatic HF with structural heart disease with prior or current symptoms of HF

Stage-D: Refractory end-stage HF despite maximal medical therapy, requiring specialized interventions

Class I: No limitation of physical activity. Ordinary physical activity does not cause symptoms of HF.

Class II: Slight limitation of physical activity. Comfortable at rest, but ordinary physical activity (e.g., long-distance walking, climbing two flights of stairs) results in symptoms of HF.

Class III: Marked limitation of physical activity. Comfortable at rest, but less than ordinary activity (e.g., short-distance walking, climbing one flights of stairs) causes symptoms of HF.

B: *LVEF* $\leq$ *30%* and *LVEDD* $\geq$ *60 mm* and *peak oxygen uptake <20 mL/min/kg* and *stable > 2 months*

Class IV: Unable to carry on any physical activity without symptoms of HF, or symptoms of HF at rest.

INTERMACS 1: Cardiogenic shock

INTERMACS 2: High dose intravenous inotropic support with/without t-MCS in instable condition

INTERMACS 3: Low dose inotropic support with stable hemodynamics

INTERMACS 4–6: Stable hemodynamics without intravenous inotropic support

INTERMACS 7: Clinical stable

STATUS 1A: On the intravenous inotropic and mechanical circulatory support for acute hemodynamic decompensation with/without mechanical ventilation following by continuous monitoring of both ventricular filling pressures, and recertification every 7th day

(a) Ventricular assist device (left, right, biventricular) <30 days

(b) Total artificial heart

(c) Extracorporeal circulatory support with/without oxygenator

(d) Counterpulsatile balloon pumping (intra-, extra-, para-aortic)

STATUS 1B: On the intravenous inotropic support or ventricular assist device >30 days

STATUS 2: Do not meet above criteria (patients on non-intravenous medical treatment at home)

HF = heart failure; LVEDD = left ventricular end-diastolic diameter; LVEF = left ventricular ejection fraction.

Table 1. Classification and interrelation of HF.

profiles that further stratify patients with advanced HF, who will be treated with a destination therapy (**Table 4**) [6]. All other causes, which can manifest in severe cardiac decompensation, should be ruled out during diagnosis.

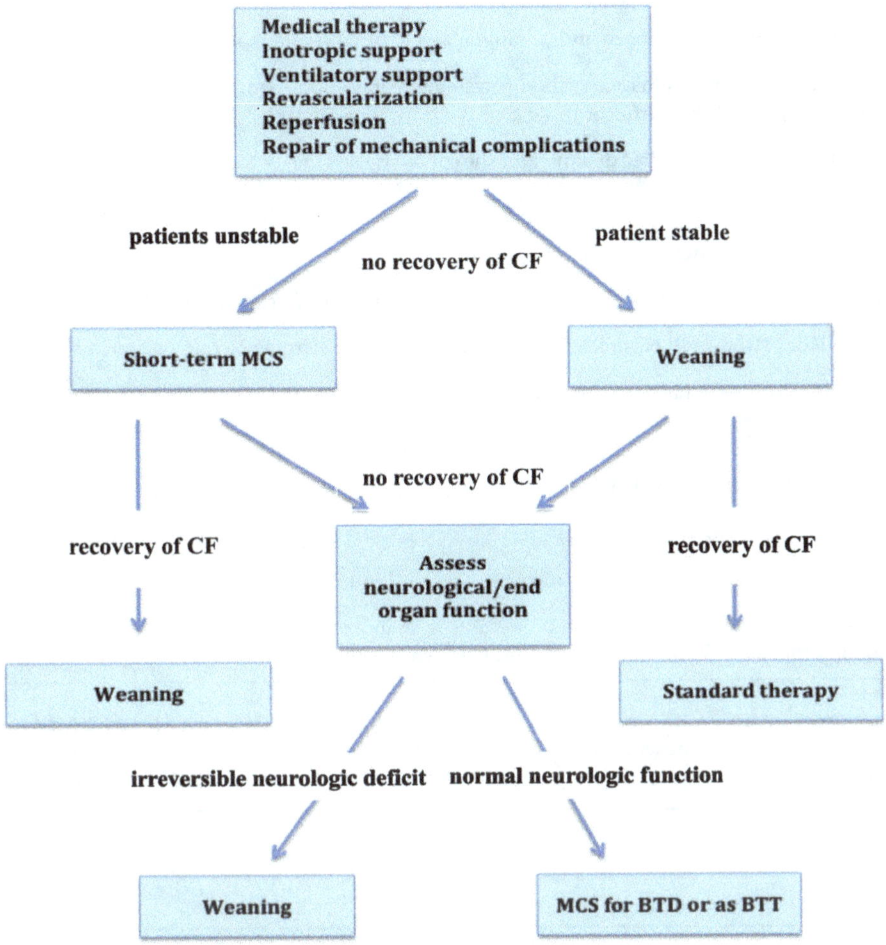

Figure 1. Management algorithm for Stage-D heart failure. BTD = bridge to destination; BTT = bridge to transplantation; CF = cardiac function; MCS = mechanical circulatory support.

Invasive treatments against HF depend on the nature and type of cardiac pathology; however, the systematic approach to their application is well defined (**Table 5**). The first step is to stabilize the patient's hemodynamics using pharmacological hemodynamic support (PHS), with full intravenous medication including inotropics, vasodilatators, inodilatators, diuretics, etc. Management of total fluid volume (1.5–2 L/day) and sodium restriction are essential to reduce congestive symptoms, although it is important to avoid hyponatremia by maintaining sodium above 132 mEq/L. Full and continuous monitoring of pre- and afterload (central venous and pulmonary artery catheterization) and CO measurements, echocardiographic examinations (transthoracic and/or transesophageal), and laboratory findings should be implemented in the intensive care unit (ICU). The second step is to carry out any percutaneous interventional support required to eliminate anatomorphologic pathologies (coronary artery stenosis, fibrotic valvular stenosis, etc.) for the purpose of maintaining the satisfactory filling pressures, myocardial contractility, and forward ejection in both circulations. The third and fourth steps apply to patients that are provided with electrical resynchronization and/or mechanical ventilatory support as needed to relieve the negative effects of electromechanical

1.	Severe symptoms of HF with dyspnea and/or fatigue at rest or with minimal exertion (NYHA class III or IV)
2.	Episodes of fluid retention (pulmonary and/or systemic congestion, peripheral edema) and/or reduced cardiac output at rest (peripheral hypoperfusion)
3.	Objective evidence of severe cardiac dysfunction shown by at least one of the following:
	a. LVEF < 30%
	b. Pseudonormal or restrictive mitral flow pattern
	c. Mean PCWP > 16 mmHg and/or RAP >12 mmHg by pulmonary artery catheterization
	d. High BNP or NT-proBNP plasma levels in the absence of noncardiac causes
4.	Severe impairment of functional capacity shown by one of the following:
	a. Inability to exercise
	b. 6-minute walk distance ≤ 300 m
	c. Peak Vo_2 < 12 to 14 mL/kg/min
5.	History of ≥ 1 HF hospitalization in past 6 months
6.	Presence of all the previous features despite "attempts to optimize" therapy, including diuretics and GDMT, unless these are poorly tolerated or contraindicated, and CRT when indicated

BNP = B-type natriuretic peptide; CRT = cardiac resynchronization therapy; GDMT = guideline-directed medical therapy; HF = heart failure; LVEF = left ventricular ejection fraction; NT-proBNP = N-terminal pro-B-type natriuretic peptide; NYHA = New York Heart Association; PCWP = pulmonary capillary wedge pressure; RAP = right atrial pressure.

Table 2. Definition of advanced heart failure.

- Repeated (≥2) hospitalizations or emergency department visits for HF in the past year
- Progressive deterioration in renal function (e.g., rise in BUN and creatinine)
- Weight loss without other cause (e.g., cardiac cachexia)
- Intolerance to ACE inhibitors due to hypotension and/or worsening renal function
- Intolerance to beta blockers due to worsening HF or hypotension
- Frequent systolic blood pressure <90 mmHg
- Persistent dyspnea with dressing or bathing requiring rest
- Inability to walk 1 block on the level ground due to dyspnea or fatigue
- Recent need to escalate diuretics to maintain volume status, often reaching daily furosemide equivalent dose >160 mg/d and/or use of supplemental metolazone therapy
- Progressive decline in serum sodium, usually to <133 mEq/L
- Frequent ICD shocks

ACE = angiotensin-converting enzyme; BUN = blood urea nitrogen; HF = heart failure; ICD = implantable cardioverter defibrillator.

Table 3. Clinical events and findings for identifying patients with advanced HF.

Profile	Profile description	Shorthand	Features	IABP	t-MCS*	Hospitalization	Life expectancy	p-MCS**	Timing
1	Critical cardiogenic shock	Crash and burn	Life-threatening hypotension and excessive inotropic/ vasopressor support, critical organ hypoperfusion, often worsening acidosis and lactate levels	Yes	Yes	Yes (ICU)	Hours	Emergent (Rescue)	<7 days
2	Progressive decline	Sliding fast	Dependent on inotropic support with/without continuing nutritional depletion, worsening renal function, inability to restore volume balance, or other major status indicator.	Yes	Yes	Yes (ICU/Ward)	Days to weeks	Urgent (salvage)	<30 days
3	Stable, but inotrope-dependent	Dependent stability	Stable blood pressure, organ function and nutrition on mild-moderate doses of continuous intravenous inotropic support after repeated documentation of failure to wean without symptomatic hypotension, worsening symptoms, or progressive organ dysfunction (usually renal).	Yes/ no	Yes/no	Yes (Ward)	Few weeks	Elective (destination)	<90 days
4	Recurrent advanced HF	Frequent flyer	Resting and/or daily living activities (dressing or bathing) symptoms of congestion (orthopnea, abdominal discomfort, nausea, poor appetite, disabling ascites, or severe lower-extremity edema), on oral therapy at home,	No	No	No	Weeks to months	Elective (destination)	>90 days
5	Exertion intolerant	House-bound	Comfortable at rest, but unable to engage in any activity, living predominantly within the house or housebound	No	No	No	Weeks to months	Yes/no	?
6	Exertion limited	Walking wounded	Comfortable at rest without evidence of fluid overload and able to do some mild activity, daily living are comfortable and minor activities outside the home, but fatigue results within a few minutes or with any meaningful physical exertion.	No	No	No	Months	Yes/no	No
7	NYHA class III B		Clinically stable with a reasonable level of comfortable activity, despite a history of previous decompensation that is not recent, able to walk more than a block.	No	No	No		No	No

*t-MCS includes IABP, ECMO, ECCS, and others;
**p-MCS includes LVAD, TAH.
HF = heart failure; ICU = intensive care unit; p-MCS = permanent mechanical circulatory support; t-MCS = temporary mechanical circulatory support; NYHA = New york Heart Association.

Table 4. INTERMACS profiles.

(I) Pharmacological hemodynamic support (PHS)

(II) Percutaneous interventional support (PIS)

- **1.** Coronary revascularization
    - **a.** Angioplasty
    - **b.** Coronary artery bypass grafting on the beating heart (CABG-BH)
        - **i.** Off-pump
        - **ii.** On-pump
- **2.** Mitral valve repair
    - **a.** Percutaneous
    - **b.** Surgical neo-chordae

(III) Electrical resynchronizational support (ERS)

(IV) Mechanical ventilatory support (MVS)

(V) Mechanical counterpulsatile hemodynamic support (MCHS)

- **1.** Intraaortic counterpulsatile support (IACP)
    - **a.** Intraaortic balloon pump (IABP)
- **2.** Extraaortic counterpulsatile support (EACP)
    - **a.** Extra-aortic balloon pump (EABP)
- **3.** Paraaortic counterpulsatile circulation (PACP)
    - **a.** Paraaortic circulatory device (PACD)
    - **b.** Pressure-unload left ventricular assist device (PULVAD)
    - **c.** Kantrowitz CardioVAD (KCV)
    - **d.** Symphony

(VI) Mechanical circulatile support (MCS)

- **1.** Temporary mechanical cardiopulmonary support (t-MCPS)
    - **a.** Cardiopulmonary bypass (CPB)
    - **b.** Extracorporeal cardiopulmonary support (ECCPS) or Extracorporeal life support (ECLS)
- **2.** Temporary mechanical circulatory support (t-MCS)
    - **a.** Extracorporeal circulatory support (ECCS)
    - **b.** Intracorporeal circulatory support (ICCS)
- **3.** Permanent mechanical circulatory support (p-MCS)
    - **a.** Ventricular assist device (VAD)
    - **b.** Total artificial heart (TAH)

(VII) Heart transplantation

- **1.** Isolated

	2. Heart and lung transplantation
(VIII)	Left ventricular structural restoration
	1. Aneurysmectomy
	2. Cardiomyoplasty
	3. Reshaping
	a. Intracardiac
	b. Extracardiac
	i. CorCap Cardiac Support Device
	ii. Paracor HeartNet Device

Table 5. Invasive treatment sequences of the severe end stage heart failure.

dyssynchrony and poor systemic oxygenation. The fifth step entails provision of hemodynamic supports using temporary mechanical circulatory support (t-MCS) devices such as counter-pulsatile circulatory support (CPCS), extracorporeal cardiopulmonary support (ECCPS), or extracorporeal circulatory support (ECCS) to maintain adequate CO for sufficient body perfusion without any congestive sign of the left and/or right HF. The sixth step consists a long-term circulatory support to obtain adequate left with or without right heart circulation for bridging to a destination therapy. The left ventricular assist device (LVAD) and total artificial heart (TAH) are permanent mechanical circulatory support (p-MCS) devices, and for the time being represent the last and best chance to bridge patients to transplantation or destination therapy. The last step is HTx with or without lung(s), which is considered the gold standard for the treatment of refractory Stage-D HF.

1. Pharmacological hemodynamic support (PHS)

Decompensation of Stage-D HF should be treated in hospital immediately, medically, aggressively, intravenously, and with a multidisciplinary approach. Nowadays, we have a lot of pharmacological treatment weapons with contractor, vasodilator, vasopressor, and inactivator effects [7]. Diuretics for congestion, antiarrhythmics for dysrhythmia, anticoagulations for thrombosis, and digoxin for right heart failure are integral parts of medical treatment (**Figure 2**). With the advent of neurohormonal blockade, tremendous progress has been made in the medical treatment of the advanced HF. Treatment of comorbid conditions such as diabetes and iron deficiency can aid clinical recovery.

Inotropic or inodilator therapy is the initial pharmacological strategy to improve myocardial contractility, increase heart rate, reduce afterload through peripheral vasodilatation, and augment CO. Dobutamine and dopamine (inotropic), and milrinone (inodilator) are the three most commonly used intravenous agents.

Dobutamine (2–20 μg/kg/min) is the most used sympathomimetic agent, and its inotropic and chronotropic effects derive from direct stimulation of β_1 adrenergic receptors, which are

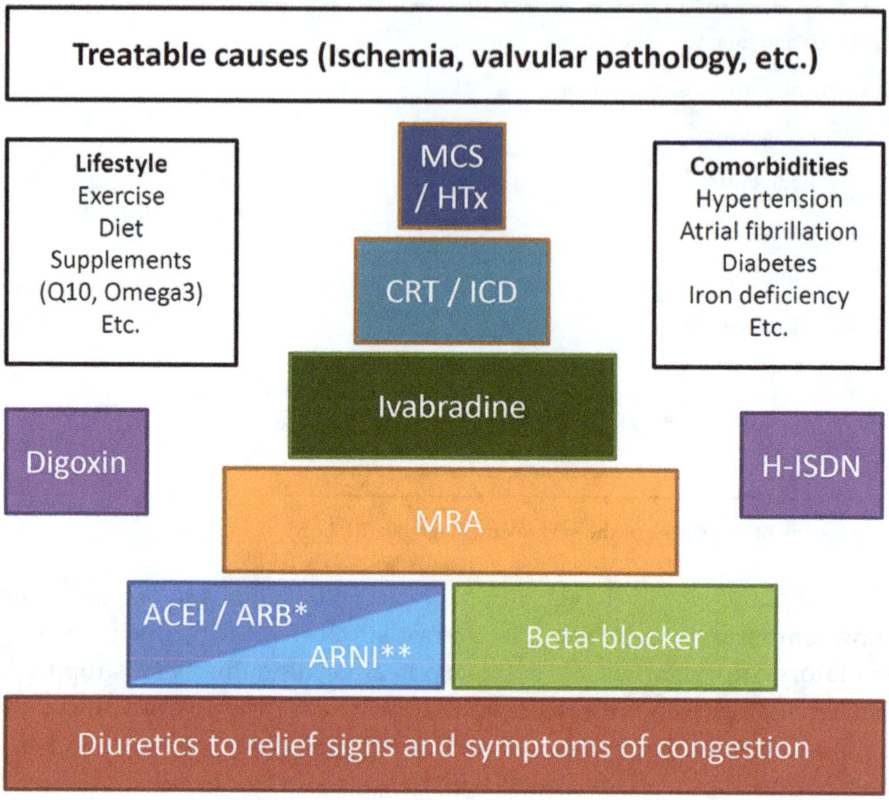

Figure 2. Current therapies for end-stage heart failure. *An ARB is recommended when an ACEI is not tolerated. **An ARNIs is recommended when both RAAS inhibitors are ineffective. ACEI = angiotensin converting-enzyme inhibitor; ARB = angiotensin receptor blocker; ARNI = angiotensin receptor neprilysin inhibitor; CRT = cardiac resynchronization therapy; ICD = implantable cardioverter defibrillator; H-ISDN = hydralazine-isosorbide dinitrate; HTx = heart transplantation; MCS = mechanical circulatory support; MRA= mineralocorticoid antagonist; omega3 = omega-3 polyunsaturated fatty acids; Q10 = coenzyme Q10.

mostly downregulated in end-stage HF patients. The main effect is inotropic, and it may increase coronary blood flow, but myocardial oxygen consumption can increase if dobutamine induces tachycardia. Tachycardia depends more on dobutamine-related cardiac output than on infusion level.

Dopamine stimulates different receptors depending on dose level: in low (diuretic) doses (0.5–3 μg/kg/min) dopaminergic receptors in the renal, mesenteric, and coronary arterial beds are stimulated; in moderate (inotropic) doses (3–10 μg/kg/min), nonselective adrenergic receptors are activated; in high (vasoconstrictive) doses (>10 μg/kg/min), especially α-adrenergic receptors are induced.

Milrinone (0.25–0.75 μg/kg/min) acts by a nonadrenergic mechanism, increasing c-AMP via phosphodiesterase III inhibition. It is preferred mostly in patients with increased PVR and/or SVR due to better vascular vasodilation than dobutamine. It is crucial to be aware of the risk of systemic hypotension, for which concomitant vasopressors should be added. Milrinone increases CO without increasing overall myocardial oxygen consumption, but does improve myocardial diastolic relaxation (lusitropic effect).

Vasopressor therapy is necessary to increase SVR, blood pressures, and mean arterial pressure, when the low cardiac output syndrome (LCOS) is serious with fairly lower systemic blood pressure. *Adrenalin* (2–10 μg/min or 0.01–0.4 μg/kg/min) is used primarily to maintain cardiac contractility and CO by counteracting bradycardia and hypocontractility. *Noradrenalin* (2–16 μg/min or 0.01–0.3 μg/kg/min) is used primarily to maintain mean systemic arterial pressure by controlling hypotension, severe vasodilatation, or vasoplegia syndrome. It is also an integral part of inodilator treatment modality to prevent systemic vasodilatation.

Vasodilator therapy is needed in most HF patients to decrease SVR and also PVR. Nitroglycerin (10–500 μg/min) and nitroprusside (10–500 μg/min) are the most commonly-used agents in cardiac surgery, but prostaglandins and nitric oxide (NO) more specifically decrease PVR and right ventricular afterload in patients with end-stage HF due to the improvement of the right ventricular dysfunction (RVD) and CO. Long-term therapy with sildenafil has demonstrated better hemodynamics in lowering PVR. In addition, endothelin receptor antagonists, such as bosentan, can also be used although they are not currently included in treatment guidelines.

Diuretics restrict the reabsorption of sodium in the renal tubes, increase urinary sodium excretion, and decrease congestive symptoms in HF patients. Loop diuretics (furosemide, bumetanide, torsemide) are preferred pharmacological agents in hospitalized patients and used intravenously. The first goal is to resolve fluid retention and congestive signs (edema, hepatomegaly, pulmonary edema, etc.), and then to prevent the recurrence of volume overload. The most common side effects of excessive diuretic usage include fluid depletion, hypokalemia, hypomagnesaemia, and azotemia. Furosemide is the most common used loop diuretic, the dose and frequency should be increased until the adequate diuresis and weight loss is maintained. Low-dose dopamine (2 μg/kg/min) infusion can improve diuresis and better preserve renal function. If the diuretic strategy is unsatisfactory or ineffective due to renal failure, ultrafiltration to remove water and small- to medium-weight solutes may be considered as a primary volume-removal therapy. After acute decompensation caused by volume overload resolves, oral diuretic therapy is started with furosemide and/or thiazides and spironolactone combination. Daily recording of body weight is the best parameter to follow diuretic treatment's effectiveness and to adjust dosage.

Renin-angiotensin-aldosterone system (RAAS) is at the core of the pathophysiology of HF, and its modulation is central to altering the disease process in HF with reduced LVEF. Blockade of RAAS can be provided by an angiotensin-converting enzyme inhibitor (ACEI), angiotensin-receptor blocker (ARB), or mineralocorticoid receptor antagonist (MRA). This inhibition can reduce blood pressure in hypertensive patients, prevent target organ damage in diabetes, and improve outcomes in HF patients [8]. This hormone system regulates protective acute stress response through inflammatory and proliferative mechanisms; however, chronic stimulation has detrimental effects including vasoconstriction, sodium and water retention, vascular smooth muscle proliferation, endothelial dysfunction, inflammation, fibrosis, and thrombosis [9]. The RAAS cascade begins with renin secretion by renal juxtaglomerular cells, continues with the conversion of hepatic angiotensinogen to the inactive angiotensin I, and finishes with conversion of angiotensin I to angiotensin II by angiotensin-converting enzyme (ACE). Angiotensin II is the strongest mediator to promote all effects above mentioned, and it stimulates the secretion of aldosterone from adrenal cortex and arginine vasopressin from posterior pituitary. Blockade of the RAAS with ACEIs has been a cornerstone of HF therapy for over 20 years, so that ACEIs decrease the formation of angiotensin II and inhibit the breakdown of bradykinin with the formation of NO and other vasodilators. Additionally, further blockade of RAAS with aldosterone antagonists and ARBs has increased the efficiency, so that ARBs bind competitively to and dissociate slowly from angiotensin type-1 receptors and blockade aldosterone secretion. MRAs cover mineralocorticoid receptors for competitive inhibition. The direct renin inhibitor (DRI) agents blockade the RAAS at the most proximal step via the inhibition of angiotensinogen conversion.

Natriuretic peptide system (NPS) counter regulates the detrimental effects of the up-regulation of RAAS, inhibits secretion of arginine vasopressin, modulates the autonomic nervous system, and antagonizes their vasopressor effects in HF [10]. There are three peptides: atrial natriuretic peptide (ANP), brain natriuretic peptide (BNP), and endothelial cell natriuretic peptide (CNP). Both ANP and BNP have similar structural, hypotensive, natriuretic, and diuretic properties. Distension of the atria and ventricles due to cardiac injury and/or overload, ventricular dysfunction, and HF stimulates the expression of ANP from atria and BNP from brain and ventricles with several effects: (1) activation of membrane-bound natriuretic peptide receptors-A leading to vasorelaxation, natriuresis, and diuresis; (2) inhibition of RAAS due to blocked of renin secretion and associated aldosterone production; (3) reduction in adverse cardiovascular changes via remodeling, apoptosis, ventricular hypertrophy, and fibrosis; and (4) enhanced myocardial relaxation. On the other hand, CNP extracted from endothelial cells and brain acts only as a vasodilator without potent diuretic and natriuretic effects. Measurements of peptides ANP, BNP, and its inactive precursor N-terminal fragment of pro-B-type natriuretic peptide (NT-proBNP) are useful in prognosis assessment and antifailure therapy monitoring, but CNP is not measurable due to low concentrations in circulating blood. Natriuretic peptides are removed from circulation through two mechanisms: clearing by natriuretic peptide clearance receptor (NPRC and NPRC3) or inactivating by a degrading enzyme. The endothelial enzyme *neprilysin* hydrolyzes ANP rapidly and also degrades a large number of other vasodilators and vasoconstrictors although BNP is relatively resistant to its digestion. Inhibition of neprilysin (NEPi) with *sacubitril* (1) increases concentrations of circulating vasodilators (ANP, adrenomedullin, and bradykinin), but also circulating vasopressors (angiotensin II, endothelin I); (2) augments plasma ANP and BNP levels leading to enhanced natriuretic-diuretic-vasodilator effects, lower preloads, and inhibition of fibrosis; (3) inhibits renin secretion and angiotensin I to II conversion, but that is not a complete inhibition effect on the RAAS. However, blocking neprilysin alone does not effect a complete inhibition of RAAS, which is stimulated by the activated sympathetic nervous system (SNS) leading to increasing renin secretion and ACE activation of angiotensin I to II. These opposing effects neutralize each other and therefore NPS inhibitors alone exert little effect on hemodynamics. This problem is solved by dual blockade of RAAS by ARB and NPS by NEPi. The combined molecule of sacubitril (NEPi) and valsartan (ARB) is a first drug (LCZ696) in class angiotensin receptor neprilysin inhibitor (ARNi), and represents a new treatment modality by blocking the angiotensin type-1 receptor and inhibiting the natriuretic peptide system concurrently [11]. Valsartan does not inhibit the breakdown of bradykinin, with decreasing angioedema risk; however, inhibition of angiotensin II action prevents vasopressor effects. This combination favors NPS activation and RAAS blockade, as well as residual angiotensin II effects from the SNS [12].

Digoxin is the oldest cardiac drug still in contemporary use, and can be useful in patients with persistent severe end-stage HF (LVEF <25%, cardiothoracic ratio >55%, New York Heart Association (NYHA) class III or IV) undergoing guideline-directed medical therapy, and especially symptomatic patients being treated with neurohormonal antagonists [13]. Digoxin has been used as the first line of pharmacological treatment for HF until the understanding of HF pathophysiology changed in recent decades, which leads to the shift from inotropic support to neurohormonal modulation [14]. The effect is regardless of the rhythm, etiology of HF, or concomitant therapy. Digoxin binds for the sarcolemmal Na^+-K^+-ATPase pump to blocking and impeding Na^+ extrusion outside, accumulated intracellular Na^+ decreases the transmembrane sodium gradient, and as a consequence suppresses the activity of the Na^+-Ca^{++}-exchanger, raising the intracellular Ca^{++} concentration and effecting more forceful contraction. Digoxin is the only inotrope known to improve LVEF and CO and also to reduce PCWP without tachycardia and/or hypotension. The beneficial effect of the drug occurs even at low maintenance dosage (serum digoxin concentration 0.5–0.9 ng/mL; 0.125 mg/day) with positive inotropic but negative chronotropic (4–7 beats/min in sinus rhythm) properties. The hemodynamic effects of digoxin are not attenuated by chronic administration, because Na^+-K^+-ATPase is not upregulated. In noncardiac tissue, digoxin acts as a neurohormonal modulator by increasing parasympathetic tone and dampening activation of the SNS (sympatholytic) and RAAS.

2. Percutaneous interventional support (PIS)

Cardiac decompensation is usually a consequence of myocardial ischemia and/or mechanical complications, or chronic remodeling. Acute HF develops after ischemic damage or acute hemodynamic compromise of chronic HF with well-known structural pathologies during medical follow-up. These patients may not improve with medical therapy; however, correction of underlying pathologies such as coronary artery disease, valvular stenosis, or regurgitation can result in significant improvement in functional status. Before mechanical circulatory treatments, all applicable interventional therapies must be evaluated and performed confidentially. First of all, percutaneous revascularization is the initial step in managing inadequate oxygen delivery due to stenotic or occluded coronary arteries, and that must be followed by percutaneous palliative mitral valve repair if it is necessary. Significant mitral regurgitation (MR) resulting in inadequate forward ejection of the LV can cause intractable left heart failure (LHF), even if total stroke volume seems enough to produce adequate CO. The goal of palliative percutaneous interventions for these pathologies is to maintain and sustain adequate left ventricular filling and forward ejection. If these treatment strategies are successful, patients have the chance to get better and postpone mechanical hemodynamic and/or circulatory support; however, inoperable or untouchable patients should be considered for destination therapy.

2.1. Coronary revascularization

Ischemic myocardium or acute coronary syndrome decreases significantly ventricular contractile function due to oxygen supply/demand imbalance. Hibernating, stunning, or infarction reduces LVEF, causes left ventricular remodeling, and exacerbates mitral valve dysfunction. Coronary angiography shows stenotic or occluded coronary territory, but stress echocardiography, nuclear imaging, and magnetic resonance imaging examinations show whether there are viable tissues and/or valvular dysfunction requiring corrective interventions, as well as for surgical treatment despite higher procedural risks. Coronary revascularization can salvage and improve the myocardium histologically and functionally, but these strategies usually fail to improve myocardial recovery due to nonviable myocardium.

2.1.1. Angioplasty

Any severe atherosclerotic plaque, plaque rupture, or thrombotic occlusion reduces oxygen delivery to the myocardium, which results acute LHF. Persistent angina is also a common symptom (approximately 30%) in patients with ischemic CMP despite medical therapy, which increases major cardiac events by one third [15]. Percutaneous coronary intervention via balloon angioplasty associated with or without stent implantation is the first-stage therapy for coronary artery disease causing severe cardiac decompensation due to massive ischemia in high-risk patients with well-known compensated HF associated with or without mechanical complications of myocardial infarction, particularly MR. Coronary revascularization could aid in recovery of myocardial dysfunction if the affected myocardium consists of viable tissue, and MR may also be improved. Myocardial reserve after angioplasty also results in contractile improvement and favorable left ventricular remodeling in patients with LVD, and it also decreases HF symptoms (angina, functional class, BNP levels) [16, 17]. Partially or fully viability or transmural scar within the infarct should be identified by any test (scintigraphy, magnetic resonance, etc.) in this group of patients, because improvement in oxygen supply will abate ischemia burden [18, 19]. Transmural distribution of the postinfarction scar, which spreads from the subendocardium to the subepicardium without intermittent viability, does not provide any benefit by angioplasty. Although surgical coronary revascularization is superior to medical therapy in patients with HF [20], there is no real superiority of surgery over angioplasty [21]. Contrarily, the positive benefit of percutaneous revascularization of the viable region is a significant improvement in the LVEF and LVESV in the LHF patients. New designed clinical trials will give more detailed results regarding angioplasty performed in HF [22]. Unstable or hemodynamically instable patients with significant HF symptoms must be undertaken in catheter laboratory with a t-MCS to prevent sudden decompensation or cardiac arrest. The most preferable device to maintain adequate CO during percutaneous procedures is intraaortic balloon pump (IABP), which can be supported or replaced by a percutaneous temporary device (Impella, TandemHeart, etc.).

2.1.2. Coronary artery bypass grafting

Patients with severe HF and coronary artery disease suitable for coronary artery bypass grafting (CABG) are at higher risk for surgical morbidity and mortality. Paradoxically, those patients who derive the greatest clinical benefit from CABG and are also at the greatest operative risk, which leads clinicians to hesitate to refer these patients for CABG [23]. Despite the fact that bypass surgery can create potential risks for HF patients, significantly viable tissue should be revascularized by on- or off-pump CABG [24]. Minimal invasive CABG procedures are an option, but dilated left ventricular cavity with or without right ventricular enlargement complicates off-pump CABG due to hemodynamic instability during the elevation of the heart for circumflex or right coronary artery anastomoses [25]. Single vessel bypass to the dominant left anterior descending territory can be useful in symptomatic multivessel disease patients, and this approach can cause a limited improvement in the LVEF and clinical status [26]. But, in the case of unsuitable pathology and anatomic structure of the coronary artery territory, viable tissue should be identified before surgery. Single coronary artery revascularization could be performed percutaneously or off-pump surgically [27]. On-pump CABG could be more harmful due to aortic cross clamping, but enrichment of cardioplegia with different agents may be protective [28].

2.2. Mitral valve repair

Functional MR due to LVD and remodeling is a common complication in dilated or ischemic CMPs, and severe symptomatic MR requires an invasive corrective intervention to prevent poor prognosis and to improve clinical status. However, the effectiveness of repair of MR in these situations is often compromised because it does not reverse the underlying cause of the CMP. While surgical mitral valve repair is the conventional treatment for MR, it is controversial in end-stage HF patients due to high surgical risk and lack of randomized trials about survival benefit. Because severe functional MR clearly increases the mortality as an independent predictor but mitral valve repair does not improve mid- and long-term survival in patients with end-stage HF, most major guidelines recommend against isolated mitral valve surgery in these patients, although surgery is generally recommended if aortic valve or coronary artery bypass graft surgery is also being performed [29]. Ideal candidates should have less fibrotic spherical ventricle with more contractile reserve, patients with irreversible pulmonary hypertension and severe right ventricle dysfunction would be unlikely to benefit from intervention [30]. Transcatheter mitral valve repair or implantation alternatives are currently preferred in high-risk patients not eligible for surgery [31]. Percutaneous mitral valve implantation seems to be the best solution to eliminate MR in end-stage HF patients with significant MR caused by severe annular enlargement [32].

2.2.1. Percutaneous mitral valve repair

Newly developed percutaneous mitral valve repair techniques can be useful in patients, who cannot be referred for surgical therapy (**Table 6**) [33]. In contrast to the positive effect of percutaneous mitral valve repair techniques in patients with severe MR-associated nonfailed hearts, mitral valve repairing is offered without targeting of full coaptation of mitral valve in end-stage HF patients. It is usually anatomically impossible to fully repair the mitral valve completely due to severe annular enlargement and/or thethering of the leaflets caused by left

Percutaneous mitral valve repair	
Leaflet	
Edge-to-edge (leaflet plication)	MitraClip
	MitraFlex
Space occupier (leaflet coaptation)	Percu-Pro
Leaflet ablation	Thermocool
Annulus	
Indirect approaches	
Coronary sinus annuloplasty	Carillon
	Monarc
	Viacor
Asymmetrical approach	St Jude annulus reshaping device
	NIH-cerclage technology
Direct approaches	
Percutaneous mechanical cinching	Mitralign suture-based plication
	Accucinch GDS millipede ring system
Percutaneous energy-mediated cinching	QuantumCor
	ReCor
Hybrid	Mitral solution
	MiCardia
Chordal implants	
Transapical artificial chord	NeoChord
	MitraFlex
Transapical-Transseptal	Babic
Left ventricle	
LV remodelling	Mardil-BASE
	iCoapsys
Percutaneous mitral valve implantation	
Right mini-thoracotomy	Endovalve-Herrmann prosthesis
Transapical	Lutter prosthesis
Transseptal	CardiaQ prosthesis

Table 6. Percutaneous mitral interventions.

ventricular enlargement, as well as it can be very devastating for failed hearts. Therefore, percutaneous mitral valve repair techniques are palliative, but also preparative interventions to improve patients' clinical status and hemodynamics before destination therapies like LVAD or HTx.

The MitraClip is a a novel technology for percutaneous treatment of MR, although its utility in patients with end-stage HF is somewhat limited [34]. This leaflet plication technology is based on the surgical Alfieri technique, which brings the anterior and posterior leaflets together with a suture, creating a "double orifice" mitral valve. The device is inserted by way of the femoral vein and utilizes a 24F guidewire to gain transseptal access to the left atrium (LA). It is essential to place the V-shaped clip at the main MR site between the anterior and posterior leaflet with the guidance of transesophageal echocardiography. The first clip may not solve the problem, but decreases degree of regurgitation from massive to severe or moderate-severe, and additional clip(s) could be applied to significantly reduce degree of regurgitation to moderate or lower. At least 50% reduction in the MR performed by mitral clips could be accepted as a successful procedure, while more than 75% without mitral stenosis could cause effective correction. This new device has shown benefit in outcomes for patients without HF, but it is unable to improve the clinical course in end-stage HF patients due to an immediate deterioration of left ventricular function, further aggravation of afterload mismatch, and progressive LHF [35]. MitraClip is a good alternative to surgery in functional MR refractory to medical and/or resynchronization therapy in patients with adequate anatomy, but not in patients who are considered inoperable due to high surgical risks [36]. It can be considered an important clinical option in the multidisciplinary treatment of HF, but postprocedural MR increases midterm cardiac mortality [37]. To increase utilization of the MitraClip treatment, this new approach must be used in selective cases or as an earlier step before the destination therapy. The first 30 days have an acceptable course, but after that the frequency of adverse events increases, especially early recurrence/persistence of MR [38].

The Carillon is a percutaneous coronary sinus-based mitral annuloplasty device designed to treat functional MR in end-stage HF patients [39]. This device consists of self-expandable nitinol distal and proximal anchors connected by a nitinol bridge, which are placed in the great cardiac vein and proximal coronary sinus located behind the posterior mitral annulus. Tension applied on the system results in cinching of the posterior periannular tissue, and displacement of the posterior mitral leaflet toward the anterior leaflet to reduce anterior-posterior (septal-lateral) dimension improves their coaptation and reduces functional MR [40]. Residual MR is not frequently observed in patients without HF, and it can decrease significantly in the first 3 months [41]. However, LVD associated with significant mitral annular enlargement results in significant MR, but also, mitral valve thethering complicates MR. This pathologic course could not be reversed completely by percutaneous mitral annuloplasty devices. This technique reduces functional MR significantly, increases functional capacity and quality of life, as well as induces improvement of left ventricular remodeling [42]. The major limitations to use this kind of devices are the significant distance between coronary sinus and mitral annulus, closed anatomic neighborhood of coronary arteries, and annular calcifications.

2.2.2. Surgical mitral valve repair

Surgical mitral valve correction is seldom preferred because of the high risks associated with the operation. On-pump surgery is usually not recommended, and severe MR with clinical deterioration can be the first indication for LVAD implantation. Transapical correction using NeoChord has been popularized in degenerative MR, and the new devices facilitate transapical implantation of neo-chordae on the beating heart without cardiopulmonary bypass (CPB) [43]. This approach is useful in isolated mitral valve leaflet(s) prolapse with lower operative risk [44]. However, no high-quality studies have investigated the possibility of implantation in severe HF situations with LVD and mitral leaflet thethering. This approach could be preferred in severe MR caused by chordal rupture without adding of ring annuloplasty. However, patients with a LVD and a significant MR have significant mitral annular dilatation without mitral valve prolapses, and in such cases MR can be corrected only via a prosthetic ring percutaneously. Otherwise, severe HF associated with significant MR is one of the best candidates for LVAD destination therapy.

3. Electrical resynchronizational support (ERS)

Electromechanical dyssynchrony is common in end-stage HF patients and can be found at different levels within the heart. Electrical dyssynchrony is evidenced by QRS prolongation (≥120 ms) and has a prevalence of 15–30% in HF population. Electrical dyssynchrony, and the subsequent abnormal mechanical activation, results in cellular, structural, hemodynamic, and ultimately clinical adverse effects [45]. Left bundle branch block results in a shorter diastolic time interval and longer isovolumetric contraction and relaxation times, which impair pump function because of abnormal electrical and mechanical properties, as well as functional MR. These effects can be ameliorated by resynchronizing the failing heart by means of pacing in the right atrium (RA) and both ventricles (biventricular pacing). Cardiac resynchronization therapy restores the appropriate timing of the cardiac contraction pattern and thereby not only reduces cellular, hemodynamic, and structural maladaptations to dyssynchrony, but also ultimately improves functional status, reduces hospitalization, and improves survival.

4. Mechanical ventilatory support (MVS)

Even when cardiac dysfunction is the only reason for HF syndrome, increased PVR raises respiratory effort and increased SVR reduces systemic output, decreasing pre- and afterload and increasing oxygenation, which results hemodynamic stability. The most common supportive approach in end-stage HF patients with respiratory failure is mechanical ventilation under general anesthesia. Intubation is usually the first step to maintain hemodynamic stability through decreased respiratory effort and adrenergic stimulation. Increasing oxygenation and use of vasodilator inhalation decrease adverse responses and PVR, which is the main treatment strategy for the right ventricular failure (RVF). Supportive mechanical hemodynamic approaches prevent unnecessary and prolonged mechanical ventilation, which can be a significant risk factor for ventilator-dependent infections. Elective intubation is also required for percutaneous mitral valve repair.

5. Mechanical countèrpulsatile hemodynamic support (MCHS)

In severe cases of decompensated HF, pharmacological hemodynamic support cannot usually achieve complete hemodynamic stability and maintain adequate blood supply to end-organs and tissues in the decompensated HF. End-stage HF patients with severe ventricular decompensation are frequently referred to ICUs for hemodynamic support. After full monitoring and assessment of hemodynamic parameters, the required appropriate medications are used to solve symptoms and signs of LCOS; however, full medication can heal patients for once, but then healing degrades and pharmacologic bridge to transplantation cannot stabilize patients, and hence mechanical counterpulsatile hemodynamic support (MCHS) becomes necessary.

5.1. Intraaortic counterpulsatile support (IACPS)

Counterpulsatile devices for MHS improve patient status by same physiologic effects, but with different mechanisms (**Table 7**) [46]. The principle of counterpulsation is to produce diastolic augmentation. Prediastolic inflation coincided with T-P interval on electrocardiogram provides increase in peak diastolic aortic pressure (aortic uploading) to enhance coronary perfusion during ventricular relaxation and filling. Presystolic deflation coincided with QRS-T interval on electrocardiogram, which is always triggered by R wave, assures decreasing in end-diastolic aortic pressure (aortic unloading) to facilitate intraaortic impedance reduction during ventricular contraction and ejection. These devices are usually used for short-term supportive therapy in early postoperative period to wean patients from CPB. There are several positive effects of counterpulsation on systemic hemodynamics and left ventricular mechanoenergetics, but the main goal is to increase CO without bypassing the heart or the related ventricle [47]. Second application area in end-stage HF patients is to stabilize hemodynamics and to gain time for keeping patients alive or bridging to a more durable therapy. The first step

	Intraaortic	**Paraaortic**
Insertion	Percutaneously	Surgically
Incision	Sliding technique or local incision	Intraoperatively or left thoracotomy
Placement way	Peripheral	Semicentral
Placement area	Suprarenal thoracoabdominal aorta	Thoracal descending aorta
Capacity	30–50 mL	20–100 (or more) mL
Working principle	Volumetric	Circulatory
Working space	Intraluminal	Extraluminal
Working risk	Systolic occlusive	Nonocclusive
Inflation/deflation	Diastole/systole	Diastole + systole
Coronary perfusion	Optimum/steal	Optimum
Stroke work	Decreasing (+)	Decreasing (+++)
Cardiac output	Increasing	Increasing

Table 7. Comparison of counterpulsatil devices.

is to stabilize the end-stage HF patients using IABP for up to 2 weeks and if the patients are hemodynamically stabilized (no need for inotropes, no peripheral organ malfunction, CVP ≤ 10 mmHg, mean arterial pressure ≥ 65 mmHg) but could not wean from IABP, then they can be transitioned to a more effective counterpulsatile or t-MCS devices as a bridge to recovery or to end-stage therapy (p-MCS device or HTx).

Intraaortic balloon pump (IABP) is the most preferred, well-tolerated, and most cost-efficient method among mechanical supportive approaches with significant hemodynamic improvements in patients with unstable hemodynamic status (**Table 8**) [48]. But the frequency of IABP

(I) Therapeutic

- **A.** Preoperatively
  - **1.** Unstable myocardial ischemia
    - **a.** acute coronary syndrome
    - **b.** intractable coronary ischemia
    - **c.** severe left main disease
    - **d.** malign ventricular arrhythmia
  - **2.** Cardiogenic shock
    - **a.** myocardial infarction
    - **b.** mechanical complications of AMI (MR, VSD, LVR)
    - **c.** myocarditis
    - **d.** sepsis
  - **3.** Cardiomyopaties
  - **4.** Procedural support during coronary angiography
  - **5.** Stabilization for surgery
    - **a.** cardiac surgical patients (LCOS, VSD, severe MR)
    - **b.** noncardiac surgical patients
- **B.** Intraoperatively
  - **1.** Off-pump CABG
  - **2.** On-pump CABG on the beating heart
  - **3.** LVAD implantation
- **C.** Postoperatively
  - **1.** Failure to separate from CPB
  - **2.** LCOS

(II) Bridging

- **A.** Heart transplantation
- **B.** Left ventricular assist device

	C.	Total artificial heart
(III)	Diagnostic	
	A.	Reversibility of pulmonary (PAH, PVR)

AMI = acute myocardial infarction; CABG = coronary artery bypass grafting; CPB = cardiopulmonary bypass; IABP = intraaorrtic balloon pump; LCOS = low cardiac output syndrome; LVAD = left ventricular assist device; LVR = left ventricular rupture; MR = mitral regurgitation; PAH = pulmonary arterial hypertension; PVR = pulmonary vascular resistance; VSD = ventricular septal defect.

Table 8. Indications for IABP.

usage in the end-stage HF patients has broadened in last decade due to the increase in the usage of t-MCS devices to bridge to HTx or LVAD implantation. The main indications for IABP are to increase myocardial perfusion in critical uncontrolled coronary artery stenosis preoperatively and to improve CO in severe LHF postoperatively [49]. The purpose of this indication is to decrease afterload and consequently to facilitate unloading of the LV, especially LHF complicated with significant MR. Intraaortic balloon pumping relies on the principle of diastolic counterpulsation, which causes a reduction in left ventricular afterload and an increase in aortic diastolic and consequently coronary artery perfusion pressures. Because the descending aorta has a particular diameter the balloon catheter should have a limited volume, which are two types for adults: 40 mL (26 cm length and 1.5 cm diameter) and 50 mL (27 cm length and 1.8 cm diameter). Even the hemodynamic effect of this capacity affects the myocardial oxygen supply/demand ratio favorably due to the decreasing peak systolic wall stress and contractile work of the LV, the net effect will be an increase in forward LVEF, CI, and CO (**Table 9**). However, when IABP support has only limited positive impact on cardiac hemodynamics, it cannot maintain adequate cardiac output in patients with decompensated severe left HF or reduce clinical symptoms and hemodynamic signs. In such cases, this hemodynamic supportive strategy must be complemented by more advanced MCS devices [50].

Therapeutic usage of IABP is well known and accepted treatment strategy to reverse or prevent moderate LCOS owing to hibernating or stunned myocardium after acute coronary syndrome, during percutaneous cardiac interventions, along malign ventricular arrhythmias, and after mechanical complications of myocardial infarction [51]. High-risk patients undergoing cardiac operations may be also protected against adverse outcomes [52, 53]. Pharmacological and mechanical hemodynamic supports remedies pre- and afterload deterioration through improved CO, coronary perfusion, and improved end-organ perfusion. The latter effect is the main curative treatment strategy to terminate and reverse organ dysfunctions, which increase pre- and postoperative mortality and morbidity. The significant life-saving benefit of IABP support on the early mortality is well known; however, the benefit on either 30-day or 1-year all-cause mortality is dubious in end-stage HF patients due to insufficiency to achieve and sustain adequate CO. Therefore, a more effective MCS device should be utilized if IABP could not achieve adequate CO in a couple of days (<7 days) or immediately when any decompensation develops on the IABP treatment.

Prophylactic long-term usage of counterpulsation to optimize cardiac output and RV function as a bridge to HTx or long-term LVAD implantation is a growing area of application (**Table 10**) [54].

Decrease	
Systolic blood pressure	up to 10%
Presystolic aortic pressure (afterload)	up to 30%
LV systolic pressure (wall tension)	up to 20%
Isometric phase of LV contraction	
LV energy utilization (myocardial oxygen consumption; TTI)	
LVEDV + LVEDP (preload)	
PCWP	
Increase	
Diastolic blood pressure	
LV mechanical performance	
EF	up to 5%
CI	up to 20%
CO	up to 30% (0.5-1 L/min)
LV energy obtainment (myocardial oxygen supply; DPTI)	
Endocardial Viability Ratio improvement	DPTI/TTI > 1
(<0.7 indicates severe myocardial ischemia)	
LV contractility and active relaxation	
Coronary blood flow	
Cerebral, renal, mesenteric, and pulmonary blood flow	
Mean arterial pressure (in shock)	

CI = cardiac index; CO = cardiac output; DPTI = diastolic pressure time index; EF = ejection fraction; LV = left ventricular; LVEDP = left ventricular end-diastolic pressure; LVEDV = left ventricular end-diastolic volume; PCWP = pulmonary capillary wedge pressure; SV = stroke volume; TTI = tension time index.

Table 9. Effects of counterpulsation on hemodynamics mechanoenergetics.

Predestinative usage of IABP improves and stabilizes clinical status of potential recipients suffering from multi-organ hypoperfusion and ischemia, which are significant predictors for adverse outcome after HF surgery, to obtain good postoperative results [55]. Prophylactic IABP implementation decreases left ventricular preload and therefore RV upload, which could

Outcome	Recovery	Destination
Bridge to recovery (BTR)	Biventricular or left ventricular	Discharge
Bridge to candidacy (BTC)	Bi- or univentricular	Additional mechanical interventions
Bridge to destination (BTD)	Right ventricular	LVAD
Bridge to transplantation (BTT)	None	Heart ± lung transplantation

IABP = intraaortic balloon pump; LVAD = left ventricular assist device.

Table 10. Potential outcomes of long-term IABP support in chronic heart failure.

terminate hepatic congestion and dysfunction. On the other hand, IABP support improves renal and gastrointestinal blood supply with significant recovery of dysfunctional organs [56]. This strategy can reduce HF symptoms, signs, and laboratory findings (serum total bilirubin and creatinine, plasma BNP levels), especially in the first 48 hours significantly. The most important point is the optimal timing of IABP insertion, which must be earlier as possible, before end-organ dysfunction exceeds the threshold of reversibility, and prophylactic usage must be continued for a minimum of 2 weeks to get effective results. However, long-term IABP support can cause several major complications including acute limb ischemia, severe bleeding, embolic events, infection, and sepsis. When IABP support could not sustain and/or maintain stable hemodynamics, it should be enhanced by implementing more durable devices.

Diagnostic usage is a controversial strategy that could present a significant, favorable alteration in pulmonary arterial pressure and PVR. This improvement could facilitate decisions regarding LVAD implantation or HTx in end-stage HF patients with moderate PVR (6-8 Woods). These patients are not considered to be ideal candidates for HTx according to the guidelines, but they must be investigated whether they could be eligible for initial or postimplant (after LVAD) HTx, or just for destination therapy. More effective left ventricular unloading via IABP also decreases LVEDV, which is the main stimulator for reducing pulmonary venous and consequently pulmonary arterial pressure, and effects a significant reduction in PCWP and CVP initially, as well as in creatinine and total bilirubin concentrations. Two-week application is necessary to see reversibility of PVR, because the positive effect of IABP could be negatively balanced or withdraw after the first week. In this case, PVR will not improve after heart transplant, and mid-term outpatient pharmacologic (sildenafil) and/or mechanical (LVAD) PVR-lowering therapy will be the preferred strategy, with follow-up re-catheterization after 3–6 months to evaluate PVR. Adequate reduction in PVR (<6 Woods) makes these patients potential candidates for HTx. If reduced PVR is sustained, patients will be included in urgent waiting list for HTx (Status 1B) without any additional criteria.

Support with IABP is started after standard maximal pharmacological thresholds (adrenalin or noradrenalin >0.15 μg/kg/min) fail to restore hemodynamic stability. The balloon catheter is usually passed percutaneously into the descending thoracic aorta through the femoral artery, but alternative routes, such as the axillary, the subclavian, or the brachial arteries, can be preferred if the femoral artery is not suitable for usage, as well as the ascending aorta could be preferred surgically [57]. Support with IABP is not a complication-free procedure and the most common complications are peripheral arterial injuries (rupture, perforation, bleeding, dissection, embolism, etc.), which is best avoided by sliding technique under ultrasonographic visulation, or complications of distal tissue malperfusion (extremities' ischemia), which is best prevented by the sheatless application of balloon catheters [58].

As the patient's cardiac performance improves, the IABP support must be removed step by step. First of all, all inotropic medication should be lowered (dobutamine or dopamine dose ≤5 μg/kg/min) parallel to hemodynamic stability, cardiac output, and mixt venous oxygen saturation changes. The next step to reduce balloon augmentation by one of two different methods: decreasing counterpulsation intervals or slow, step-wise deflation. Because a stagnation of the balloon catheter within the blood stream can cause microclots on its surface, decreasing of augmentation levels seems more complication-free. Deflating the balloon catheter simultaneously decreases MCHS; a 50% reduction over 12 to 24 hours is a good indicator of successful weaning, terminating with the removal of the catheter.

5.2. Extraaortic counterpulsatile support (EACPS)

Extraaortic balloon pump (EABP), C-Pulse, is a new, counterpulsatile, nonblood-contacting device that involves placement of an inflatable cuff with a polyurethane balloon and polyester wrap around the ascending aorta for the management of end-stage HF patients, who remain symptomatic despite IABP therapy with optimum PHS [59]. C-Pulse is designed to provide permanent, long-term, continuous partial MCHS for end-stage HF patients [60]. The cuff inflates inwardly causing thumb-print deflection of the outer curvature of the ascending aorta, which creates a pressure across the aortic wall ranging from 6 to 25 mmHg. Approximately 20–30 mL of ascending aortic blood volume can be displaced per beat, depending on the cuff size and aortic diameter. The implantation is achieved via midline sternotomy, without cardiopulmonary bypass. There is no any deterioration in the aortic valve and aortic regurgitation, no intimal disruption and only minor thickening of the adventitia on microscopy [61].

5.3. Paraaortic counterpulsatile circulation support (PACPCS)

Paraaortic blood pump (PABP) or *paraaortic circulatory device (PACD)* has been produced to enhance the hemodynamic effect and also to expand the indications of counterpulsation [62]. The first use in humans was disappointing, with large volume (100 mL) and on the ascending aorta implantation. Decreasing the device volume [63] and redesigning it so as to avoid the ascending aorta [64] were successful in decreasing initial systolic hypotensive symptoms and improving hemodynamic success, and for this reason it has been suggested that PABP may be more capable of efficiently supporting end-stage HF patients than IACPS or EACPS approaches. The IACPS systems should have limited dimensions and that is why IABP with limited capacity is preferred mostly in patients with moderate cardiac failure. However, IABP is unsatisfactory in patients with severe LVD, in whom systolic aortic pressure is lower than 70 mmHg. On the other hand, EACPS systems require a disease-free ascending aorta with appropriate length and therefore EABP can be used only in IABP-contraindicated patients with moderate cardiac failure because of nonblood contacting extravascular working principle. However, it needs a midline sternotomy incision and limited capacity related to the size of the ascending aorta could reduce device efficiency. If it is predicted that IABP or EABP may not provide enough stroke volume, blood pressure, and effective support in patients with moderate or more advanced LCOS (CMPs, myocarditis, etc.), PABP may provide better support. Additionally, PABP support must be preferred longer than a couple weeks in patients with severe LVF because it provides higher stroke volume, fewer vascular complications (ischemia, amputation, etc.), allows mobilization, and may be a better bridge to LVAD implantation or HTx [65]. There are several devices to provide PACP, but their usage is limited in special patient population or animal studies [66]. Partial unloading of the failed LV may interrupt the progressive hemodynamic deterioration of HF and improve quality of life in patients with earlier stages of HF. This partial support provided by PACDs may reduce native ventricular workload, augment myocardial blood flow, support positive myocardial remodeling, and prevent RVF [67, 68]. They do not require CBP support during implantation, and a major branch artery is usually the preferred site for in- and outflow graft anastomosis. These devices preserve heart integrity, unload the LV, decrease its energy consumption, enhance native left ventricular functional performance, and retain pulsatility of flow. Recovery occurs usually within the first 3–6 months on mechanical assistance (bridge to recovery). The other philosophy about PACDs is to maintain arterial wall physiology with natural counterpulsatile flow.

6. Mechanical circulatory support (MCS)

End-stage HF is usually treated, healed, and stabilized by pharmacologic and/or mechanical hemodynamic support, but advanced HF is characterized by increasing frequency of intervals of decompensation, rehospitalization, and reintervention. If the MHS is insufficient for the recovery of LCOS, MCS is required to maintain CO (**Table 11**). Temporary MCS devices increase arterial blood circulation with or without extracorporeal oxygenation to provide an adequate CO, which acts as a parallel or serial artificial circulation to the physiologic circulation pattern. Permanent mechanical pumps provide a parallel artificial circulation of failed ventricles or entirely assume the pump function of the resected heart. Short-term devices are extracorporeal or paracorporeal pumps located outside the body, whereas durable devices are intracorporeal pumps implanted inside the body. The definitions of circulatory supports are dependent on cardiac chambers and oxygenation (**Table 12**).

	Counterpulsation	Short-term VAD	Long-term VAD
LVEF	<40%	<30%	<25%
LVD	No	Yes/no	Yes
Systolic ABP	<90 mmHg	<80 mmHg	<80 mmHg
Mean ABP	<60 mmHg	<50 mmHg	<50 mmHg
CVP	≥15 mmHg	≥18 mmHg	≥20 mmHg
Mean PCWP	≥15 mmHg	≥18 mmHg	≥20 mmHg
CI	≤2.2 L/min/m^2	≤2 L/min/m^2	≤1.8 L/min/m^2
SVR			>2100 Dynes/cm/sec
Inotropic agents with high doses	≤2	≥2	>2
IABP	No	Yes	Yes
Urine output	<0.5 mL/kg/h	<0.5 mL/kg/h	<20 mL/h
Metabolic asidosis	Yes/no	Yes/no	Yes
HRF	No	Yes/no	Yes/no
Application stage	First	Second	Second or last

ABP = arterial blood pressure; CI = cardiac index; CVP = central venous pressure; HRF = hepatorenal failure; IABP = intraaortic balloon pump; LVD = left ventricular dilatation; LVEF = left ventricular ejection fraction; MCS = mechanical circulatory support; PCWP = pulmonary capillary wedge pressure; SVR = systemic vascular resistance; VAD = ventricular assist device.

Table 11. Hemodynamic indication criteria for MCS in patients suffered heart failure.

Ventricular contribution: to decrease ventricular unloading and work index
• *Ventricular assist*: ventricular outloading through the left ventricular cavity directly (after mitral valve)
• *Ventricular support*: ventricular unloading through the left atrium (before mitral valve)
Cardiac relinquishment: to circulate out-of-heart uni- or biventricularly
• *LV-bypass*: no-loading of the left ventricular
• *RV-bypass*: no-loading of the right ventricle
• *BV-bypass*: no-loading of both ventricles
With external oxygenator: to oxygenate blood in the external circulatory circuit
• *va-ECCPS*: veno-arterial circulatory assistance with external oxygenation
• *va-a-ECCPS*: venoatrial-arterial circulatory assistance with external oxygenation
• *aa-ECCPS*: atrio-arterial circulatory assistance with external oxygenation
• *vp-ECCPS*: veno-pulmonary circulatory assistance with external oxygenation
BV = biventricular; ECCPS = extracorporeal cardiopulmonary support; LV = left ventricular; MCS = mechanical circulatory support; RV = right ventricular.

Table 12. Definitions of MCS in heart failure.

After full implementation of pharmacological and MHS therapies, most acute failed hearts after cardiogenic shock, interventional coronary revascularization, or surgical or percutaneous cardiac procedures can recover from LCOS within hours (peroperatively) or days (postoperatively). When this primary treatment strategy does not work or fails during a situation of intractable decompensated HF, MCS devices are the only life-saving instruments. These devices can be also used as a bridge to keep patients alive if weaning from CPB is not possible or when intractable LCOS does not recover. Consecutive or combined usage of these devices with or without extracorporeal oxygenation could be also an effective, maybe, an essential preference to get a successful outcome [69].

The working mechanism of MCS devices in HF syndrome is very simple: sucking circulatory blood under negative pressure and ejecting it into the systemic or pulmonary arterial circulation. The inflow cannula (temporary) or inlet tube (permanent) is inserted in the relevant ventricle and the outflow cannula (temporary) or outlet graft (permanent) is connected to the ventricle-associated main artery. These devices have two different action principles: pulsatile or continuous flow. Devices working by pulsatile flow have a blood-compatibility chamber and a moveable diaphragm separating the chamber into the blood and air spaces. The blood space is connected to the aorta or main pulmonary artery through a graft forced with a prosthetic valve. The air space is connected to a compressor-console providing power for counterpulsation through inflation and deflation. Devices working by nonpulsative flow have a blood-compatibility compartment and a frictionless turnable rotor directing input flow to the related circulation.

Pulsatility is the indispensable principle of the native, physiological, durable, regulated, and protective circulation in human. Pulsatile flow has several benefits for maintaining natural life (**Table 13**). The superiority of pulsatility over continuous flow has not yet been definitively demonstrated, but several studies have addressed adverse nonphysiological transformation in the vascular bed, inequable neuroendocrine responses, and device-related complications from mechanical continuous circulation. More complicated extracorporeal devices are required to produce pulsatile flow, while pulsatile intracorporeal devices require more space than centrifugal pumps if used for uni- or biventricular support; however, only total artificial hearts produce the true pulsatile flow as prosthetic HTx.

There are two main types of extracorporeal pumps with different working mechanisms (**Table 14**). Pulsatile pumps are often used in biventricular failure and in pediatric patients [70]. Nonpulsatile pumps are mostly preferred for CPB and MCS. Roller pumps, which generate forward blood flow by roller compression, rate of rotation, and the length of the compression raceway, are useful for

Transmission of energy to the microcirculation
Reduction critical capillary closing pressure
Augmentation of lymphatic flow
Improvement of tissue perfusion
Amelioration of cellular metabolism
Alleviation of vasoconstrictive reflexes
Diminution of acidosis
Regulation of neuroendocrine responses

Table 13. Physiologic effects of pulsatile flow.

(I)	Pulsatile flow pumps		
	1.	Abiomed	
	2.	Thoratec paracorporeal ventricular assist device	
	3.	Excor	
(II)	Nonpulsatile flow pumps		
	1.	Roller pumps	
	2.	Centrifugal pumps	
		a.	Medtronic Bio-Medicus
		b.	Maque Rotaflow
		c.	Levitronix CentriMag
		d.	TandemHeart
	3.	Axial pumps	
		a.	Impella

MCS = mechanical circulatory support.

Table 14. Devices for temporary MCS.

CPB during open heart surgery, but not for circulatory support due to hemolysis and tubing wear. Extracorporeal continuous flow pumps are useful for CBP as well as extended t-MCS with fewer adverse effects than roller pumps. Intracorporeal devices are designed with a smaller structure using two separate pump mechanisms: axial flow pumps have a pump rotor parallel to the blood path, and centrifugal pumps have an impeller rotor perpendicular to the blood path. The rotor is magnetically levitated, and rotation is achieved without friction or wear, thus minimizing blood trauma, mechanical failure, and heat generation. These devices work by an external motor-driven system, direct-drive system, or self-bearing system. In direct-drive system, the impeller becomes the motor rotor supported by a separate levitation system. In self-bearing system, both the drive and the levitation coils share the same stator core [71].

Because the duration of their usage could be limited, the decision for the destination goal should take into hemodynamic, hematologic, and neurologic courses. Even though the gold standard therapy for end-stage HF is HTx, this is possible in only a small number of patients due to limited organ availability. These devices are generally used to maintain adequate organ perfusion for several days, but more time could be required before a final decision is made (**Table 15**). Bridging to curative treatments should be life-saving and any device could be effective, but do not hesitate to change the treatment stages and devices.

Designed to assist the native heart, MCS devices are differentiated by the implant duration [short-term (<10 days), mid-term (10–90 days), long-term (>90 days)], indication [temporary (bridge therapy) versus permanent (destination therapy)], type (cardiopulmonary versus circulatory), approach (percutaneous versus surgical), location (extracorporeal versus intracorporeal), flow characteristic [pulsatile versus continuous), pump mechanism (volume displacement, axial, centrifugal), and the ventricle(s) supported (left, right, biventricular) [72].

6.1. Temporary mechanical cardiorespiratory support (t-MCRS)

Acute decompensation of cardiac functions requires emergent circulatory support when pharmacological treatment and/or counterpulsatile support are ineffective or when weaning from CPB fails (**Table 16**). There are several options for t-MCS, which can be applied percutaneously or centrally, but right ventricular and respiratory functions are decision-making factors [73]. Sufficient oxygenation by the lungs suspends usage of external oxygenator, but associated RVF necessitates its usage. Temporary cardiorespiratory support (t-MCRS) devices are designed to rapidly reestablish adequate organ perfusion and oxygenation. Biventricular t-MCRS is the most common approach to maintain adequate CO and oxygenation in the presence of severe RVF; however, univentricular t-MCRS can be the preferred approach in the absence of significant RVF. An ideal device should support adequate flow, maximal hemodynamics, sufficient oxygenation, and avoid need for anticoagulation with its serious related serious complications (**Table 17**). After echocardiography fails to reveal a surgically correctable cause, a temporary mechanical device is considered for MCS according to several hemodynamic data (**Table 11**). Daily follow-up with transthoracic and/or transesophageal echocardiography is mandatory to evaluate biventricular function, regional wall motion abnormalities, valvular mechanics, septal malformations, and extracardiac compression, as well as native heart recovery. On the other hand, the stabilized patient should also undergo daily evaluation for end-organ functions, hematologic and infectious conditions, and neurologic status.

Bridge to recovery (BTR): *Salvage therapy.* Clinical situation consists of either acute developed cardiogenic shock or acutely decompensated Stage-D HF. Acute huge myocardial infarction with or without mechanical complications, acute myocarditis, and postcardiotomy syndrome after cardiac surgery cause acutely developed myocardial dysfunction, which can be refractory to optimal treatment via PHS and counterpulsatile MHS despite viable myocardium. Any reason can worsen and decrease stable Stage-D HF into unstable condition with severe LCOS. The myocardium could be recovered by MCS devices via unloading the left ventricular in a couple of hours or days (<4–7 days), and after that patients should be put into advanced bridging therapies. Daily echocardiographic examinations are guiding and following practices to investigate the reverse remodelling of the failed myocardium. During this period, the main goal is to keep patients alive.

Bridge to decision (BTD): *Rescue therapy.* Acutely cardiac failure subsequent to myocardial infarction or cardiac operations, or acutely decompensation of Stage-D HF requires optimal treatment via MHS and/or MCS devices (1) to keep patients alive, and then (2) to maintain vital functions due to mechanical supported cardiac output, and finally (3) to gain time for decision to the most appropriate curative or egress treatment solution for related patients. Clinicians have a couple of days (<14 days), but not more than one week, to evaluate each patient separately with his/her own cardiac pathology and to decide the next step(s). During this period, the main goal is to let the heart in rest and no-load, and also to keep extracardiac organs in normal functions.

Bridge to wean (BTW): *Separation therapy.* Improvement in cardiac functions and healing of acute decompensation of acute or chronic HF improves patient's status and makes it possible to disconnect mechanical devices. After the hemodynamics recover completely in several days or weeks (<30 days), weaning protocol is started via reducing all pharmacological agents to their minimum dosages, improving respiratory functions, and decreasing mechanical support levels. Patients should be followed with daily echocardiography and pulmonary arterial catheterization (wedge pressure, mixt venous oxygen saturation). During this period, the main goal is to keep patients noncardiacly complication-free.

Bridge to curative surgical and/or percutaneous interventions (BTI): *Supportive therapy.* Associated curable cardiac pathologies (CAD, MR, postinfarct VSD, etc.) could be treated to improve cardiac functions and to prevent new decompensations. The hemodynamically stable condition gained by MCS devices enables clinicians (1) to revascularize ischemic myocardium, (2) to repair these structural mechanical complications, (3) to rescue the acute failed heart, (4) to recovery myocardial dysfunction, and (5) to bridge to weaning or advanced treatments. During this period, the main goal is to keep extracardiac organs in normal functions, and also to provide hemodynamic with or without respiratorial support during procedures.

Bridge to bridge (BTB): *Exchange therapy.* Short-term mechanical supportive devices cannot provide adequate flow and facilitate further improvement in the clinical status of patients, as the result patients cannot be weaned from MCS. The preferred MCS type should be switched more a failed-oriented type of MCS or more durable approach. Weaning from right ventricular and/or pulmonary support make it possible to disconnected venous cannulas or oxygenator from the circuit (bridge from va-a-ECCPS to aa-ECCS).

Bridge to candidacy (BTC): *Preparatory therapy.* Switching from t-MCS to p-MCS due to the necessity of the long-term follow for successful recovery is necessity for the decision (1) to wean from the device, (2) to use the device as the destination therapy, or (3) to take the patients into the transplantation list. The reversibility of the elevated PVR or the prolonged healing of damaged myocardium requires a prolonged treatment period (>30 days), usually a couple of months, but not more than six months. Long-term predicted recovery should be verified by invasive tests a significant reduction in PVR. During this period, the main goal is to keep patients in their daily lives.

Bridge to destination (BTD): *Continuity therapy.* Long-term mechanical support is a durable treatment alternative to HTx in with Stage-D HF patients, who are not eligible for transplantation due to extracardiac diseases, irreversible elevated PVR, advanced age, or donor inability. Left ventricular assist devices may prolong and improve the quality of life.

Bridge to transplantation (BTT): *Curative therapy.* Irreversible myocardial function is the main indication for HTx in the decompensated or device-dependent Stage-D HF. Progressive lengthening of waiting times on transplantation lists can be an indication for LVAD implantation, but this reason is most pertinent to bridge to destination therapy. On the other hand, there is no widely accepted guideline to show the indication and timing for a mechanical supportive device placement as a bridge treatment. The true indications for this therapy are (1) patients with implanted p-MCS devices with/without complications, (2) unrecoverable patients supported with t-MCS devices, and (3) borderline patients on the bridge to candidacy protocol.

Table 15. Bridging from live-saving t-MCS to advanced therapy modalities.

Acute myocarditis
Acute huge myocardial infarction with/without mechanical complications
Cardiogenic shock
Cardiopulmonary arrest
Postcardiotomy syndrome
Acutely decompensation of Stage-D heart failure
Intractable decompensation of end-stage cardiomyopathies
Intractable ventricular tachycardia in end-stage cardiomyopathies
Bridge to destination therapy or heart transplantation
Postimplant right ventricular failure

Table 16. Indications of t-MCS for heart failure.

Decrease preload
Decrease pulmonary capillary wedge pressure
Not increase afterload
Augment cardiac output
Increase coronary perfusion
Improve peripheral tissue perfusion
Provide adequate oxygen delivery

Table 17. The primary hemodynamic goals of t-MCS.

6.1.1. Cardiopulmonary bypass (CPB)

The first used life-supportive approach is CBP with a roller or centrifugal pump for circulatory assistance and an oxygenator for respiratory reinforcement during open heart surgery. This shortest extracorporeal circulation has several parts resulting in hemolysis, especially the cardiotomy suction and venous reservoir. Failing to wean from bypass after cardiac procedures enforces to prolong circulatory support via CPB. Because this approach is not suitable for short-term or longer circulatory support, CPB has been used only for ultrashort-term (<1 day) circulatory assistance. The main differences of CBP circuit are the drainage of venous blood, typically by gravity, into venous reservoir of the heart-lung machine, and aspiration of blood from the surgical field into the reservoir. Both of these can cause also inflammatory and humoral responses, thrombosis and bleeding problems. The rest of the supportive mechanism is similar with the other t-MCPS devices: to pump venous blood through an oxygenator for gas exchange, and therefrom into the arterial circulation. This basic extracorporeal perfusion system can be used for partial or total circulatory and respiratory support, or partial support of the LV. Modern membrane oxygenators add up to 470 mL of O_2 and remove up to 350 mL of CO_2 per minute at

1–7 L of flow with resistances of 12–15 mmHg per liter blood flow. Preferable pumps are centrifugal ones consisting of a vaned impeller or nested smooth plastic cones, which propel blood by centrifugal force when they rotate rapidly. Centrifugal pumps produce forward pressure of up to 900 mmHg, but only half as much of negative pressure, and therefore, less cavitation and fewer gaseous microemboli. Flow rate should be set to maintain mean arterial pressure at ≥70 mmHg at 35 to 37°C, with a hematocrit of 30%. This flow rate provides and maintains adequate body perfusion, with higher mixed venous oxygen saturation >60%.

It is meaningful to use CBP as a mechanical support only in the theater for *ultrashort-term (several hours)* assistance, but advanced technology provides more appropriate devices for short- and long-term MCPS. There are several side effects of CBP that preclude its usage as a short- and long-term cardiopulmonary support. The main problem is left ventricular distention and lack of unloading during CPB support, which will be prevented by insertion of a vent catheter into the LA or LV. The second limitation is the necessity of full dose heparinization to gain an activated clotting time greater than 400 seconds during extracorporeal circulation to prevent thrombo-embolic events, which usually causes bleeding problems. The third possible hazard is massive air embolism due to the integrity of the extracorporeal circuit. The fourth side effect is generalized inflammatory reactions, which result in a number of undesired pathophysiologic cascades. The fifth negative damage is possible lung injury, which is inevitable during CPB support due to increased pulmonary capillary permeability, interstitial lung water, and adverse inflammatory responses.

6.1.2. Extracorporeal life or cardiopulmonary support (ECLS or ECCPS)

The casually accepted term for these support strategies is ECMO, but the true definition must be extracorporeal cardiopulmonary support (ECCPS) while using for treatment in decompensated Stage-D HF or extracorporeal life support (ECLS) while using for similar support in acute cardiogenic shock. Although the unsuitability of CBP for short- or long-term ECLS has been established, its principles have been applied to never small, durable, practical, integrated, and mobile devices that are practical for providing ECLS in all appropriate circumstances. The principal aim of ECLS is to provide acute temporary ECCPS globally as a bridge to more durable therapy in patients with cardiorespiratory failure refracted to maximal conventional therapy [74]. For extracorporeal membrane oxygenation (ECMO), an oxygenator is inserted in the extracorporeal circuit for gas exchange before returning patient's venous blood to the patient's arterial circulation, which is driven by a centrifugal pump. They are suitable for t-MCS, but single or multiple replacement of the failed oxygenator with a new one can allow prolongation of ECCPS to more than 1 month if myocardial recovery is the desired and expected goal. If pulmonary functions are well or pulmonary recovery occurs during ECCPS, the external oxygenator is not necessary and it must be disconnected from the circuit to provide acute or prolonged temporary extracorporeal circulatory support (ECCS) for the LHF or RHF. Double established ECCSs could be used separately for biventricular HF patients with unimpaired respiratory functions.

The devices designed for short-term ECCPS have a number of advantages in comparison with CPB (lower dose of heparin, a continuous circuit, etc.). A hollow-fiber membrane oxygenator with an integrated heat-exchange system operated by a centrifugal pump provides circulatory, respiratory, and thermatory supports. These pumps are totally nonocclusive and afterload-dependent, and when myocardial recovery occurs, physiological circulation overtakes artificial circulation, manifesting as reduced device flow. These pumps do not create excessive output pressure (so as not to rupture the circuit) or significant negative input pressure (so as to avoid cavitation and microembolus). Using this system, ECCPS flow is maintained between 4 and 6 L/min by providing a pump speed of between 3000 and 3500 rpm, with higher pump speed risking mechanical trauma to blood cells. The heat exchanger provides normothermia during ECCPS, which is mandatory for physiologic body functions. A biocompatible heparin-coated bypass circuit provides an antithrombotic surface to reduce or eliminate the necessary dose of heparin and inflammatory responses. Because roller pumps cause hemolysis beyond 4 and 5 hours of usage, continuous flow pumps are preferred for ECCPS.

The real problem with ECCPS in end-stage HF patients is how to protect and unload one or both ventricles. Conventional ECLS bypasses both ventricles through the venous drainage and arterial inflow, and physiologically, that will unload the RV without unloading the LV due to the increased afterload. In the borderline depressed LV or during the recovering process of LVF, both a remarkable drop in preload and a certain rise in afterload reduce left ventricular wall stress, produce smaller LVEDV, augment coronary perfusion, and ultimately improve left ventricular contractility. However, if the heart is dilated and/or contracting poorly, a markedly increased afterload handicaps any offset in both LVEDV and LVESV by blocking the opening of the aortic valve. Theoretically, left ventricular wall stress and myocardial oxygen consumption remain increased and inhibit the recovery of the failed LV. The first goal should therefore be to unload the LV using IABP and/or left atrial venting. The second target is to deliver the highly oxygenated blood directly to the coronary and cerebral circulations. Adding an IABP device to support left ventricular systolic function (by reducing afterload) and coronary perfusion (by increasing aortic diastolic pressure) is an integral part of ECLS therapy. Although ECLS balances hemodynamics, the insertion of IABP aggrandizes coronary and cerebral perfusion effects and also maintains aortic valve opening more effectively.

Establishment of ECCPS could be central or peripheral: central approach is superior due to better left ventricular unloading and the avoidance of peripheral vascular complications; however, peripheral cannulation permits later decannulation without reopening the chest. Both approaches are effective for managing cardiorespiratory failure with uni- or biventricular dysfunction associated with respiratory dysfunction (**Table 18**).

Central ECCPS is established through cardiac cannulation and is usually preferred for the failure of weaning from the bypass in the theater or postcardiotomy syndrome that develops in the ICU. The preference of central cannulation is based on several physiological hemodynamic requirements that allow shorter myocardial recovery for the acutely decompensated heart: effective biventricular unloading, highly adequate blood flow, sufficient tissue oxygenation, and easy transition from the cardiopulmonary support to left ventricular circulatory support. This approach is superior to peripheral ECCPS due to better coronary, cerebral, and upper extremities perfusion and easy insertion of left atrial vent. Central ECCPS is established via central cannulations used during cardiac surgery for postcardiotomy syndrome, or via full

ECLS- strategy	Bypass	Type	Establishment between	Approach
A. ECCPS (with ECMO)				
va – ECCPS	*bv-bypass*	*veno-aortic* *veno-arterial*	RA – Ao femoral and/or jugular vein – femoral or subclavian artery	Median sternotomy Peripheral percutaneous
va-a-ECCPS	*bv-bypass*	*biatria-aortic* *venoatrio-aortic* *venoatrio-arterial*	(RA + LA) – Ao (femoral vein + LA) – Ao (femoral vein + LA) – femoral or subclavian artery	Median sternotomy Median sternotomy Peripheral percutaneous
aa – ECCPS	*lv-bypass*	*atrio-aortic* *atrio-arterial*	LA – Ao LA – femoral/subclavian artery	Median sternotomy Peripheral percutaneous
vp – ECCPS	*rv-bypass*	*atrio-pulmonaric* *venopulmonaic*	RA – PA femoral and/or jugular vein – PA	Median sternotomy Peripheral percutaneous
B. ECCS (without ECMO)				
lv – ECCS	*lv-bypass*	*atrio- or ventriculo-aortic* *atrio- or ventriculo-arterial*	LA – or LV – Ao LA – or LV – femoral or subclavian artery	Median sternotomy Mini-thoracotomy
rv– ECCS	*rv-bypass*	*atrio-pulmonaric* *veno-pulmonaric*	RA – PA femoral and/or jugular vein – PA	Median sternotomy Mini-thoracotomy
bv– ECCS	*bv-bypass*	separately lv- and rv-ECCS		

ECCPS = extracorporeal cardiopulmonary support; ECCS = extracorporeal circulatory support; ECLS = extracorporeal life support; ECMO = extracorporeal membranous oxygenation; bv = biventricular; lv = left ventricular; rv = right ventricular; Ao = aorta; LA = left atrium; LV = left ventricle; PA = pulmonary artery; RA = right atrium.

Table 18. Temporary ECLS strategies for end-stage HF patients.

or limited sternotomy incision (reverse-T upper hemisternotomy). Both cannulas are taken out from the mediastinum below the xiphoid or through the jugulum. A new design of a biventricular assistance circuit including an oxygenator-bypass line (Kırali circuit) assists and provides the improvement of life-saving HF therapy from the sophisticated immovable t-MCPS circuit to the simplest mobile t-MCS circuit (va-a-ECCPS).

Peripheral ECCPS is established through peripheric cannulation and usually preferred as a rescue approach in nonsurgical patients suffered from acute cardiogenic shock or decompensated HF. Any perfusion strategy creating a right to left shunt requires an oxygenator in the circuit. Peripheral ECCPS is generated through the femoral artery (peripheral or upstream) or the axillary artery (periphero-central or downstream). Femoral access is more commonly used in patients requiring urgent ECLS due to rapidity of insertion and avoidance of sternotomy. The most important drawback is the left ventricular afterload mismatch and inadequate left ventricular decompression, which will cause pulmonary edema in patients with very low native CO and severe MR. To assist left ventricular unloading, IABP is used concomitantly to reduce afterload and facilitate aortic valve opening. Failure of aortic valve opening may provoke catastrophic results such as intracardiac thrombosis with or without clot embolism, worsening of LVF, coronary malperfusion, and pulmonary edema. Several percutaneous alternative approaches can be used to unload the LV during peripheral ECCPS: transaortic left ventricular unloading, transseptal left atrial decompression, atrial septostomy, and transapical left ventricular drainage. On the other hand, coronary and upper body hypoxia can occur if myocardial recovery occurs and lung function remains poor, or as mostly seen, if pump flow is reduced. Peripheral cannulation depends on the arterial structure and size, the presence of any occlusive pathology, and deficiencies in distal perfusion. A distal perfusion cannula is inserted in the selected artery distal to the inflow cannula and connected to the inflow cannula to perfuse distally to prevent extremities from ischemic complications. The same problem may develop in venous system, and a small cannula inserted into distal vein is connected into the outflow cannula to facilitate distal drainage.

Extracorporeal cardiopulmonary support is achieved using an ECMO system as described above. They can be designed according to uni- or biventricular support, and also the system must be prepared for weaning from biventricular and respiratory support step by step (**Figure 3**).

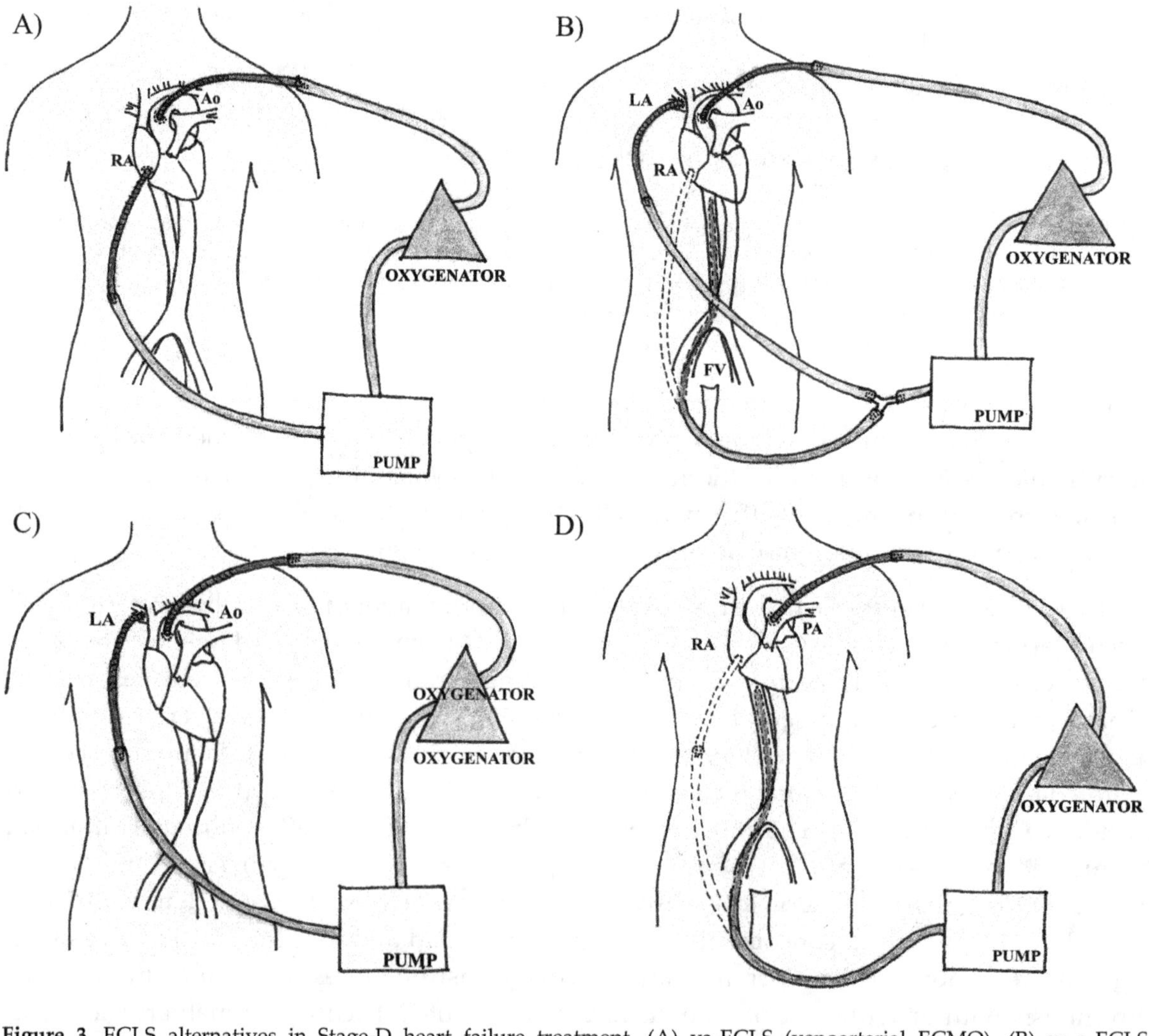

Figure 3. ECLS alternatives in Stage-D heart failure treatment. (A) va-ECLS (venoarterial ECMO). (B) va-a-ECLS (venoatrio-arterial ECMO). (C) aa-ECLS (atrio-arterial ECMO). (D) vv-ECLS (veno-venous ECMO). Ao = aorta; FV = femoral vein; LA= left atrium; RA = right atrium.

The ECCPS system can be created with several ways for different indications (**Table 18**).

va-ECCPS (va-ECMO) (biventricular bypass circuit) is the conventional ECMO system with biventricular bypass circuit by which a centrifugal pump drives blood from the patient's venous circulation through an externalized membrane oxygenator for gas exchange before returning the blood to the patient's arterial circulation. This approach is usually implemented percutaneously at the bedside in all emergent situations, in order to rescue patients suffering from fatal cardiac failure; however, a final decision about the most beneficial durable strategy should be made within a couple days (<7 days). If weaning does not seem possible, it is more appropriate to convert patients to a longer sustainable ECCPS circuit or to switch to an ECCS design.

va-a-ECCPS (va-a-ECMO) (biventricular unloading circuit; Kırali circuit) is a new format of a biventricular assistance circuit including biatrial drainage cannulas and an oxygenator-bypass line (Kırali circuit) assists and provides the improvement of life-saving HF therapy from the sophisticated immovable t-MCPS circuit to the simplest mobile t-MCS circuit (**Figure 4**); particularly it is meaningful in patients with expected RV and respiratory recovery in a couple of weeks (<1 month). This biventricular unloading circuit includes a centrifugal pump that drives blood from the patient's both atria through an externalized membrane oxygenator for gas exchange before returning to the patient's arterial circulation. This circuit has two venous cannulas: the first venous cannula (a multistage venous ECMO 28F cannula) is inserted percutaneously into the femoral vein or directly into the RA for venous drainage, and the second venous cannula (a malleable one-stage venous cannula ranged between 22F and 28F) is placed into the LA at first for left heart venting (drainage), and then for left heart bypassing (unloading). An arterial cannula (an arterial ECMO cannula ranged between 15F and 19F) is inserted into the distal ascending aorta or aortic arch, and the distal end of the cannula is placed distal to cerebral branches. Both left heart cannulas with or without the RA cannula are taken out below the sternal incision and the sternum is closed to prevent bleeding and to allow mobilization. Each outflow line has its own tap that allows blood sampling to follow blood gas and pulmonary recovery, and can be controlled by partial or total clamping to manage adequate blood drainage from each atrium according to the related ventricular dysfunction/ recovery cascade. Peripheral venous cannulation is preferred for periods of brief support (<1 week) because decannulation of the percutaneously inserted femoral venous cannula is simple. If RV recovery is expected to take more than a week, then right atrial venous cannulation should be performed centrally or a small drainage cannula is inserted distal to the outflow cannula at the femoral vein to prevent peripheral venous complications. Daily echocardiographic examination introduces RV recovery, and frequently follow-up blood samples from the left atrial inflow line propound the pulmonary recovery. Weaning from the external oxygenator should be completed in ≥4 days, and the external oxygenator should remain in the circuit for the purpose of emergent actuation in case of unexpected respiratory failure during this weaning period.

Weaning from va-a-ECCPS protocol in end-stage HF patients is simpler than others and does not require reopening of the sternum or establish a new circuit and disconnection steps should be made long enough to observe any pulmonary complications or recurrence of respiratory failure (**Table 19**). Decannulation of peripheric venous cannula is very simple when RV

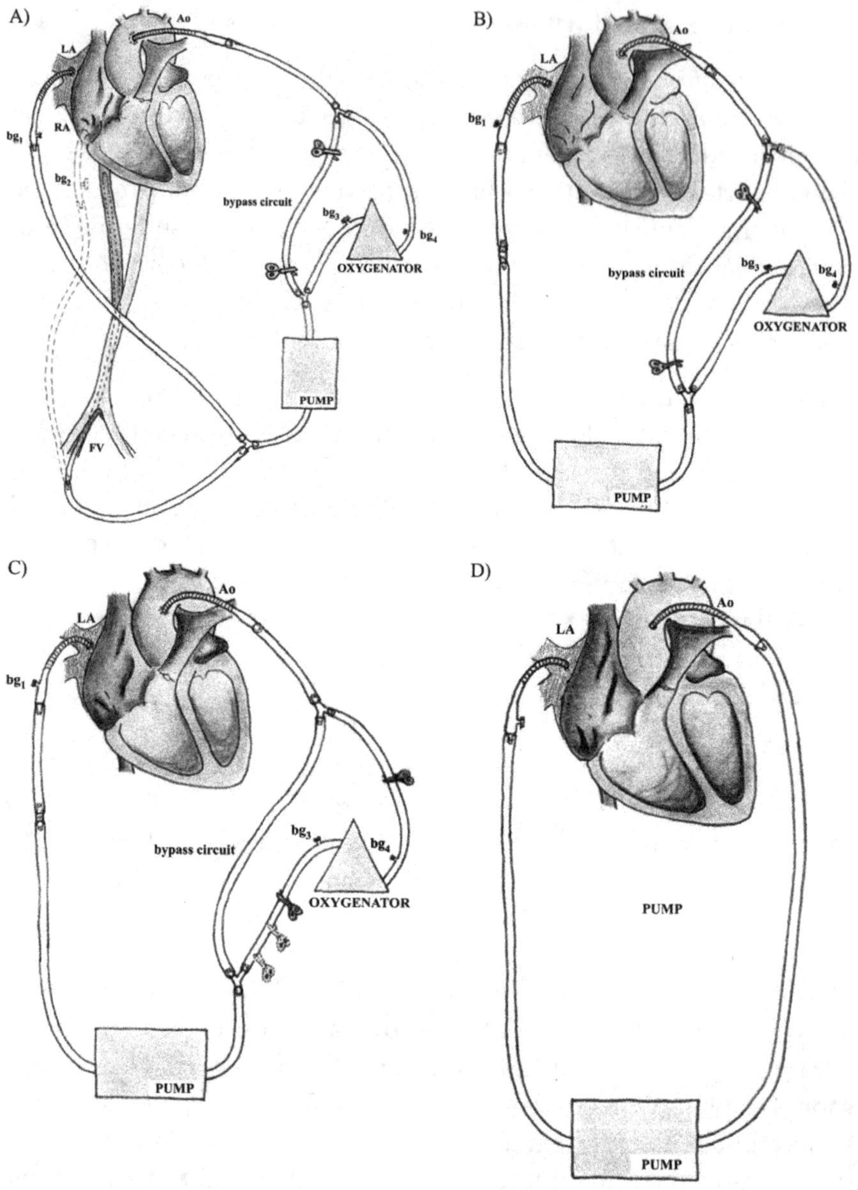

Figure 4. Venoatrial-arterial ECLS support (Kırali Circuit for biventricular unloading). (A) The circuit is constituted between both atria and the arterial circulation for right heart, pulmonary, and left heart bypass. Left ventricular unloading is necessary for left heart bypass, right ventricular unloading is necessary for right heart bypass and as well as pulmonary bypass. Blood samples from bg_1 (pulmonary gas exchanges) and bg_2 (mixt venous) show oxygen saturations in patients, and bg_3 (preoxygenator) and bg_4 (postoxygenator) gas exchanges; whereas arterial blood sample shows true body oxygenation. (B) After right heart recovery, right heart bypass line is removed from the circuit to get pulmonary and left heart bypass. (C) After pulmonary recovery, oxygenator bypass circuit is actuated to decrease oxygenator support. (D) After pulmonary recovery, oxygenator is removed from the circuit to get isolated left heart bypass. Ao = aorta; bg = blood gas sample; FV = femoral vein; LA= left atrium; RA = right atrium.

recovery is completed, and at this first stage, the circuit is converted to left heart bypass system supported with external oxygenator after removing right ventricular support (aa-ECCPS). After pulmonary recovery, the oxygenator could be removed from the circuit. First, the

First step	To convert va-a-ECCPS to aa-ECCPS after sufficiently recovery of the RV.
Second step	To reduce the oxygen delivery by respirator (res-FiO_2) till 35–40%, while the oxygen delivery by external oxygenator (oxy-FiO_2) is stabilized at 40%.
Third step	To open the oxygenator bypass line and to direct the left atrial blood flow through both oxygenator inflow lines nonocclusively with a flow ratio 3:1 (bypass line/on line) depending on membrane resistance, after blood samples from the left atrial cannula show effective native pulmonary oxygenation (left atrial oxygen saturation >95%) at least one day.
Fourth step	To reduce oxy-FiO_2 until the air ratio (21%) or disconnect the external oxygenator from oxygen gas supply, after patient's oxygenation does not collapse at least one day.
Fifth step	To begin weaning from mechanical ventilation and to extubate the patient, after arterial oxygen saturation is maintained at a level higher than 95% with res-FiO_2 40% at least one day.
Sixth step	To disconnect the external oxygenator from the circuit and to switch aa-ECCPS to aa-ECCS, after arterial oxygenation does not retrogress after extubation at least one day.

Table 19. Disconnection steps from the external oxygenator.

oxygenator bypass line is taken over pump flow step by step, and the full declamping of this line allows approximately three times more blood flow than those passing through the oxygenator due to resistance of membrane. This strategy reduces oxygenator support and enables native lungs to oxygenate most part of the pump blood flow. Finally, oxygenator is switched off and disconnected, and at this stage, the circuit is converted to left heart bypass system without oxygenator (aa-ECCS). The last stage and the simplest LV-ECCS system allows patients to be discharged from the ICU and mobilized at the ward, and provides hemodynamically stable bridging to destination therapies (LVAD or HTx).

This stage of cardiopulmonary circuit used for ECCPS provides several benefits (**Table 20**). This new strategy is independent of recovery durations, and unless any fatal complication occurs, the supportive therapy can be extended for weeks until a destination treatment could be performed, because it is easier to exchange failed oxygenator and/or pump head with a new one in this strategy, converting from "ECCPS to ECCS" or reverse, and from "va-a to aa" or reverse. The presence of the functionally significant MR facilitates left ventricular unloading through the left atrial cannula, but it can increase pulmonary congestion if the pump flow is not increased to sustain and maintain PCWP < 18 mmHg and CVP < 12 mmHg. In this circumstance, wean protocol from LV-ECCS should be started after mitral valve recovery or any percutaneous or transapical mitral valve repair intervention. The presence of the competent mitral valve, which does not facilitate left ventricular unloading due to blocking regurgitant flow, and the increased afterload, which does not enable left ventricular ejection, impair LV recovery. The best solution is provided by arterial pulsation augmenting LV unload via aortic valve opening during all left heart bypass steps.

aa-ECCPS (aa-ECMO) (left ventricular bypass circuit) is a univentricular ECMO system in which the left heart bypass circuit uses a centrifugal pump to drive blood from the LA through an external membrane oxygenator for gas exchange before returning to the patient's arterial circulation. This approach is preferred in patients with LVF and respiratorial insufficiency without RVF, who could not be managed with full mechanical ventilation, or can be a part of va-a-ECCPS.

Stage	Bridging	Established	Converting to	Benefits
Initial	Bridge to recovery	t-MCS MRS	va-a-ECCPS MRS	Effectively providing of biventricular support and gas exchange through a single pump configuration; Decompression of the left heart, reducing the LV wall stress, better coronary and body perfusion, minimizing oxygen consumption
First	Bridge to RV recovery	va-a-ECCPS MRS	aa-ECCPS MRS	Decreasing PAP, PCWP, RV afterload; Improvement of the RV; Disconnection of RV support
Second	Bridge to pulmonary recovery	aa-ECCPS MRS	aa-ECCS MRS	Decreasing LAP, pulmonary unloading; Improvement of gas exchange and adequate oxygenation; Facilitating of pulmonary recovery; disconnection oxygenator
Third	Bridge to decision	aa-ECCS MRS	aa-ECCS spontaneous ventilation	Significantly decreasing of LVEDV and LVEDP; extubation
Fourth	Bridge to bridge	aa-ECCS	aa-ECCS	Possibility of weaning, listing for HTX, or candidate for durable therapy; Mobilization in ICU
Fifth	Bridge to candidacy	aa-ECCS	wean or p-MCS	Mobilization at ward
Sixth	Bridge to destination therapy	aa-ECCS	LVAD or HTx	Destination treatment

aa = atrio-aortic; ECCPS = extracorporeal cardiorespiratory support; ECCS = extracorporeal circulatory support; HTx = heart transplantation; ICU = intensive care unit; LAP = left atrial pressure; LV = left ventricular; LVAD = left ventricular assist device; LVEDP = left ventricular end-diastolic pressure; LVEDV = left ventricular end-diastolic volume; p-MCS= permanent mechanical circulatory support; t-MCS = temporary mechanical circulatory support; MRS = mechanical respiratory support; PAP = pulmonary arterial pressure; PCWP = pulmonary capillary wedge pressure; RV = right ventricular; va-a = venoatrio-aortic.

Table 20. Bridging effects of va-a-ECCPS in Stage-D HF patients.

vp-ECCPS (vp-ECMO) (right ventricular bypass circuit) is a univentricular ECMO system in which the right heart bypass circuit uses a centrifugal pump to drive blood from the patient's vena cava or the RA through an external membrane oxygenator for gas exchange before returning to the patient's pulmonary circulation. This approach is preferred in patients with RVF and respiratorial insufficiency without LVF, who could not be managed with full mechanical ventilation. The more preferred indication can be postimplant RVF accompanied by respiratory failure.

6.2. Temporary mechanical circulatory support (t-MCS)

Most patients requiring MCS are candidates for t-MCRS, but there are some conditions that do not require ECMO support. Patients whose pulmonary function is sufficient with spontaneous or mechanical ventilation may be able to avoid or wean from oxygenator use during MCS for decompensated HF. Patients with isolated univentricular failure can mostly be treated with counterpulsatile devices, but if hemodynamic parameters do not improve more aggressively t-MCS should be performed using an ECCS system to assist the failed ventricle. Another alternative is intracorporeal circulation support (ICCS), which can be preferred in cases of cardiogenic shock or left ventricular unloading during va-ECCPS.

6.2.1. Extracorporeal circulation support (ECCS)

Isolated left or right heart ECCS is provided by a centrifugal pump; however, an external oxygenator may be implanted in the circuit if any acute respiratory decompensation develops (switch from ECCS to ECCPS). The ECCS is mostly preferred in decompensated CMPs with LVF or refracted LVD to keep patients alive until destination treatments. Another indication for weaning patients from ECCPS-based t-MCPS to ECCS-based t-MCS, by removing the oxygenator from the circuit in patients suffering from acute severe postcardiotomy syndrome. In both situations, moribund patients should be treated and followed very carefully, and HTx should not be considered unless the patients show significant recovery from multisystem organ failure. The ECCS system can be used many weeks to improve clinical status of patients. Limited recovery with appropriate t-MCS could encourage surgeons to implant more permanent LVADs to eliminate external lines and pumps, but t-MCS is also an acceptable treatment modality to maximize patient survival, for mobilize patients, to provide better rehabilitation, and to prepare them for transplantation. Temporary ECCS can be created surgically central for LV support or percutaneously peripheral for RV support (**Table 18**).

aa-ECCS or left-to-left ECCS (left heart bypass system) between the LA and aorta (or arterial circulation) is the preferable approach to sustain the end-stage HF patients with irreversible LVF, but preserved right ventricular and pulmonary function. Any of the several types of centrifugal pumps is chosen for long-term left ventricular ECCS (for several weeks), because all of them have similar technologic principles. The inflow cannula is connected to the pump, and the outflow cannula is inserted into the arterial circulation. The inflow cannula is usually inserted in the LA. Left atrial insertion of a malleable venous cannula ranging from 22 to 28F is performed through the left atrial wall just at the interatrial groove, not on the right pulmonary veins like as in left atrial vent insertion, because the drainage cannula is big enough to injury the walls of the pulmonary vein. Similar to standard mitral valve surgery, a limited Sondergaard's plane is dissected approximately 2 cm from the junction of both right pulmonary veins at the left atrial wall. Then, two pledgeted sutures are used to fix the cannula and prevent bleeding. After the removal of the cannula, the dissected tissues support the sutures like a pillow to block bleeding. Left ventricular cannulation is not commonly chosen when the LV is not dilated in postcardiotomy syndrome, or when the left ventricular apex is to be left untouched for permanent LVAD implantation. Two pure-string sutures are placed on the apex, and after the apex is incised. Tubbs dilatators are used to enlarge the vent hole for the venous cannula, and finally the cannula is secured with purse-string sutures. The outflow cannula is inserted into the distal ascending aorta or aortic arch, and a longer ECMO arterial cannula ranging from 15 to 19F is placed. The distal edge of the cannula locates distal to the cerebral arteries in order to avoid cerebral embolic complications. This system is preload-dependent, with an ideal PCWP maintained between 18 and 20 mmHg and CVP between 8 and 12 mmHg, and they should be monitored. Lower dose heparin infusion is necessary (ACT < 200 seconds) to prevent any thromboembolic complication. Absolute contraindications are aortic insufficiency that is any more than mild in degree, or intracardiac septal defects.

vp-ECCS or right-to-right ECCS (right heart bypass system) between the RA (or vena cava through the femoral vein) and pulmonary artery is rarely a preferred approach for isolated RVF because the normally functioning LV can take on most of the right ventricular work. The main indication of right heart bypass systems is acute postimplant RVF after LVAD implantation. Permanent LVADs are increasingly used worldwide, and the most commonly observed cardiac complication is RVF after implantation [75]. Therefore, special attention should be devoted to the evaluation of the right ventricular function when patients are assessed for LVAD implantation. The outflow cannula is inserted either into the RA or in the femoral vein, and the inflow cannula is placed into the pulmonary artery, either directly or through a tubular graft extending outward from the second intercostal space.

TandemHeart is approved for ultrashort-term MCS and as a life-saving approach (as aa-ECCS) in the catheterization lab. Percutaneous t-MCS (TandemHeart) could be a more practical alternative due to not reopening the patient's chest. This system could be also used for vp-ECCS, and as well as for ECCPSs. The device consists of a small hydrodynamic centrifugal pump. It is a very versatile system providing easy deployment and discontinuation. For aa-ECCS, the left atrial cannulation is performed through a femoral vein and delivered across the atrial septum, and positioning is facilitated and confirmed by fluoroscopy or TEE guidance. Outflow is directed into the common femoral or axillary artery. Excellent left atrial decompression is obtained as long as the inflow cannula is approximately positioned. The standard percutaneous transseptal approach includes 21F inflow cannula and 17F arterial outflow cannula. However, larger cannulas could be used during surgically implantation and the size of the inflow cannula regulates pump flow between 4 and 8 L/min. Anticoagulation with low dose heparin to keep ACT below 200 s is sufficient while patients are on support. The atrial septum should be repaired when an LVAD is implanted. The most undesirable aspect of this device is that it requires complete immobilization of the patient.

6.2.2. Intracorporeal circulation support (ICCS)

Percutaneous t-MCSs are developed to unload the LV for better recovery and to maintain adequate CO in nonsurgical patients suffering from acute decompensated HF (acute cardiogenic shock), especially at bedside in the ICU or immediately in the catheterization laboratory [76]. A second application is short-term support of circulation during high-risk percutaneous or surgical cardiac interventions (coronary revascularization, mitral valve repair, etc.) in very sick patients without HF [77, 78]. The third indication could be transaortic left heart unloading in patients suffering from postcardiotomy syndrome treated with peripheral va-ECMO. The fourth clinical usage area is acute decompensation of end-stage HF to improve end-organ functions and to bridge to advanced HF treatments [79].

Impella is an axial-flow pump with three flow options (models 2.5 with flow 2.5 L/min, 5 with flow 5 L/min, CP with flow range between 3 and 4 L/min) and is suggested for t-MCS lasting up to five days [80]. This device is inserted percutaneously into the LV through the aortic valve. Models 2.5 and CP are implemented using 12F or 14F sheaths, respectively; however, model 5 requires surgical cut-down for a 21F catheter. The tip of the device is a pigtail that provides stabilization for the device in the LV. The pigtail connects by a cannula to a pump with a motor housing, intake (below the aortic valve) and output (above the aortic valve) areas, and a pump pressure monitor. The Impella device pumps blood directly from the LV into the proximal aorta, thereby unloading the LV, increasing cardiac output, and improving mean arterial pressure, while reducing LVEDP, myocardial workload, and oxygen consumption [81]. The device is dependent on the left ventricular preload, and hence on satisfactory right ventricular function and adequate CVP (8–12 mmHg).

6.3. Permanent mechanical circulatory support (p-MCS)

Use of long-term MCS devices has grown more rapidly than expected in recent years due to disproportionately low number of donor hearts. Advanced technological improvements in permanent MCS, especially LVADs, increase patients' survival and quality of life. Whereas t-MCS devices are implanted as a short-term rescue treatment to keep patients alive as a bridge to more durable long-term MCS devices, p-MCS devices are implanted as a long-term survival and/or bridging treatment to HTx. In the last years, p-MCS has been accepted as a destination therapy for Stage-D HF, and several types of permanent supportive devices could be used for uni- or biventricular assistance. The indication interval has changed in the recent years and will change even more in the future, so that patients in better condition will be referred to LVAD therapy earlier for the purpose of achieving better outcomes. Patients with relative contraindication such as higher PVR, obesity, or tobacco usage may be switched to eligible transplantation candidates over time. Compared with pulsatile flow devices, continuous flow technology has led to notable improvements in survival and reduction of adverse events, as well as in renal and hepatic function as a result of hemodynamic support.

6.3.1. Ventricular assist device (VAD)

The best technological developments happened in HF therapies, especially surgically. The benefits of different surgical treatment options are depend on underlying causes, and coronary revascularization, valve interventions, or defect repairs can achieve the recovery in early-stage HF. The variety and efficiency of options for surgical intervention decreases with advanced stages, and new surgical strategies must be used to keep patients alive and to provide them with better quality of life. The last step of Stage-D HF surgery is HTx. On the other hand, LVAD implantation has been accepted as a new therapy option for Stage-D HF as destination therapy for older or those who are not otherwise suitable for HTx. Usage of LVAD is promising, will continue to grow, and has become a standard therapy for advanced HF as a bridge to recovery, as a destination therapy, and as a bridge to HTx [82].

A shift from the concept of TAH as heart replacement, toward the development of single-chamber pumps provided the impetus for development of p-MCS devices. In the past decade, ventricular assist device (VAD) systems showed a substantial progress in miniaturization, durability, reliability, and noise emission (**Table 21**) [83]. These devices ensure an adequate and regulable additional blood flow in parallel with the particular ventricle. They can be used either as an isolated LVAD or right ventricular assist device (RVAD) or biventricular VAD. *First generation* VADs were either pneumatically or electrically driven membrane pumps, generating hydrodynamically pulsatile flow with artificial heart valves as the inlet and outlet. *Second generation* VADs with reduced size consists of a rotary pump

Device type	Name	Assist	Mechanism
1st generation extracorporeal pulsalite devices	Thoratec PVAD	BV	Pneumatic pump
	Excore (Berlin Heart)	BV	Pneumatic pump
1st generation intracorporeal pulsatile devices	Thoratec IVAD	BV	Implantable version of Thoratec pVAD
	HeartMate IP, HM VE, XVE	LV	Pneumatic, electric vented pump
	Novacor	LV	Pulsatile
2nd generation continuous axial flow devices	EvaHeart LVAS	LV	thromboresistant coating
	Micromed DeBakey VAD	LV	Axial flow pump
	Jarvik 2000 Flowmarker	LV	Axial flow, intracardiac located small pump
	HeartMate II	LV	Axial flow pump
3rd generation continuous centrifugal pumps	Arrow CorAide	LV	
	ReliantHeart HeartAssist 5	LV	Axial, child version is FDA approved.
	Incore (Berlin Heart)	LV	Magnetically suspended axial flow
	Ventr-assist (Ventracor)	LV	Hydrodynamically suspended rotor
	Duraheart	LV	Magnetically suspended centrifugal pump
	HeartWare HVAD	BV	Miniature hydromagnetically suspended rotor
	HeartMate III	LV	Magnetically suspended centrifugal pump
	HeartWare MVAD	BV	development-stage miniature device
Total artificial heart	Abiocor	-	Pulsatile, motor driven hydraulic system
	CardioWest (Syncardia)	BV	Pulsatile, pneumatic pump, mechanical valves
	Carmat	BV	Pulsatile, pneumatic pump, biological valves

Table 21. The characteristics of long-term devices.

(impeller) with axial-flow design electromagnetically generating continuous flow without prosthetic valves, air vents, and compliance chambers. *Third generation* VADs eliminate bearings by using either hydrodynamic or electromagnetic suspension of an impeller. They employ a radial pump with both suspension mechanisms for contact-free rotation of an impeller that centrifugally generates continuous flow to reduce mechanical wear and trauma to blood cells.

Successful long-term outcomes after LVAD implantation are highly dependent on the timing of surgery (**Table 4**) and HF criteria (**Table 11**). If the LVAD is implanted too late, the outcome may worsen due to end-organ damage caused by prolonged HF (e.g. from poor nutritional status, low serum albumin, impaired liver- and renal function, markers of RHF). Long-term survival is best for patients with INTERMACS level 3 to 5, and worse for patients with INTERMACS level 1. With third generation LVADs (HeartWare or HeartMate III), early and mid-term survival has improved (>85% for 6 months and 1 year) with lower complication rates.

Five-year survival is approximately 60% with HeartWare device [84]. Absolute contraindications for LVAD implantation are obstructive or restrictive CMPs, irreversible lung or liver damage, active infection, aortic regurgitation, and severe RVF. Relative contraindications are increased risk of bleeding, cerebral ischemia, irreversible kidney damage, and prior implantation of mechanical aortic valve prosthesis [85].

6.3.2. *Total artificial heart (TAH)*

Total replacement of the biventricular-failed heart with a total prosthetic heart is unlikely to see widespread usage due to the extraordinarily aggressive nature of the surgery. Several complicating factors can constrain the implantation of these devices: patient characteristics, device size, implantation timing and location, and the need for extensive surgery. Implantation of LVAD alone could aid these patients because of its ability to partially right ventricular functions, and this advantage makes the LVAD approach generally preferred over TAH in patients with biventricular failure. The usage of TAH devices is restricted to the patient's in whom LVAD is not feasible due to infiltrative or restrictive CMPs, cardiac malignancies, nonsurgical postinfarction ventricular septal defect, intractable ventricular arrhythmias, and cardiac graft failure [86]. The device has two artificial ventricles lined with polyurethane, and ejects blood via a four-layer, moving diaphragm driven pneumatically or hydraulically [87]. The ventricle cuffs are sutured to patient's atria and outflow grafts to the aorta and pulmonary artery. The device has four mechanical or biological valves maintaining unidirectional flow. The implanted device is powered by a loud and very heavy external compressor. Thrombosis, thromboembolic events, postoperative bleeding, or infections are significant and relatively frequent complications. The other dissuasive structure can be double drivelines tunneled under the skin, but the drive unit can be set inside the patients' body. Both artificial ventricles alternately eject blood to balance left and right heart CO. There are certain sizing criteria for TAH implantation: chest antero-posterior distance >10 cm, body surface area >1.7 m^2, cardiothoracic ratio >0.5, and LVEDD >66 mm.

7. Cardiac transplantation

Heart transplantation is the only curable and durable treatment option for HF, especially with new immunosuppression therapies, improved clinical management, and pharmaceutical development for refractory or end-stage HF. The most common indication is dilated CMP (50%), and the second is ischemic CMP (35%), but retransplantation ratio has not changed (3%) in the last decade. Once patients are approved for HTx, they are listed according to the medical urgency status and severity of the illness (**Table 22**). Worldwide, a steady decline in heart transplantation has been observed over the last 15 years due to a one-third decrease in the availability of donor organs, while the numbers of patients awaiting heart transplant has doubled. About 15–20% of patients listed for transplantation die before a suitable organ becomes available and more than 30% of patients awaiting HTx require an appropriate MCS to bridge to transplant. The median waiting time for HTx in several countries is

Code status	Description

1A	- Patients in the intensive care unit with inotropic support + mechanical support (ECMO, ECCS) ± respiratorial support + a pulmonary artery catheter for hemodynamic monitoring
	- LVAD patients with
	  - life-threatening ventricular arrhythmia
	  - right ventricular failure
	  - device malfunction/mechanical failure, thromboembolism, infection
	  - RVAD
	- LVAD < 30 days
	- TAH

1B	Patients who are on inotropic support but not meeting 1A criteria Patients have a ventricular assist device longer than 30 days
2	Patients who are waiting at home on medical therapy
7	Patients who are on hold because of an intervening medical illness, making them inappropriate candidates for transplantation

Table 22. Transplantation urgency code status.

approximately 6 to 9 months and depends on several factors, including listed status, body weight, blood group, and differences between recipient and donor. Potential transplant recipients can have decompensated HF requiring high-dose pharmacological treatment and/or MCS, symptomatic Stage-D HF under optimal medical therapy, asymptomatic advanced HF with a peak VO_2 of less than 15 mL/kg/min, or recurrent arrhythmias despite interventions. Maximal VO_2 is the most noninvasively valuable test for better evaluation of potential recipients, and a peak VO_2 of less than 12 mL/kg/min indicates a poor prognosis. The most variable relative contraindication among centers is the age limit; however, transplant guidelines extend the eligibility to 70 years of age, leading individual centers to determine their own age cut-off. Malignancy, impaired lung and renal functions can increase morbidity and impair prognosis. Patients with presenting fixed PAH are associated with high early mortality, and should be considered for combined heart-lung transplantation. Nevertheless, it has been shown that a continuous flow LVAD may help to reduce PVR, so that the patient becomes eligible for subsequent cardiac transplantation. The number of HTx recipients on MCS has doubled and reached 45% of total HTx candidates in the last decade (>50% in 2014): LVAD 85.2%, RVAD 7.2%, TAH 3.1%, and ECMO 2.9% [88]. Patients implanted with a LVAD on status 1A because of device complications or a 30-day elective grace period or on Status 1B will be priority to receive the organ unless they are deemed nontransplantation candidate (Status 7). It has been reported that approximately more than 50% patients were in Status 1A, and one-half patients had LVAD with in Status 1A (70%) or 1B (30%) at the time of HTx; whereas one-third of the patients in Status 1A had LVAD, o which 50% had device complications, and one-fifth patients in Status 1B had LVAD [89].

Early (<30 days) mortality ranges from 5% to 10% usually due to primary graft failure (35.3%), multiple organ failure (21.6%), and infection (14.3%); and 1-, 2-, 3-, 4-, 5-, 10-, and 15-year cumulative survival rates are 82, 78, 75, 72.5, 69.5, 52, and 34.4%, respectively [88]. A decline in 1-year overall survival after HTx from 85 to 76% in the EuroTransplant region has been observed, presumably because of increasing donor age and recipient comorbidity [90]. Early mortality and long-term survival rates in recipients assisted by ECMO are worse than those assisted by LVAD: early mortality is 35 versus 5%, and 1-, 2-, 3-, 4-, and 5-year survival rates are 60 versus 89%, 54 versus 86%, 51.5 versus 82%, 51.5 versus 81%, and 51.5 versus 76%, respectively [88]. The one-year survival after HTx is similar in patients with LVAD (89%), but complicated postimplant recipients have worse, 3-year survival than noncomplicated postimplant recipients (78 versus 85%) [89]. Long-term survival is dependent on several factors, but the availability of the donor hearts from younger male donors with shortest ischemic times is identified as the most significant factor improving long-term survival [91]. The median survival is at least 13.5 years for patients who survive the first year. Survival is lower in patients with valvular cardiomyopathy, congenital heart disease, or following retransplantation, and for those requiring pretransplant MCS. Additionally, patients who are sicker prior to transplant have worse survival outcomes [92]. Cardiac allograft vasculopathy is among the primary causes of death after the first year of HTx, and it is the most important limiting factor in long-term survival, along with neoplasms, with an incidence of 8% in the first year, 30% in 5 years, and 50% in 10 years [93].

Heart transplantation surgery is not a complex procedure, and surgical implantation techniques are the easiest part of HTx. The main problem with HTx is cold ischemic time to donor heart transportation, which should be <4 hours without continuous coronary perfusion or >4 hours with coronary perfusion via special equipment. The ideal cold ischemic time is shorter than 2 hours. Second problem is immunosuppression to prevent organ rejection, which is the main risk factor for graft failure preoperatively and early postoperatively (<1 year), and thereafter cardiac allograft vasculopathy is the major problem after the first posttransplant year. Third problem is increased PVR and it should be managed aggressively, because the unprepared donor RV may be unable to overcome this increased afterload. The standard technique is orthotopic HTx. The great arteries are transected at the sinotubular junctions, whereas the LA is insiced along the atrioventricular groove, leaving left atrial cuff for anastomosis. For biatrial technique, the RA is prepared with the same manner; however, for bicaval technique, both vena cavae are transected at their right atrial junctions. Bicaval anastomosis is a more common approach for implantation of the donor heart rather than biatrial technique [94]. The advantages of bicaval technique are reducing the right atrial size, preserving atrial conduction pathways, decreasing the risk of tricuspid regurgitation, and avoiding permanent pacemaker need [95]. Annuloaortic ectasia with the ascending aorta aneurysm could be managed by the replacement of the recipient ascending aorta during HTx [96].

Author details

Kaan Kırali[1,2]*, Özge Altaş Yerlikhan[1] and Hakan Hançer[1]

*Address all correspondence to: imkbkirali@yahoo.com

1 Department of Cardiac Transplantation and Ventricular Assist Device, Kartal Koşuyolu YIEA Hospital, Istanbul, Turkey

2 Department of Cardiovascular Surgery, Faculty of Medicine, Sakarya University, Sakarya, Turkey

References

[1] Yancy CW, Jessup M, Bozkurt B, Butler J, Casey DE, Drazner MH, Fonarow GC, Geraci SA, Horwich T, et al. 2013 ACCF/AHA guideline for the management of heart failure. JACC 2013;62(16):e147–239.

[2] Metra M, Ponikowski P, Dickstein K, et al. Advanced chronic heart failure: a position statement from the Study Group on Advanced Heart Failure of the Heart Failure Association of the European Society of Cardiology. Eur J Heart Fail 2007;9:684–94.

[3] Hunt SA, Abraham WT, Chin MH, et al. 2009 Focused update incorporated into the ACC/AHA 2005 guidelines for the diagnosis and management of heart failure in adults: a report of the American College of Cardiology Foundation/American Heart Association Task Force on Practice Guidelines. J Am Coll Cardiol 2009;53:e1–90.

[4] Russell SD, Miller LW, Pagani FD. Advanced heart failure: a call to action. Congest Heart Fail 2008;14:316–21.

[5] Kinugawa K. How to treat stage D heart failure? When to implant left ventricular assist devices in the era of continuous flow pumps? Circ J 2011;75(9):2038–2045.

[6] Stevenson LW, Pagani FD, Young JB, Jessup M, Miller L, Kormos RL, Naftel DC, Ulisney K, Desvigne-Nickens P, Kirklin JK. INTERMACS profiles of advanced heart failure: the current picture. J Heart Lung Transplant 2009;28(6):535–541.

[7] Naegele M, Flammer AJ, Enseleit F, Ruschitzka F. Medical therapy of heart failure with reduced ejection fraction: current evidence and new developments. Swiss Med Ekly 2016;146:w14295.

[8] Mentz RJ, Bakris GL, Waeber B, McMurray JJ, Gheorghiade M, Ruilope LM, Maggioni AP, Swedberg K, Piña IL, Fiuzat M, O'Connor CM, Zannad F, Pitt B. The past, present and future of renin-angiotensin aldosterone system inhibition. Int J Cardiol 2013;167 (5):1677–1687.

[9] Gradman AH. Evolving understanding of the renin–angiotensin–aldosterone system: pathophysiology and targets for therapeutic intervention. Am Heart J 2009;157:S1–6.

[10] Jhund PS, McMurray JJV. The neprilysin pathway in heart failure: a review and guide on the use of sacubitril/valsartan. Heart 2016;102(17):1342–1347.

[11] Yancy CW, Jessup M, Bozkurt B, Butler J, Casey DE, Colvin MM, Drazner MH, Filippatos G, Fonarow GC, et al. 2016 ACC/AHA/HFSA focused update on new pharmacological therapy for heart failure: an update of the 2013 ACCF/AHA guideline for the management of heart failure. JACC 2016;68(13):1476–1488.

[12] Braunwald E. The Path to an angiotensin receptor antagonist-neprilysin inhibitor in the treatment of heart failure. J Am Coll Cardiol 2015;65(10):1029–1041.

[13] Ambrosy AP, Butler J, Ahmed A, Vaduganathan M, van Veldhuisen DJ, Colucci WS, Gheorghiade M. The use of digoxin in patients with worsening chronic heart failure: reconsidering an old drug to reduce hospital admissions. J Am Coll Cardiol 2014;63 (18):1823–1832.

[14] Konstantinou DM, karvounis H, Giannakoulas G. Digoxin in heart failure with a reduced ejection fraction: a risk factor or a risk marker? Cardiology 2016;134(3):311–319.

[15] Mentz RJ, Broderick S, Shaw LK, Chiswell K, Fiuzat M, O'Connor CM. Persistent angina pectoris in ischaemic cardiomyopathy: increased rehospitalization and major adverse cardiac events. Eur J Heart Fail 2014;16(8):854–860.

[16] De Luca L, Olivari Z, Farina A, Gonzini L, Lucci D, Di Chiara A, Casella G, Chiarella F, Boccanelli A, Di Pasquale G, De Servi S, Bovenzi FM, Gulizia MM, Savonitto S. Temporal trends in the epidemiology, management, and outcome of patients with cardiogenic shock complicating acute coronary syndromes. J Heart Fail 2015;17(11):1124–1132.

[17] Hoebers LP, Claessen BE, Elias J, Dangas GD, Mehran R, Henriques JP. Meta-analysis on the impact of percutaneous coronary intervention of chronic total occlusions on left ventricular function and clinical outcome. Int J Cardiol 2015;187:90–96.

[18] Cardona M, Martín V, Prat-Gonzalez S, Ortiz JT, Perea RJ, de Caralt TM, Masotti M, Pérez-Villa F, Sabaté M. Benefits of chronic total occlusion coronary percutaneous intervention in patients with heart failure and reduced ejection fraction: insights from a cardiovascular magnetic resonance study. J Cardiovasc Magn reson J 2016;18(1):78.

[19] Petrucci E, Balian V, Bocchieri A. Real-time assessment of myocardial viability in the catheterization laboratory using the intracoronary electrograms recorded by the PTCA guidewire in patients with left ventricular dysfunction: comparison with delayed-enhancement magnetic resonance imaging. JACC Cardiovasc Interv 2014;7(9):988–996.

[20] Jolicœur EM, Dunning A, Castelvecchio S, Dabrowski R, Waclawiw MA, Petrie MC, Stewart R, Jhund PS, Desvigne-Nickens P, Panza JA, Bonow RO, Sun B, San TR, Al-

Khalidi HR, Rouleau JL, Velazquez EJ, Cleland JG. Importance of angina in patients with coronary disease, heart failure, and leftventricular systolic dysfunction: insights from STICH. J Am Card Coll 2015;66(19):2092–2100.

[21] Adachi Y, Sakakura K, Wada H, Funayama H, Umemoto T, Fujita H, Momomura S. Determinants of left ventricular systolic function improvement following coronary artery revascularization in heart failure patients with reduced ejection fraction (HFrEF). Int Heart J 2016 Sep 28;57(5):565–72.

[22] King's College, London. Study of efficacy and safety of percutaneous coronary intervention to improve survival in heart failure (REVIVEDBCIS2). 2015. Available at: http://clinicaltrials. gov/show/NCT01920048. Accessed August 30, 2015.

[23] Wrobel K, Stevens SR, Jones RH, Selzman CH, Lamy A, Beaver TM, Djokovic LT, Wang N, Velazquez EJ, Sopko G, Kron IL, DiMaio JM, Michler RE, Lee KL, Yii M, Leng CY, Zembala M, Rouleau JL, Daly RC, Al-Khalidi HR. Influence of baseline characteristics, operative conduct, and postoperative course on 30-day outcomes of coronary artery bypass grafting among patients with left ventricular dysfunction: results from the Surgical Treatment for Ischemic Heart Failure (STICH) Trial. Circulation 2015;132(8):720–730.

[24] Kırali K, Rabus MB, Yakut N, Toker ME, Erdoğan HB, Balkanay M, Alp M, Yakut C. Early- and long-term comparison of the on- and off-pump bypass surgery in patients with left ventricular dysfunction. Heart Surg Forum 2002;5(2):177–181.

[25] Ömeroğlu SN, Kırali K, Güler M, Toker ME, İpek G, Işık Ö, Yakut C. Midterm angiographic assessment of coronary artery bypass grafting without cardiopulmonary bypass. Ann Thorac Surg 2000;70(3):844–849.

[26] Kırali K, Mansuroğlu D, Kayalar N, Güzelmeriç F, Alp M, Yakut C. Markers of myocardial ischemia in the evaluation of the effect of left anterior descending coronary artery lesion and collateral circulation on myocardial injury in 1-vessel off-pump coronary bypass surgery. Heart Surg Forum 2003;6(3):143–148.

[27] Şişmanoğlu M, Sarıkaya S, Onk OA, Adademir T, Aksoy E, Kırali K. Treatment of left anterior descending coronary artery stenosis: stent or surgery. Asian Cardiovasc Thorac Ann 2013;21(5):528–532.

[28] Uyar İ, Mansuroğlı D, Kırali K, Erentuğ V, Bozbuğa NU, Uysal G, Yakut C. Aspartate and glutamate-enriched cardioplegia in left ventricular dysfunction. J Card Surg 2005;20 (4):337–344.

[29] Nishimura RA, Otto CM, Bonow RO, et al. American College of Cardiology/American Heart Association Task Force on Practice Guidelines. 2014 AHA/ACC guideline for the management of patients with valvular heart disease: a report of the American College of Cardiology/American Heart Association Task Force on Practice Guidelines. J Am Coll Cardiol 2014;63(22):e57–185.

[30] Di Salvo TG, Acker MA, Dec GW, Byrne JG. Mitral valve surgery in advanced heart failure. J Am Coll Cardiol 2010;55(4):271–282.

[31] Ramlawi B, Gammie JS. Mitral valve surgery: current minimally invasive and transcatheter options. Methodist Debakey Cardiovasc J 2016;12(1):20–26.

[32] Taramasso M, Kuwata S, Biefer HRC, Nietlispach F, Maisano F. Percutaneous mitral valve repair and replacement: complementary or competitive techniques? EuroIntervention 2016;12:Y97–101.

[33] Chiam PTL, Ruiz CE. Percutaneous transcatheter mitral valve repair: a classification of the technology. J Am Coll Cardiol Intv 2011;4(1):1–13.

[34] Stewart MH, Jenkins JS. The evolving role of percutaneous mitral valve repair. Ochsner J 2016;16(3):270–276.

[35] Neuss M, Schau T, Schoepp M; Seifert M, Hölschermann F, Meyhöfer J, Butter C. Patient selection criteria and midterm clinical outcome for MitraClip therapy in patients with severe mitral regurgitation and severe congestive heart failure. Eur J Heart Fail 2013;15(7):786–795.

[36] Maisano F, Godino C, Giacomini A, Denti P, Buzzatti N, Arendar I, Colombo A, Alfieri O, La Canna G. Patient selection for MitraClip therapy impaired left ventricular systolic function. Minerva Cardioangiol 2011;59(5):455–71.

[37] De Bonis M, Taramasso M, Lapenna E, Denti P, La Canna G, Buzzatti N, Pappalardo F, Di Giannuario G, Cioni M, Giacominni A, Alfieri O. MitraClip therapy and surgical edge-to-edge repair in patients with severe left ventricular dysfunction and secondary mitral regurgitation: mid-term results of a single-centre experience. Eur J Cardiothorac Surg 2016;49(1):255–262.

[38] Philip F, Athappan G, Tuzcu EM, Svensson LG, Kapadia SR. MitraClip for severe symptomatic mitral regurgitation in patients at high surgical risk: a comprehensive systematic review. Catheter Cardiovasc Interv 2014;84(4):581–590.

[39] Lipiecki J, Siminiak T, Sievert H, Müller-Ehmsen J, Deen H, Wu JC, Schandrin C, Kalmucki P, Hofmann I, Reuter D, Goldberg SL, Haude M. Coronary sinus-based percutaneous annuloplasty as treatment for functional mitral regurgitation: the TITAN II trial. Open Heart 2016 Jul 8;3(2):e000411.

[40] Jerzykowska O, Kalmucki P, Woloszyn M, Smuszkiewicz P, Firek L, Sinimiak T. Echocardiographic evaluation of percutaneous valve repair in patients with mitral regurgitation using the CARILLON™ system. Kardiol Pol 2010;68(1):57–63.

[41] Klein N, Pfeiffer D, Goldenberg S, Klein M. Mitral annuloplasty device implantation for non-surgical treatment of mitral regurgitation: clinical experience after the approval studies. J Invasive Cardiol 2016;28(3):115–120.

[42] Schofer J, Siminiak T, Haude M, Herrman JP, Vainer J, Wu JC, Levy WC, Mauri L, Feldman T, Kwong RY, Kaye DM, Duffy SJ, Tübler T, Degen H, Brandt MC, Van Bibber R, Goldberg S, Reuter DG, Hoppe UC. Percutaneous mitral annuloplasty for functional mitral regurgitation results of the CARILLON Mitral Annuloplasty Device European Union Study. Circulation 2009;120(4):326–333.

[43] Seeburger J, Rinaldi M, Nielsen SL, Salizzoni S, Lange R, Schoenburg M, Alfieri O, Borger MA, Mohr FW, Aidietis A. Off-pump transapical implantation of artificial neo-chordae to correct mitral regurgitation: the TACT trial (Transapical Artificial Chordae Tendinae). J am Coll Cardiol 2014;63(9):914–919.

[44] Jensen H, Jensen MO, Waziri F, Honge JL, Sloth E, Gron MF, Nielsen SL. Transapical neochord implantation: is tension of artificial chordae tendineae dependent on the insertion site? J Thorac Cardiovasc Surg 2014;148(1):138–143.

[45] Ståhlberg M, Lund LH, Zabarovskaja S, Gadler F, Braunschweig F, Linde C. Cardiac resynchronization therapy: a breakthrough in heart failure management. J Intern Med 2012;272(4):330–343.

[46] Lu PJ, Lin PY, Yang CFJ, Hung CH, Chan MY, Hsu TC. Hemodynamic and metabolic effects of para- versus intraaortic counterpulsatile circulation supports. ASAIO J 2001;57(1):19–25.

[47] Kontogiannis CD, Malliaras K, Kapelios CJ, Mason JW, Nanas JN. Continuous internal counterpulsation as a bridge to recovery in acute and chronic heart failure. World J Transplant 2016;6(1):115–124.

[48] Parissis H, Graham V, Lampridis S, Lau M, Hooks G, Mhandu PC. IABP: history-evolution-pathophysiology-indications: what we need to know. J Cardiothorac Surg 2016;11 (1):122.

[49] Kırali K, Güler M, Erentuğ V, Dağlar B, Balkanay M, Akıncı E, Ipek G, Işık Ö, Yakut C. Intraaortic balloon pump: 15-years experience with 765 patients. Turkish J Cardiovasc Thorac Surg 1999;7(5):353–357.

[50] Mizuno M, Sato N, Kajimoto K, Sakata Y, Minami Y, Munakata R, Hagiwara N, Takano T. Intra-aortic balloon counterpulsation for acute decompensated heart failure. Int J Cardiol 2014;176(3):1444–1446.

[51] Kapelios CJ, Terrovitis JV, Siskas P, Kontogiannis C, Repasos E, Nanas JN. ounterpulsation: a concept with a remarkable past, an established present and a challenging future. Int J Cardiol 2015;172(2):318–325.

[52] Pilarczyk K, Boening A, Jacob H, Langebartels G, Markewitz A, Haake N, Heringlake M, Trummer G. Preoperative intra-aortic counterpulsation in high-risk patients undergoing cardiac surgery: a meta-analysis of randomized controlled trials. Eur J Cartiothorac Surg 2016;49(1):5–17.

[53] Sá MP, Ferraz PE, Escobar RR, Martins WN, Nunes EO, Vasconcelos FP, Lima RC. Prophylactic intra-aortic balloon pump in high-risk patients undergoing coronary artery bypass surgery: a meta-analysis of randomized controlled trials. Coron Artery Dis 2012;23(7):480–486.

[54] Norkiene I, Ringaitiene D, Rucinskas K, Samalavicius R, Baublys A, Miniauskas S, Sirvydis V. Intra-aortic balloon counterpulsation in decompensated cardiomyopathy

patients: bridge to transplantation or assist device. Interact Cardiovasc Thorac Surg 2007;6(1):66–70.

[55] Imamura T, Kinugawa K, Nitta D, Hatano M, Kinoshita O, Nawata K, Kyo S, Ono M. Prophylactic intra-aortic balloon pump before ventricular assist device implantation reduces perioperative medical expenses and improves postoperative clinical course in INTERMACS profile 2 patients. Circ J 2015;79(9):1963–1969.

[56] Bezerra CG, Adam EL, Baptista ML, Ciambelli GS, Kopel L, Bernoche C, Lopes LNGD, Macatrao-Costa MF, Falcao BAA, Lage SG. Aortic counterpulsation therapy in patients with advanced heart failure: analysis of the TBRIDGE registry. Arq Bras Cardiol 2016;106 (1):26–32.

[57] Sarıkaya S, Adademir T, Özen Y, Aydın E, Başaran EK, Şahin M, Rabuş MB, Kırali K. Alternative non-femoral accesses for intra-aortic balloon pumping. Perfusion 2015;30 (8):629–635.

[58] Erentuğ V, Bozbuğa N, Izgi A, Eren E, Kırali K, Balkanay M, Ipek G, Akıncı E, Alp M, Yakut C. Traumatic vascular complications due to intra-aortic balloon pump support. Ulus Travma Derg 2004;10(1):28–33.

[59] Legget ME, Peters WS, Milsom FP, et al. Extra-aortic balloon counterpulsation: an intraoperative feasibility study. Circulation 2005;112(Supp l):I26–31.

[60] Solanki P. Aortic counterpulsation: C-pulse and other devices for cardiac support. J Cardiovasc Transl Res 2014;7(3):292–300.

[61] Hayward CS, Peters WS, Merry AF, Ruygrok PN, Jansz P, O'Driscoll G, Larbalestier RI, Smith JA, Ho B, Legget ME, Milsom FP. Chronic extra- aortic balloon counterpulsation: first-in-human pilot study in end-stage heart failure. J Heart Lung Transplant 2010;29 (12):1427–1432.

[62] Nanas JN, Lolas CT, Charitos CE, Nanas SN, Margari ZJ, Agapitos EV, et al. A valveless high stroke volume counterpulsation device restores hemodynamics in patients with congestive heart failure and intractable cardiogenic shock awaiting heart transplantation. J Thorac Cardiovasc Surg 1996;111(1):55–61.

[63] Terrovitis JV, Charitos CE, Tsolakis EJ, Dolou P, Pierrakos CN, Siafakas KX, Nanas JN. Superior performance of a paraaortic counterpulsation device compared to the intraaortic balloon pump. World J Surg 2003;27(12):1311–1316.

[64] Shi C, Zhou DD, Liu G, Zhang L, Meng JJ, Geng Y, Liu XG. The left ventricular assist effect and biocompatibility study of a novel para-aortic counterpulsation device. Eur Rev Med Pharmacol Sci 2015;19(10):1869–1865

[65] Zhang JM, Liu XC, Liu ZG, Zhao L, Yang L, Liu TW,He GW. Comparison of effects of extra-thoracic paraaortic counterpulsation to intraaortic balloon pump on circulatory support in acute heart failure. J Cardiothorac Surg 2015;10:173.

[66] Jeevanandam V, Jayakar D, Anderson AS, Martin S, Piccione W Jr, Heroux AL, Wynne J, Stephenson LW, Hsu J, Freed PS, Kantrowitz A. Circulatory assistance with a permanent implantable IABP: initial human experience. Circulation 2002;106(12 Suppl 1):I183–I188.

[67] Marinakis S, Nanas Y, Sarchosi S, Kontogiannis C, Kapelios C, Tachliabouris G, Charitos C, Nanas J, Malliaras K. A novel implantable counterpulsation assist device, the PULVAD, induced superior left ventricular pressure unloading compared to the intraaortic balloon pump in a bovine model of acute heart failure. Eur J Heart Fail 2015;17(Suppl 1):196.

[68] Giridharan GA, Bartoli CR, Spence PA, Dowling RD, Koenig SC. Counterpulsation with symphony prevents retrograde carotid, aortic, and coronary flows observed with intra-aortic balloon pump support. Artif Organs 2012;36(7):600–606.

[69] Mishra S. Upscaling cardiac assist devices in decompensated heart failure: choice of device and its timing. Indian Heart J 2016;68(Suppl 1):S1–4.

[70] Nair PK, Kormos RL, Teuteberg JJ, Mathier MA, Bermudez CA, Toyoda Y, Dew MA, Simon MA. Pulsatile left ventricular assist device support as a bridge to decision in patients with end-stage heart failure complicated by pulmonary hypertension. J Heart Lung Transplant 2010;29(2):201–208.

[71] Loforte A, Montalto A, Ranocchi F, Monica PLD, Casali G, Lappa A, Contento C, Musumeci F. Levitronix CentriMag third-generation magnetically levitated continuous flow pump as bridge to solution. ASAIO J 2011;57(4):247–253.

[72] Sen A, Larson JS, Kashani KB, Libricz SL, Patel BM, Guru PK, Alwardt CM, Pajaro O, Farmer JC. Mechanical circulatory assist devices: a primer for critical care and emergency physicians. Crit Care 2016;20(1):153.

[73] Gilotra NA, Stevens GR. Temporary mechanical circulatory support: a review of the options, indications, and outcomes. Clin Med Insights Cardiol 2014;8(Suppl 1):75–85.

[74] Shekar K, Mullany DV, Thomson B, Ziegenfuss M, Platts DG, Fraser JF. Extracorporeal life support devices and strategies for management of acute cardiorespiratory failure in adult patients: a comprehensive review. Crit Care 2014;18(3):219.

[75] Meineri M, Van Rensburg AE, Vegas A. Right ventricular failure after LVAD implantation: prevention and treatment. Best Pract Res Clin Anaesthesiol 2012;26(2):217–229.

[76] Ergle K, Parto P, Krim SR. Percutaneous ventricular assist devices: a novel approach in the management of patients with acute cardiogenic shock. Ochsner J 2016;16:243–249.

[77] Palacios IF. Left ventricular assistant device Impella 2.5 usage for patients undergoing high-risk PCI. Catheter Cardiovasc Interv 2012;79(7):1135–1137.

[78] Szafron B, Smoczyński RH, Drobiński D, Pawlak A, Wojciechowski D, Liszka IM, Witkowska A, Kaliciński Z, Gil R, Suwalski P. Impella LD microaxial pump supporting

combined mitral and coronary surgery in a patient with dilated cardiomyopathy. A short bridge to recovery? Kardiochir Torakochirurgia Pol 2015;12(1):56–59.

[79] Bansal A, Bhama JK, Patel R, Desai S, Mandras SA, Patel H, Collins T, Reilly JP, Ventura HO, Parrino E. Using the minimally ınvasive Impella 5.0 via the right subclavian artery cutdown for acute on chronic decompensated heart failure as a bridge to decision. Ochsner J 2016;16(3):210–216

[80] Sarkar K, Kini AS. Percutaneous left ventricular support devices. Cardiol Clin 2010;28 (1):169–184.

[81] Rihal CS, Naidu SS, Givertz MM, Szeto WY, Burke JA, Kapur NK, Kern M, Garratt KN, Goldstein JA, Dimas V, Tu T. Society for Cardiovascular Angiography and Interventions (SCAI); Heart Failure Society of America (HFSA); Society of Thoracic Surgeons (STS); American Heart Association (AHA), and American College of Cardiology (ACC). 2015 SCAI/ACC/HFSA/STS clinical expert consensus statement on the use of percutaneous mechanical circulatory support devices in cardiovascular care: endorsed by the American Heart Association, the Cardiological Society of India, and Sociedad Latinoamericana de Cardiolog´ıa Intervencionista; affirmation of value by the Canadian Association of Interventional Cardiology-Association Canadienne de Cardiologie d'Intervention. J Am Coll Cardiol 2015;65(19):e7–26.

[82] Englert JA 3rd, Davis JA, Krim SR. Mechanical circulatory support for the failing heart: continuous-flow left ventricular assist devices. Ochsner J 2016;16(3):263–269.

[83] Prinzing A, Herold U, Berkefeld A, Krane M, Lange R, Voss B. Left ventricular assist devices: current state and perspectives. J Thorac Dis 2016;8(8):E660–666.

[84] Schmitto JD, Zimpfer D, Fiane AE, Larbalestier R, Tsui S, Jansz P, Simon A, Schueler S, Strueber M. Long-term support of patients receiving a left ventricular assist device for advanced heart failure: a follow-up analysis of the Registry to Evaluate the HeartWare Left Ventricular Assist System. Eur J Cardiothorac Surg 2016;50(5):834–838.

[85] Jurkiewicz BS, Szczurek W, Suliga K, Rempega G, Rajwa P. Mechanical circulatory support in heart failure. Kardiochir Torakochirurgia Pol 2016;13(2):130–134.

[86] Samak M, fatullayev J, Sabashnikov A, Zeriouh M, Rahmanian PB, Choi YH, Wippermann J, Wahlers T, Schmack B, Ruhparwar A, Dohmen PM, Karck M, Popov AF, Simon AR, Weymann A. Past and present of total artificial heart therapy: a success story. Med Sci Monit Basic Res 2015;21:183–190.

[87] Gerosa G, Scuri S, Iop L, Torregrossa G. Present and future perspectives on total artificial hearts. Ann Cardiothorac Surg 2014;3(6):595–602.

[88] Lund LH, Edwards LB, Dipchand AI, Goldfarb S, Kucheryavaya AY, Levvey BJ, Meiser B, Rossano JW, Yusen RD, Stehlik J. The Registry of the International Society for Heart and Lung Transplantation: Thirty-third Adult Heart Transplantation Report—2016; focus theme: primary diagnostic indications for transplant. J Heart Lung Transplan 2016;35 (10):1158–1169.

[89] Trivedi JR, Rajagopal K, Schumer EM, Birks EJ, Lenneman A, Cheng A, Slaughter MS. Differences in Status 1A heart transplantation survival in the continuous flow left ventricular assist device era. Ann Thorac Surg 2016;102:1512–1516.

[90] Smits JM. Actual situation in Eurotransplant regarding high urgent heart transplantation. Eur J Cardiothorac Surg 2012;42(4):609–611.

[91] Sareyyüpoğlu B, Kırali K, Göksedef D, Rabuş MB, Tuncer A, Erentuğ V, Mansuroğlu D, Yakut C. Factors associated with long-term survival following cardiac transplantation. Anatol J Cardiol 2008;8(5):360–366.

[92] Katz JN, Waters SB, Hollis IB, Chang PP. Advanced therapies for end-stage heart failure. Curr Cardiol Rev 2015;11(1):63–72.

[93] Lund LH, Edwards LB, Kucheryavaya AY, Dipchand AI, Benden C, Christie JD, Dobbels F, Kirk R, Rahmel AO, Yusen RD, Stehlik J. The Registry of the International Society for Heart and Lung Transplantation: Thirtieth Official Adult Heart Transplant Report—2013; focus theme: age. J Heart Lung Transplant 2013;32(10):951–964.

[94] Kara İ, Mansuroğlu D, Kırali K, Güler M, Ömeroğlu SN, Eren E, Balkanay M, Alp M, İpek G, Işık Ö, Yakut C. Early-term results of bicaval and biatrial techniques in orthotopic heart transplantation. Turk Gogus Kalp Dama 2012;20(2):223–229.

[95] Kara İ, Kırali K, Yakut C. A comparison of the results of the bicaval and biatrial surgical technique in orthotopic heart transplantation: a review and meta-analysis. Turk Gogus Kalp Dama 2012;20(3):672–681.

[96] Kırali K, Eren E, Mataracı İ, Çevirme D. Combined orthotopic heart transplantation and prophylactic ascending aorta replacement in a Marfan patient. Turk Gogus Kalp Dama 2011;19(3):434–436.

9

Cirrhotic Cardiomyopathy

Coskun Celtik, Nelgin Gerenli,

Halil Haldun Emiroglu and Nimet Cındık

Abstract

Cirrhotic cardiomyopathy (CCMP) is a functional disorder characterized by electrophysiologic disturbances and diastolic and/or systolic dysfunction in patients with chronic liver disease, especially those with ascites and portal hypertension. This disorder is a well-defined entity in adults, but pediatric data are limited. Clinical and laboratory findings are generally latent. The diagnostic criteria are prolonged QT on electrocardiography due to metabolic and extrahepatic causes, in addition to some abnormal echocardiography findings. If echocardiographic findings are normal and only specific prolonged QT is present, this disorder is named as "latent CCMP"; otherwise, it is "manifest CCMP." This disorder is important because it may lead to problems such as cardiac failure and dysrhythmia before or after liver transplantation. Moreover, it may worsen the prognosis.

Keywords: cirrhosis, portal hypertension, cardiomyopathy, prolonged QT, liver

1. Introduction

Portal hypertension (PHT) is an important disorder that increases morbidity and mortality rates. Many hemodynamic changes related to PHT occur in the human body. The majority of these changes are associated with hyperdynamic circulation, which is characterized by elevated heart rate and cardiac output accompanied by vasodilatation in the splanchnic area and systemic circulation and decreased systemic vascular resistance [1–9]. Moreover, disturbances of the autonomic nerve system and baroreceptors and the increased arterial compliance in patients with cirrhosis aggravate the condition [10–12]. Hemodynamic changes that occur in portal hypertension are shown in **Table 1**.

Cardiovascular disorders associated with cirrhosis were first defined in alcoholic cirrhotic patients, in 1953 by Kowalski and Abelmann, but for many years, it was thought that these disorders were associated with chronic alcohol intake [10–12]. Similar disturbances were described in patients with cirrhosis who had hemochromatosis in some later research, but this time the changes were associated with hemochromatosis [13]. Consequently, cirrhotic cardiomyopathy was not known in those years.

Systemic circulation	
Plasma volume ↑ Total blood volume ↑ Noncentral blood volume ↑ Central arterial blood volume → ↓ (↑)	Cardiac flow (→) ↑ Arterial blood tension → ↓ Heart rate ↑ Systemic vascular resistance ↓
Heart	
Left atrial volume ↑ Left ventricle volume → (↓) Right atrial volume → ↑ ↓ Right ventricle volume → ↑ ↓	Right atrial tension → ↑ Right ventricle end-diastole tension → Pulmonary arterial tension → ↑ Pulmonary capillary wedge tension → Left ventricle end-diastole tension →
Pulmonary circulation	
Pulmonary blood flow ↑	Pulmonary vascular resistance ↓ (↑)
Renal circulation	
Renal blood flow ↓	Renal vascular resistance ↑
Cerebral circulation	
Cerebral blood flow ↓ →	
Skin, muscular, and skeletal circulation	
Skin blood flow → ↑	Muscular and skeletal circulation → ↑ ↓

↑, increased; ↓, decreased; →, not changed

Table 1. The hemodynamic changes due to cirrhotic portal hypertension [6].

Caremelo et al. first described cirrhotic cardiomyopathy in 1986. The authors demonstrated cardiac function disturbances due to cirrhosis in an experimental rat model and suggested the cirrhotic cardiomyopathy hypothesis. Their hypothesis was supported by subsequent research, and cardiac disorders due to cirrhosis and portal hypertension were named "cirrhotic cardiomyopathy" in 1989 [1–12, 14]. Although the name "hepatocardiac syndrome" was proposed by some authors instead of "cirrhotic cardiomyopathy," this term was not accepted [14].

2. Definition

Cirrhotic cardiomyopathy (CCMP) is defined as a functional disorder characterized by electrophysiologic disturbances and diastolic and/or systolic dysfunction in patients with cirrhotic PHT. Even though similar hemodynamic changes have been defined in long-term non-cirrhotic PHT, the development of CCMP in such patients has not been reported. Therefore, this term is usually used for patients with cirrhosis [10, 15–18].

3. Pathogenesis

In general, arterial vasodilatation, central hypovolemia, and hyperdynamic circulation which occur as a result of cirrhosis and portal hypertension lead to the development of CCMP together with hepatorenal syndrome and hepatopulmonary syndrome (**Figure 1**) [11, 19–23]. Effects of vasoactive agents are very important in pathogenesis of CCMP. Experimentally, some changes were defined in CCMP, such as downregulation of the density of β receptors, impaired β-adrenergic signaling, alternations of calcium-ion channels, and alternations in plasma membrane fluidity in cardiomyocytes. In addition, the increased serum bile acids, cytokines, and endotoxins have been shown to create negative effects on cardiomyocytes [9–12, 14, 22].

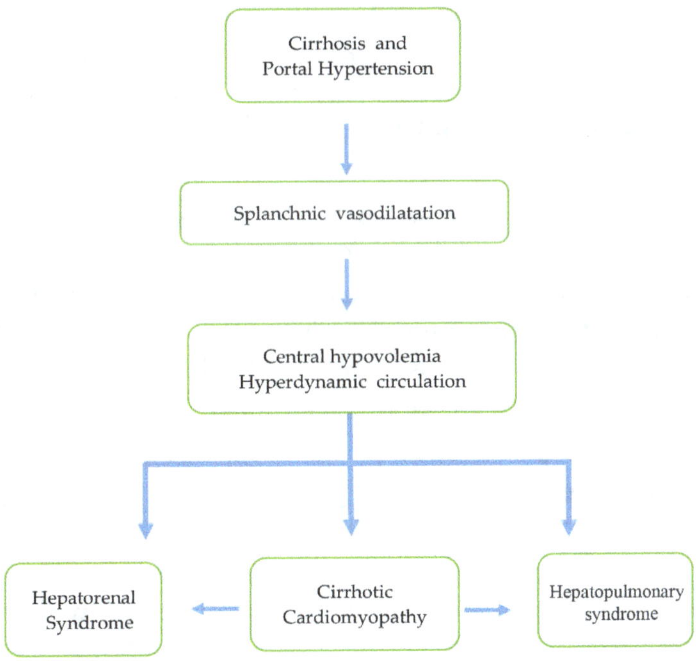

Figure 1. Cirrhotic cardiomyopathy pathogenesis.

Vasoconstrictor substances are high in the early stages of PHT, and vasodilator substances gradually increase in advanced stages; the balance tips in favor of vasodilators and a receptor insensitivity develops against vasoconstrictors [10–12, 19, 23–30]. As a result of these events, arterial vasodilatation results and the severity of PHT increases [19, 23–30].

The splanchnic vasodilatation that develops in PHT is combined with a hyperkinetic systemic circulation, low arterial tension, decreased peripheral resistance, and increased cardiac flow.

Although total plasma volume increases, as a result of collection of blood in the splanchnic area, effective blood capacity cannot be achieved, and central hypovolemia develops. After these changes, activation of the sympathetic nervous system and renin-aldosterone system occurs; vasopressin release from the hypothalamus increases, which results in fluid and salt retention [30–33].

The vasoconstrictor and vasodilator substances in the pathogenesis PHT become effective together. The most important vasoconstrictor substances are norepinephrine, angiotensin II, vasopressin, thromboxane (TX), and leukotrienes. The effects of these substances are related with activation of the sympathetic nervous system and renin-angiotensin-aldosterone system. Researches have shown that portal venous tension can be decreased using alpha-adrenergic antagonists (prazosin), beta-adrenergic antagonists (propranolol), angiotensin-II antagonists, cyclooxygenase isoenzyme blockers, and TX antagonists. Results of these researches support the pathogenesis [22, 29–34].

Endothelin (ET) can show vasoconstrictor or vasodilator effects according to the type. Endothelins are classified as ET-1, ET-2, and ET-3 according to their region in the body. ET-1 is mainly found in endothelial cells, the kidney, and the brain and ET-2 in the small intestine and kidney, and ET-3 is found in the blood. ET-1 and ET-2 create a vasoconstrictor effect, whereas ET-3 has a vasodilator effect. These two opposite effects are associated with the induction of nitric oxide and prostacyclin release. The most potent vasoconstrictor substance in the body is ET-1, and it is reported that this substance is very effective in the development of PHT complications [22, 29–34].

Nitric oxide (NO) is another very potent substance in the pathogenesis of PHT. NO is synthesized from arginine by nitric oxide synthetase (NOS) and causes vasodilatation by increasing cyclic guanosine monophosphate. NO initially increases to compensate against the elevated vasoconstrictor agents in the early stage of PHT, but secondary systemic and splanchnic vasodilatation develops because of excessive NO production. This event is a result of stimulation of NOS by cytokines such as TNF-alpha, which increases in cirrhosis [22, 30–36].

The other important vasodilator substances in the pathogenesis of PHT are carbon monoxide (CO), hydrogen sulfide (H_2S), prostaglandins, glucagon, and endocannabinoids. CO formed through the heme-oxygenase system is a weaker vasodilator agent than NO, but it is important for regulation of intrahepatic vascular tone. H_2S is formed by intestinal microbiota and increases the effects of other vasodilator substances and PHT severity [22, 30–36].

Prostaglandins are endogen vasodilators produced in the endothelium and are important for hyperdynamic circulation. Prostacyclin is produced from the vascular endothelium. It leads to vasodilatation, which increases the level of intracellular cyclic adenosine monophosphate (c-AMP) through the activation of adenylate cyclase. In recent studies, it was shown that indomethacin, a prostacyclin inhibitor, decreased the hyperdynamic circulation and balanced the vasoconstrictor effect [22, 30–36].

Glucagon is a hormone released from the pancreas. Glucagon levels increase as a result of low hepatic clearance and stimulation of pancreatic alpha cells in patients with cirrhosis. Glucagon also has the effect of reducing endogenous vasoconstrictor activity in addition to having a vasodilator effect. The use of somatostatin and synthetic glucagon analogs for PHT therapy has been proposed in some studies; however, these agents may constitute a risk because they can aggravate the splanchnic vasodilatation in advanced stages [22, 30–36].

Endocannabinoids such as anandamide are vasodilator substances that increase in PHT, worsen hepatic microcirculation, and accelerate apoptosis. These substances act by stimulating CB1 and CB2 receptors in the vascular endothelium. It has been reported that endogen cannabinoids show a negative inotropic effect on myocardial contractions, and therefore these substances are very important for the development of cirrhotic cardiomyopathy [39–41]. These negative effects can be blocked by CB-1 receptor antagonists (AM251) [22, 30–40].

4. Clinical finding and diagnosis

Cirrhotic cardiomyopathy (CCMP) represents a condition in which no real cardiac disease is present but a functional cardiac abnormality exists. With time, CCMP progresses to the chronic phase. In a resting state, there is no real disease, but with stress, the cardiac muscle does not contract appropriately and and/or electrophysiologic abnormalities appear [10–12]. There is no exact classification for CCMP and the criteria proposed by Moller et al. are still used (**Table 2**). These data are taken from an adult studies, pediatric data are very limited [41–45]. The most important points from these criteria are (1) at rest, normal, or increased left ventricular contractibility; (2) abnormal systolic contraction or diastolic relaxation with pharmacologic, physiologic, or surgical stress; and (3) cardiac electrical abnormalities [10, 11].

Diagnosis of CCMP in children with cirrhosis is difficult, because invasive methods are life-threatening and noninvasive tests are unreliable for them. In recent years, a new article was published in which CCMP criteria for children were reviewed [45]. According to this literature, a prolonged QT interval on electrocardiography (ECG) is an important finding after all non-liver causes are excluded, and shows latent cardiomyopathy due to cirrhotic changes. If there is the presence of echocardiographic abnormalities, this event is a manifest CCMP [45].

Cirrhotic cardiomyopathy is a latent disease in which there is no abnormality except under stress conditions. In such patients, there is no cardiac disease till end-stage disease. At end stage, infrequent arrhythmias or cardiac insufficiency may be seen. If these findings exist in an early cirrhotic stage, other causes of cardiomyopathy such as infections, metabolic disorders, endocrinopathies, ischemic or toxic causes, and genetic and systemic diseases should be investigated [46].

Cirrhotic cardiomyopathy is more likely dilated cardiomyopathy where some stress factors cause cardiac dysfunction. With stress, the clinical status of the patient deteriorates and decompensation may exist. These stress factors are exercise, infection, positional changes, feeding, paracentesis with high volumes, changes in intravascular volume, the use of vasoconstrictor drugs, transjugular intrahepatic portosystemic shunts (TIPS), or surgical procedures such as minor operations or liver transplantation [10–12]. Exercise tolerance in patients with cirrhosis is abnormal due to cardiac function abnormalities, and this correlates with the patient's Child score [47].

Systolic dysfunction criteria	Supporting criteria
• Inadequate cardiac flow to pharmacologic agents, exercise, blood volume changes • Resting ejection fraction under 55 % **Diastolic dysfunction** • E/A ratio <1,0 (corrected according to age) • Prolonged deceleration time (>200 milliseconds) • Prolonged isovolumetric relaxation time (>80 milliseconds)	• Electrophysiologic abnormalities • Abnormal chronotropic response • Electromechanical uncoupling/dyssynchronism • Prolonged QT intervals • Expended left atrium • Increased myocardial mass • Increased BNP and pro-BNP levels • Increased troponin I levels

BNP, brain natriuretic peptide; E/A ratio, the ratio between the early (E) and late atrial (A) phases of ventricular velocity

Table 2. Diagnostic criteria of cirrhotic cardiomyopathy.

There is a relationship between CCMP and hepatorenal syndrome (HRS), which has been reported in many articles published in recent years, so patients with HRS are at more risk [5, 25, 48].

Cardiac functions in patients with liver cirrhosis are determined by physical examination, ECG, and telecardiography besides of echocardiography. Cardiac functions such as systolic, diastolic, and electromechanical functions should be evaluated in suspected CCMP. ECG is sufficient for determining electrophysiologic function. Systolic and diastolic functions are checked using M-Mod, two- and three-dimensional echocardiocardiography, and spectral and tissue Doppler echocardiocardiography. Cardiac magnetic resonance imaging, radio nuclear angiography, and myocardial perfusion techniques are more advanced methods. Many times, for a diagnosis of CCMP, the findings on ECG and echocardiocardiography are enough.

Firstly, systolic function worsens in the late stage of CCMP. After then, the diastolic functions gradually decay. Diastolic dysfunction is best shown with echocardiographic measurement of the E/A ratio. Deceleration time (DT) and the isovolumetric relaxation time (IVRT) also are used. The E/A ratio results from blood velocity from the left atrium to the left ventricle, the velocity of which during early systole causes the E wave and the same flow causes the A wave during late diastole.

The measurement of E and A waves is expressed as cm/sec and best is done from mitral valve projection. A normal E/A ratio in healthy individuals until the age of 50 years is 1–2 cm/s, but in older people, it decreases below 1 cm/s. An E/A ratio in healthy individuals aged less than 50 years below 1 cm/s shows diastolic dysfunction. However, the restrictive pattern can be observed in advanced stages depending on the severity of the disorder in the patients with CCMP; the E/A ratio may reverse in these cases and may be determined >2 [10, 11, 49] (**Figure 2**).

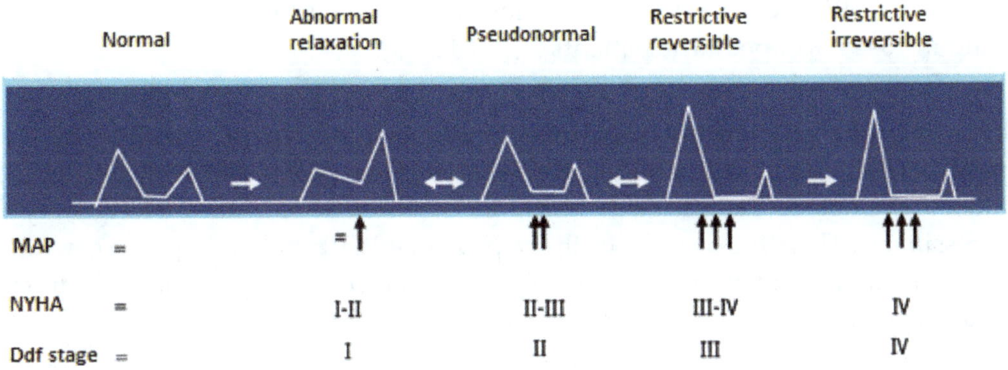

Figure 2. Diastolic dysfunction stages [49]. MAP, mean atrial pressure; NYHA, New York Heart Association; Ddf stage, diastolic dysfunction stage.

Indicator	Normal pattern	Abnormal relaxation (stage I)	Pseudonormal pattern (stage II)	Restrictive pattern (stages III–IV)
E/A	>1	<1	1–2	≥2
DT (msn)	160–210	>220	150–200	<150
IVGT (msn)	70–90	>95	60–95	<60

DT, deceleration time; E/A, transmitral early diastolic flow (E)/transmitral late diastolic flow (atrial) (A) ratio; IVGT, isovolumetric relaxation time (msn).

Table 3. Echocardiographic stages of left ventricular diastolic dysfunction [49].

There are different stages in CCMP. Clinical findings differ according to stage (**Table 3**). The E/A ratio worsens according to the severity of hepatic disease and it is worse in patients with ascites than in patients with non-ascites and normal persons. The E/A ratio improves after paracentesis and this event supports that ascites is the negative effect on cardiac functions [50–53]. There are no publications on these themes in children. There is no definitive normal value for the E/A ratio in children, but in some publications, it is proposed to be between 1.7 and 2.5 cm/s.

Electrical conduction abnormalities and arrhythmias can be seen in the patients according to severity of cirrhosis [8, 9] [54–58]. There are three types of electrophysiologic abnormalities caused by cirrhosis: (1) prolonged QT on ECG, (2) inadequate response to chronotropic stress, and (3) electromagnetic dyssynchronism [10, 11, 14]. The prolonged QT on ECG means a corrected QT interval (QTc) is longer than 0.440 value [41, 54, 55]. Prolonged QT shows abnormal myocardial repolarization as a sign of CCMP [10–12, 56–58]. QT prolongation proportionally increases with cirrhotic stage [56]. Prolonged QT on ECG is frequently seen in patients with CCMP. The rate of determination of prolonged QT is 30–60 % in adults with CCMP and in 18–45 % of pediatric patients [5, 41, 44, 56].

Actually, a prolonged QT interval may cause life-threatening arrhythmias [55], but in many patients with CCMP, despite a prolonged QT interval, no significant clinical problem and arrhythmia are not observed. Cardiac arrhythmias in cirrhotic patients are frequently related to vasopressin use. There is no evidence that a prolonged QT interval in patients with CCMP causes life-threatening arrhythmias. Probably, some compensatory mechanisms in cirrhotic patients prevent the disturbances and the disease occurs latent until end stage.

5. Treatment

Treatment consists of preventing stress exposure in patients with CCMP; rest and oxygen supplementation are important [10, 59]. There is no need for pharmacotherapy when there is no cardiac insufficiency. Drugs have adverse effects and pharmacotherapy response is weak in patients with CCMP. In recent years, aldosterone antagonists, cannabinoid receptor antagonists, and spironolactone have been used, but only the effectiveness of beta-blockers has been proved [10, 35, 59]. Beta-blockers can decrease QT wave duration [10, 32, 33]. Diagnosis of CCMP at an early stage is important. Early diagnosis and proper treatment with cardioprotective agents are important for decreasing complications during and after liver transplantation. There are no exact data on prognosis for liver transplantation in patients with CCMP. Data from the past showed that CCMP worsens in the early period after liver transplantation, and later cardiac functions and cardiac electromechanical dysfunctions improve gradually by supplying hemodynamic stabilization of the patient [10, 59–64]. Liver transplantation can be a definitive treatment for CCMP. New pharmacologic agents are needed to help these patients because many patients do not have the chance to receive a transplant.

Author details

Coskun Celtik[1*], Nelgin Gerenli[1], Halil Haldun Emiroglu[2] and Nimet Cındık[3]

*Address all correspondence to: cceltik2001@yahoo.com

1 Pediatric Gastroenterology, Health Sciences University, Istanbul Umraniye Training and Research Hospital, Istanbul, Turkey

2 Pediatric Gastroenterology, Selcuk University, Faculty of Medicine, Konya, Turkey

3 Pediatric Cardiology, Health Sciences University, Istanbul Umraniye Training and Research Hospital, Istanbul, Turkey

References

[1] Baik SK, Lee SS. Cirrhotic cardiomyopathy; causes and consequences. *J Gastroenterol Hepatol*, 2004;19(7): 185–190, DOI: 10.1111/j.1440-1746.2004.03639.x.

[2] Mandell MS, Tsou MY. Cardiovascular dysfunction in patient with end-stage liver disease. *J Clin Med Assoc*, 2008;71(7): 331-335, DOI: 10.1016/S1726-4901(08)70134-5.

[3] Liu H., Lee S. Cardiopulmonary dysfunction in cirrhosis. *J Gastroenterol Hepatol*, 1999;14(6): 600-608. DOI: 10.1046/j.1440-1746.1999.01920.x.

[4] Lee, R., Glenn T., Lee S. Cardiac dysfunction in cirrhosis. *Best Pract Res Clin Gastroenterol*, 2007;21(1): 125-140. DOI: 10.1016/j.bpg.2006.06.003.

[5] Baik S, Fouad T, Lee S. Cirrhotic cardiomyopathy. *Orphanet J Rare Dis*, 2007;2(15): 1-8. DOI: 10.1186/1750-1172-2-15.

[6] Møller S., Henriksen J. Cardiovascular dysfunction in cirrhosis. Pathophysiological evidence of a cirrhotic cardiomyopathy. *Scand J Gastroenterol*, 2001;36(8): 785-794. DOI: 10.1080/00365520120972.

[7] Liu H., Song D., Lee S. Cirrhotic cardiomyopathy. *Gastroenterol Clin Biol*, 2002;26(10), 842-847. DOI: GCB-10-2002-26-10-0399-8320-101019-ART4.

[8] Blendis L., Wong F. Is there a cirrhotic cardiomyopathy? *Am J Gastroenterol*, 2000;95, 3026-3028. DOI: 10.1111/j.1572-0241.2000.03306.x.

[9] Hamoudi WA, Lee SS. (2006): Cirrhotic cardiomyopathy. *Ann Hepatol*, 5, 132-139. PMID: 17060868.

[10] Wong, F. Cirrhotic cardiomyopathy. *Hepatol Int*, 2009;3(1), 294-304. DOI: 10.1007/s12072-008-9109-7

[11] Moller S, Henricsen JH. Cardiovascular complications of cirrhosis. *Postgrad Med J*, 2009;85,44-54. DOI: 10.1136/gut.2006.112177.

[12] Swanson KL., Krowka MJ. Pulmonary complications associated with portal hypertension. In: Sanyal AJ, Shah VH, editors. Portal Hypertension; Pathobiology, Evaluation, and Treatment, Humana Press, Totowa, 2005. p. 455-468. ISBN 1-58829-386-6

[13] Niederau C, Fischer R, Sonnenberg A, Stremmel W, Trampisch HJ, Strohmeyer G. Survival and causes of death in cirrhotic and in noncirrhotic patients with primary hemochromatosis. *N Engl J Med*. 1985;313(20),1256-1262. DOI: 10.1056/NEJM198511143132004

[14] Milani, A., Zaccaria R., Bombardieri G., Gasbarrini A., Pola P. (2007): Cirrhotic cardiomyopathy. *Dig Liver Dis*, 39, 507-515. DOI: 10.1016/j.dld.2006.12.014

[15] Sarin SK, Wadhawan M. Noncirrhotic portal hypertension and portal vein thrombosis. In: Sanyal AJ, Shah VH, editors. Portal Hypertension: Pathobiology,

Evaluation, and Treatment, Humana Press Inc, Totowa, NJ. 2005. p. 411-432. ISBN 1-58829-386-6

[16] Molina, E. & K. Reddy. Noncirrhotic portal hypertension. *Clin Liver Dis*, 2001;5(3), 769-87. PMID: 11565140

[17] Sarin SK, Kapoor D. Non-cirrhotic portal fibrosis; current concept and management. *J Gastroenterol Hepatol*, 2002;17(5), 526-534. DOI: 10.1046/j.1440-1746.2002.02764.x

[18] Okudaira M., Ohbu M., Okuda K. Idiopathic portal hypertension and its pathology. *Semin Liver Dis*, 2002;22(1), 59-72. DOI: 10.1055/s-2002-23207.

[19] Gunaratnam NT., Su GL. Pathogenesis and consequences of portal hypertension. In: Rose S, editor. Gastrointestinal and Hepatobiliary Pathophysiology, Fence Creek Publising, Madison, 1998. p.315-326. ISBN: 1-59377-181-9

[20] Møller S, Henriksen JH. Cardiovascular complications of cirrhosis. *Gut*, 2008;57(2), 268-278. DOI: 10.1136/gut.2006.112177

[21] Ma Z., Lee S. Cirrhotic cardiomyopathy; getting to the heart of the matter. *Hepatology*, 1996;24 (2), 451-459. DOI: 10.1002/hep.510240226

[22] Wiese S, Hove JD, Bendtsen F, Moller S. Cirrhotic cardiomyopathy: pathogenesis and clinical relevance. *Nat Rev Gastroenterol Hepatol*,2014; 11(3), 177–186. DOI: 10.1038/nrgastro.2013.210

[23] Treiber G., Csepregi A., Malfertheiner P. The pathophysiology of portal hypertension. *Dig Dis*, 2005;23 (1), 6-10. DOI: 10.1159/000084720

[24] Bosch J., Garcia-Pagàn JC. Complications of cirrhosis. I. Portal hypertension. *J Hepatol*, 2000; 32 (Suppl. 1), 141-156.DOI: 10.1016/S0168-8278(00)80422-5

[25] Liu H., Gaskari S., Lee S. Cardiac and vascular changes in cirrhosis; pathogenic mechanisms. *World J Gastroenterol*, 2006;12(6), 837-42. DOI: 10.3748/WJG.v12.i6.837

[26] Niederberger M., Schrier R. Pathogenesis of sodium and water retention in liver disease. *Prog Liver Dis*, 1992;10, 329-47. PMID:1296235

[27] Møller S., Bendtsen F., Henriksen J. Splanchnic and systemic hemodynamic derangement in decompensated cirrhosis. *Can J Gastroenterol*, 2001;15 (2), 94-106. DOI: 10.1155/2001/603012

[28] Møller S, Bendtsen F, Henriksen JH. Vasoactive substances in the circulatory dysfunction of cirrhosis. *Scand J Clin Lab Invest*, 2001;61, 421-429. DOI: 10.1080/00365510152567059

[29] Møller S., Henriksen JH. Cirrhotic cardiomyopathy: a pathophysiological review of circulatory dysfunction in liver disease. *Heart*, 2002;87 (1), 9-15. DOI:10.1136/heart.87.1.9

[30] Pinzani M, Vizzutti F. Anatomy and vascular biology of the cells in the portal circulation. In: Sanyal AJ., Shah VH, editors. Portal Hypertension; Pathobiology,

Evaluation, and Treatment, Humana Press Inc, Totowa, NJ, 2005, p.15-35. ISBN 1-58829-386-6

[31] Ryckman FC., Alonso MH., Tiao G. Causes and management of portal hypertension in the pediatric population. In: Sanyal AJ, Shah VH, editors. Portal Hypertension; Pathobiology, Evaluation, and Treatment, Humana Press Inc, Totowa, 2005, p.383-410. ISBN 1-58829-386-6

[32] Zambruni A, Trevisani F, Di Micoli A, Savelli F, Berzigotti A, Bracci E, Caraceni P, Domenicali M, Felline P, Zoli M, Bernardi M. Effect of chronic beta-blockade on QT interval in patients with liver cirrhosis. *J Hepatol*, 2008;48(3), 415–421. DOI: 10.1016/j.jhep.2007.11.012

[33] Henriksen JH, Bendtsen F, Hansen EF, Møller S. Acute nonselective beta-adrenergic blockade reduces prolonged frequency adjusted Q-T interval (QTc) in patients with cirrhosis. *J Hepatol*, 2004;40(2), 239–246. DOI: 10.1016/j.jhep.2003.10.026

[34] Pozzi M., Ratti L., Guidi C., Milanese M., Mancia G. Potential therapeutic targets in cirrhotic cardiomyopathy. *Cardiovasc Hematol Disord Drug Targets*, 2007;7(1), 21-26. DOI: 10.2174/187152907780059074

[35] Mallat A., Lotersztajn S. Cannabinoid receptors as therapeutic targets in the management of liver diseases. *Drug News Perspect*, 2008;21(7), 363-8. DOI: 10.1358/dnp.2008.21.7.1255306

[36] Liu H., Ma Z., Lee S. (2000): Contribution of nitric oxide to the pathogenesis of cirrhotic cardiomyopathy in bile duct-ligated rats. *Gastroenterology*, 118(5), 937-944. DOI: 10.1016/S0016-5085(00)70180-6

[37] Pacher P., Bátkai S., Kunos G. Cirrhotic cardiomyopathy: an endocannabinoid connection? *Br J Pharmacol*, 2005;146 (3), 313-314. DOI: 10.1038/sj.bjp.0706332

[38] Caraceni P., Domenicali M, Giannone F, Bernardi M. The role of the endocannabinoid system in liver diseases. *Best Pract Res Clin Endocrinol Metab*, 2009;23 (1), 65-77. DOI: 10.1016/j.beem.2008.10.009

[39] Gaskari, S., Liu H., Moezi L., Li Y., Baik S., Lee S. Role of endocannabinoids in the pathogenesis of cirrhotic cardiomyopathy in bile duct-ligated rats. *Br J Pharmacol*, 2005;146 (3), 315-23. DOI: 10.1038/sj.bjp.0706331

[40] Bátkai S., Pacher P. Endocannabinoids and cardiac contractile function; pathophysiological implications. *Pharmacol Res*, 2009;60 (2), 99-106. DOI: 10.1016/j.phrs.2009.04.003

[41] Fishberger SB., Pittman NS., Rossi AF. Prolongation of the QT interval in children with liver failure. *Clin Cardiol*, 1999; 22(10), 658-60. DOI: 10.1002/clc.4960221013

[42] Ozçay F, Tokel K, Varan B, Saygılı A. Cardiac evaluation of pediatric liver transplantation candidates. *Transplant Proc*, 2002; 34 (6), 2150-2152. DOI: 10.1016/S0041-1345(02)02886-5

[43] Polat, T., Urganci N., Yalcin Y., Akdeniz C., Zeybek C., Erdem A., Celebi A. Evaluation of cardiac function by tissue Doppler imaging in children with chronic hepatitis. *J Pediatr Gastroenterol Nutr*, 2006;43 (2), 222-227. DOI: 10.1097/01.mpg.0000228101.12326.6f

[44] Arikan C., Kilic M., Tumgor G., Levent E., Yuksekkaya HA., Yagci RV., Aydogdu S. (2009): Impact of liver transplantation on rate-corrected QT interval and myocardial function in children with chronic liver disease. *Pediatr Transplant*, 13(3), 300-306. DOI: 10.1111/j.1399-3046.2008.00909.x

[45] Celtik C, Durmaz O, Oner N, Yavuz T, Gökce S, Aydogan A, Nisli K, Emiroglu HH, Ömeroglu RE, Söküсü S. Investigation of cardiomyopathy in children with cirrhotic and noncirrhotic portal hypertension. *J Pediatr Gastroenterol Nutr*. 2015;60(2):177-81. DOI: 10.1097/MPG.0000000000000580.

[46] Towbin JA, Lowe AM, Colan SD, Sleeper LA, Orav EJ, Clunie S, Messere J, Cox GF, Lurie PR, Hsu D, Canter C, Wilkinson JD, Lipshultz SE. Incidence, causes, and outcomes of dilated cardiomyopathy in children. *JAMA*, 2006;296 (15), 1867-1876. DOI: 10.1001/jama.296.15.1867

[47] Terziyski K, Andonov V, Marinov B and Kostianev S. Exercise performance and ventilatory efficiency in patients with mild and moderate liver cirrhosis. *Clin Exp Pharmacol Physiol*, 2007;35 (2),135-140. DOI: 10.1111/j.1440-1681.2007.04751.x

[48] Ruiz-del-Arbol L, Monescillo A, Arocena C, Valer P, Ginès P, Moreira V, Milicua JM, Jiménez W, Arroyo V. Circulatory function and hepatorenal syndrome in cirrhosis. *Hepatology*, 2005;42(2), 439-447. DOI: 10.1002/hep.20766

[49] Tezel T. Evaluation of Diastolic Functions [Diyastolik fonksiyonların değerlendirilmesi]. Nobel Tıp Kitapevleri, Istanbul, Turkey 2007. p. 1-216. ISBN: 97897524205725.

[50] Moller S, Henriksen JH. Cardiopulmonary complications in chronic liver disease. *World J Gastroenterol*, 2006;12(4), 526-538. DOI: 10.3748/WJG.v12.i4.526

[51] Pozzi M, Carugo S, Boari G, Pecci V, de Ceglia S, Maggiolini S, Bolla GB, Roffi L, Failla M, Grassi G, Giannattasio C, Mancia G. Evidence of functional and structural cardiac abnormalities in cirrhotic patients with and without ascites. *Hepatology*, 1997;26(5), 1131-1137. DOI: 10.1002/hep.510260507

[52] Valeriano, V., S. Funaro, R. Lionetti, O. Riggio, G. Pulcinelli, P. Fiore, A. Masini, S. De Castro & M. Merli. Modification of cardiac function in cirrhotic patients with and without ascites. *Am J Gastroenterol*, 2000;95 (11), 3200-3205. DOI: 10.1111/j.1572-0241.2000.03252.x

[53] Finucci G, Desideri A, Sacerdoti D, Bolognesi M, Merkel C, Angeli P, Gatta A. Left ventricular diastolic function in liver cirrhosis. *Scand J Gastroenterol*, 1996;31(3), 279-284. DOI: 10.3109/00365529609004879

[54] Miller MD, Porter CJ, Ackerman MJ. Diagnostic accuracy of screening electrocardiograms in long QT syndrome I. *Pediatrics*, 2001;108 (1), 8–12. DOI: 10.1542/peds.108.1.8

[55] Friedman MJ, Mull CC, Sharieff GQ, Tsarouhas N. Prolonged QT syndrome in children: uncommon but potentially fatal entity. *J Emerg Med*, 2003;24(2), 173–179. DOI: 10.1016/S0736-4679(02)00721-7

[56] Bernardi M, Calandra S, Colantoni A, Trevisani F, Raimondo ML, Sica G, Schepis F, Mandini M, Simoni P, Contin M, Raimondo G. Q-T interval prolongation in cirrhosis: prevalence, relationship with severity, and etiology of the disease and possible pathogenetic factors. *Hepatology*, 1998;27(1), 28-34. DOI: 10.1002/hep.510270106

[57] Bal JS, Thuluvath PJ. Prolongation of QTc interval: relationship with etiology and severity of liver disease, mortality and liver transplantation. *Liver Int*, 2003;23, 243-248. DOI: 10.1034/j.1600-0676.2003.00833.x

[58] Zambruni A, Trevisani F, Caraceni P, Bernardi M. Cardiac electrophysiological abnormalities in patients with cirrhosis. *J Hepatol*, 2006;44(5), 994-1002. DOI: 10.1016/j.jhep.2005.10.034

[59] Gaskari S., Honar H., Lee S. Therapy insight; cirrhotic cardiomyopathy. *Nat Clin Pract Gastroenterol Hepatol*, 2006;3(6), 329-37. DOI: 10.1038/ncpgasthep0498

[60] Acosta F, De La Morena G, Villegas M, Sansano T, Reche M, Beltran R, Roques V, Contreras RF, Robles R, Bueno FS, Ramirez P, Parrilla P. Evaluation of cardiac function before and after liver transplantation. *Transplant Proc*, 1999;31(6), 2369–2370. DOI: 10.1016/S0041-1345(99)00383-8

[61] Myers R., Lee S. Cirrhotic cardiomyopathy and liver transplantation. *Liver Transpl*, 2000;6(4 suppl 1), 44-52. DOI: 10.1002/lt.500060510

[62] Liu H., Lee S. What happens to cirrhotic cardiomyopathy after liver transplantation? *Hepatology*, 2005; 42(5), 1203-5. DOI: 10.1002/hep.20911

[63] Torregrosa M, Aguadé S, Dos L, Segura R, Gónzalez A, Evangelista A, Castell J, Margarit C, Esteban R, Guardia J, Genescà J. Cardiac alterations in cirrhosis; reversibility after liver transplantation, *J Hepatol*, 2005;42(1), 68-74. DOI: 10.1016/j.jhep.2004.09.008

[64] Mandell MS, Lindenfeld J, Tsou MY, Zimmerman M. (2008): Cardiac evaluation of liver transplant candidates. *World J Gastroenterol*, 14(22), 3445-3451. DOI: 10.3748/wjg.14.3445

10

Infective Cardiomyopathy

Agnieszka Pawlak and Robert Julian Gil

Abstract

Both the infectious agent and development of inflammatory response to infection can lead to irreversible myocardial injury, which affects the outcome of short- and long-term prognosis. In the case of the rapid elimination of the infectious agent and rapid withholding of inflammatory process, changes in myocardium are small. If the immune response does not lead to complete elimination of infectious agent or inflammation progresses after removing the virus, chronic myocardial damage may develop. Persistence of the virus in myocardium, postinfectious immune reaction, autoimmunity, and primary cardiac damage may result in the development of progressive ventricular dysfunction, development of cardiac arrhythmias, and exacerbation of symptom. Because of the long-term consequences, it is important to diagnose infective cardiomyopathy (IC) quickly and start appropriate treatment. However, IC is still a diagnostic challenge. Infective cardiomyopathy is often underdiagnosed because of a wide spectrum of factors causing IC—infectious, toxic, immunologic, and various clinical manifestation. The processes responsible for the development of IC take place at the cellular level, which is why it is important to make the diagnosis not only based on clinical symptoms and imaging but also to confirm it with the use of histological, immunohistochemical, and molecular studies. Progress in the diagnosis and understanding of the pathomechanisms responsible for the development of IC contributed to the use of new therapeutic options. Immunosuppresive and immunomodulative treatment is still of limited use. However, in some cases of viral IC, targeted antiviral treatment can be added to the standard heart failure therapy resulting in improvement of the prognosis.

Keywords: myocarditis, infective heart disease, cardiomyoapthy

1. Introduction

Infective cardiomyopathy (IC) is a disease in which structural or/and functional heart disorders are observed as a result of present or past infection caused by various infectious agents. In the course of infective cardiomyopathy heart chambers' dilatation, heart walls' hypertrophy or restriction may occur. A relation between infection and chronic heart disease was suggested as early as 1806, when Corvisart described a cardiac inflammatory disorder that could result in progressive abnormalities of cardiac function after all the evidence of the infective agent had disappeared [1]. Because of a variety of symptoms, diagnosis of IC can be difficult [2]. Usually, the suspicion of IC is based on clinical presentation and results of noninvasive diagnostic imaging, e.g., cardiac magnetic resonance (CMR) [3]. Although endomyocardial biopsy (EMB), which can confirm myocarditis, is the gold standard in making a diagnosis, it is not often performed because of its still low availability and invasiveness. However, the interest in this method is increasing lately [2]. Although more is known about the pathophysiology of the disease, many questions remain unanswered. There are many controversions about the treatment of patients with IC, especially the most common form—viral myocarditis [3].

2. Etiology

Infective cardiomyopathy may be caused by many etiological factors including viruses, bacteria, rickettsiae, fungi, protozoa, and parasites. However, the spectrum of pathogens has changed over the decades and also varies geographically as, for example, *Trypanosoma cruzi* [4]. Moreover, it can result from noninfectious agents, such as allergic agents, autoimmunity, toxins, and drugs [5]. Etiological factors that could cause IC are presented in **Table 1**.

The most popular infective agents	
Viruses	RNA viruses: Coxsackieviruses A and B, Echoviruses, Polioviruses, Influenza A and B viruses, Respiratory Syncytial virus, Mumps virus, Measles virus, Rubella virus, Hepatitis C virus, Dengue virus, Yellow fever virus, Chikungunya virus, Junin virus, Lassa fever virus, Rabies virus, Human immunodeficiency virus-1 DNA viruses: Adenoviruses, Parvovirus B19, Cytomegalovirus, Human herpesvirus-6, Epstein-Barrvirus, Varicella-zoster virus, Herpes Simplex virus, Variola virus, Vaccinia virus
Bacteria	Staphylococcus, Streptococcus, Pneumococcus, Meningococcus, Gonococcus, Salmonella, Corynebacterium diphtheria, Haemophilus influenzae, Mycobacterium tuberculosis, Mycoplasma pneumoniae, Brucella
Spirochete	Borrelia, Leptospira
Fungi	Aspergillus, Actinomyces, Blastomyces, Candida, Coccidioides, Cryptococcus, Histoplasma, Mucormyces, Nocardia, Sporothrix
Protozoa	*Trypanosoma cruzi, Toxoplasma gondii*, Entamoeba, Leishmania
Parasites	*Trichella spiralis, Echinococcus granulosus, Taenia solium*
Rickettsiae	*Coxiella burnetti, R. rickettsii, R. tsutsugamuschi*

Source: Modified based on Ref. [2].

Table 1. Etiological factors of IC.

3. Diagnostic criteria for myocarditis

The common feature of the diseases that are called "infective heart disease" is myocarditis. Changes in myocarditis affect cardiomyocytes, interstitial tissue, vessels, and sometimes also the pericardium. Recent prospective postmortem data have implicated myocarditis in sudden cardiac death of young adults at rates of 8.6–12% [6, 7]. Furthermore, it has been identified as a cause of dilated cardiomyopathy in 9% of the cases in a large prospective series [8]. The diagnosis of myocarditis is based on histological, immunohistochemical, and immunological criteria [4].

3.1. Histological criteria—Dallas criteria

The Dallas criteria were proposed in 1986 and provided a histopathological categorization by which the diagnosis of myocarditis could be established (**Figure 1A** and **B**). Dallas criteria (acute) myocarditis requires an inflammatory infiltrate and necrosis or damage of adjacent muscle cells not characteristic of an ischemic event. Borderline myocarditis requires a less intense inflammatory infiltrate and no light microscopic evidence of myocyte destruction [8]. The histological diagnosis of myocarditis includes different forms, classified according to the type of inflammatory cell infiltrate: lymphocytic, eosinophilic, polymorphic, giant cell myocarditis, and cardiac sarcoidosis. The distribution and diffusion of the cellular infiltrate can be focal, confluent or diffuse, and mild, moderate or severe.

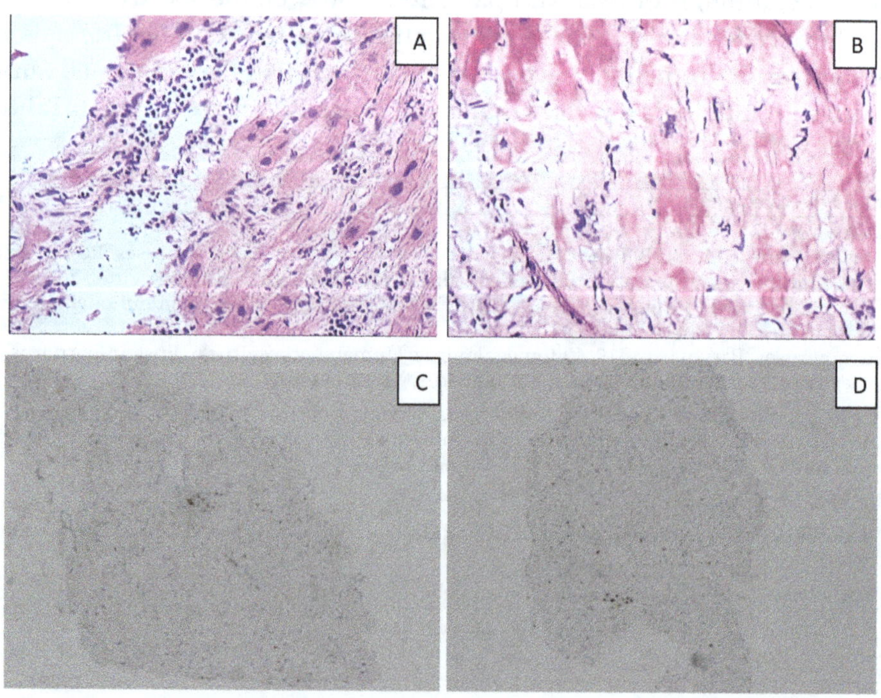

Figure 1. H&E staining, presenting numerous leucocytes (A) and myocyte damage (B). Immunohistochemical staining of leucocytes (C) and CD 3 lymphocytes (D).

3.2. Immunohistochemical criteria

The Dallas criteria are limited by the high interobserver variability in interpreting biopsy specimens (in particular with regard to borderline myocarditis) and because noncellular inflammatory processes cannot be detected (**Figure 1C** and **D**). Thus, immunohistochemistry is gaining further acceptance in the diagnosis of myocarditis. Monoclonal antibodies allow the characterization and localization of the mononuclear cell infiltrates: for example, CD3 for T cells, CD68 for activated macrophages, and human leukocyte antigen to assess HLA class II cells. With the use of these immunohistological methods, the number of EMB revealing myocarditis markedly increased. According to the World Health Organization/International Society and Federation of Cardiology Task Force on the Definition and Classification of Cardiomyopathies, EMB is considered to be inflamed by immunohistochemical detection of the inflammatory infiltration defined as: ≥14 leukocytes/mm^2 (including ≥7 cells/mm^2 CD3 + and <4 monocytes/mm^2) [2].

Histological assessment and immunohistochemical analysis of biopsy allow the determination of the presence of inflammation in the heart. In order to determine the etiology, many frequent further studies, including polymerase chain reaction (PCR), should be performed.

4. Viral infection

Viral infections are considered to be the main cause of myocarditis in Europe and in USA [9]. It is characterized by myocardial infiltrate with lymphocytes as the predominant inflammatory cell (Lymphocytic (viral) myocarditis).

With the use of molecular techniques, EMB detection of viruses is possible in up to 67% of idiopathic left ventricular dysfunction [10]. In the past, enteroviruses (especially Coxsackie B3 and B4 viruses) were assigned to be the most common cause of IC; currently, the most common viral etiologic agents are parvovirus B19 (PVB19), human herpes virus 6 (HHV 6), and cytomegalovirus (CMV) [5, 11]. It is still not known to what extent the presence of PVB19 and HHV 6 genome detected in the myocardium affects the development of inflammation. The following forms of viral heart diseases are currently distinguished based on histopathological, genetic examinations, and results of echocardiography [12] (**Table 2**):

The form of heart disease caused by viruses	Dallas and immunohistochemical criteria	The presence of viral genome	Dilatation of left ventricle
Viral myocarditis with normal ejection fraction	+	+	–
Viral inflammatory cardiomyopathy	+	+	+
Viral heart disease	–	+	+/–

Table 2. The forms of heart diseases caused by viruses based on histopathology, genetics, and echocardiography.

4.1. Parvovirus B19 (PVB19)

Parvovirus B19 is the most common cause of viral cardiomyopathy, both in the presence or without inflammation. The presence of PVB19 has been observed significantly more often in patients with an ejection fraction (EF) <45% as compared to those of EF >45% [13]. The incidence of PVB19 DNA in patients with IC ranges from 11 to 56% according to various sources [14, 15]. The presence of PVB19 is associated with a gradual deterioration of EF, and the elimination of PVB19 from the myocardium resulted in significant improvement of ventricular function [16].

4.2. Human hepresvirus 6 (HHV 6)

The genome of HHV 6, beside PVB19, is now one of the most frequently detected pathogens during EMB [11]. Its presence has been found in 11–18% of the EMB samples [10, 15]. What is important, HHV6 can activate infections caused by other viruses such Epstein-Barr virus (EBV) and PVB19 [17]. Both HHV 6, as well as PVB19, may remain in the infected cells for a lifetime. Therefore, such a high proportion of the genome of the virus among patients with IC can be associated with the previous infection [16, 18].

4.3. Enterovirus

Presently, in patients with IC, enteroviral etiology is less frequently observed. According to various sources, enteroviral RNA is found in from 3 to 53% of the patients with IC. The majority of data is related to Coxsackievirus B3 [16]. It is important that, in contrast to PVB19 and HHV 6, up to 50% of the patients with IC, spontaneous elimination of the enteroviral genome was observed, with improvement of EF [11].

4.4. Adenovirus

Currently, adenovirus genome is less often detected during EMB, and it is present in <2% of the biopsies [19]. Patients with adenovirusal IC often present only mild clinical symptoms, and the results of biopsies analyzed according to the Dallas criteria show mild myocarditis or borderline fulfill these criteria. Therefore, adenoviral IC may have been underestimated for many years [20].

4.5. Cytomegalovirus (CMV)

Currently, CMV DNA is rarely detected during EMB performed in patients with myocardial dysfunction, and the incidence is <3%; according to some sources, it is even <1% [10, 19]. However, there are reports that the presence of CMV in immunocompetent patients is associated with the occurrence of severe IC [21].

4.6. Influenza virus

The influenza virus may also be responsible for the development of IC [20, 22, 23], and its genome is detected in <1% of the patients with IC [16]. Infectious cardiomyopathy caused by influenza A virus may result in the development of heart failure, leading to patient's death or myocardial fibrosis with conduction defects [24]. The relationship between pandemic influenza virus H1N1 and IC is studied carefully. There are cases of acute IC observed mainly among young patients, which are associated with this pandemia [25].

4.7. The human immunodeficiency virus (HIV)

HIV infection may also cause myocarditis [26]. In a postmortem study of HIV-infected patients, myocarditis was established by histopathological criteria in more than 60% of the cases. However, most of these patients have discrete and unspecific abnormalities on the echocardiogram. In general, patients with advanced forms of HIV infection are subject to a high risk of developing overt myocarditis. HIV-related myocarditis is associated with a poor prognosis, especially in patients with low CD4+ counts (<400 cells/mm^3). These high-risk patients may develop severe left ventricular dysfunction, which could progress to advanced forms of dilated cardiomyopathy [27]. Nevertheless, it is still discussed, whether the virus, the medical treatment, or the coinfections are responsible for the development of IC in patients infected with HIV [27]. It is known that the IC related to HIV infection is characterized by a significantly worse prognosis than other lymphocytic IC [28].

4.8. Hepatitis C virus (HCV)

Hepatitis C virus is also considered to be the cause of IC [29]. HCV-associated cardiomyopathy can develop in genetically susceptible patients infected with HCV in whom viral, immunologic, and apotoptic mechanisms may lead to myocardial damage [30]. Hepatitis C virus not only causes myocarditis but also involved in the development of dilated cardiomyopathy, hypertrophic cardiomyopathy, and arrhythmogenic right ventricular cardiomyopathy. Frequency of HCV genomes in cardiomyopathies varies in different regions or in different populations. Major histocompatibility complex class II (MHC class II) genes may be important in the susceptibility to HCV infection and may play a role in the development of different types of cardiomyopathies. It has been suggested that interferon (IFN) treatment can be useful among these patients [31].

4.9. Clinical presentation

Infectious cardiomyopathy can be completely asymptomatic [32]. The most common symptoms in patients with IC are shortness of breath, chest pain, and palpitations [33]. Often cardiac manifestation of IC is preceded by flu-like symptoms, infection of upper respiratory tract, or gastrointestinal tract. Fatigue, shortness of breath, palpitations, and atypical chest pain may occur a few days or weeks later [34]. Infectious cardiomyopathy can result in development of fulminant heart failure [27]. Since some of the symptoms may resemble acute coronary syndrome (ACS), it is important to exclude coronary artery disease (CAD) and other diseases of the cardiovascular system [2]. In some cases, the only abnormality may be nonspecific ECG changes [27]. In some cases, laboratory examinations can reveal increased troponin I, troponin T, and CK-MB, suggesting myocardial injury [35]. There are four main clinical presentations of IC (**Table 3**):

1. Acute coronary syndrome-like
2. New onset or worsening heart failure in the absence of CAD and known causes of heart failure
3. Chronic heart failure in the absence of CAD and known causes of heart failure
4. "Life-threatening condition," in the absence of CAD and known causes of heart failure comprising

Clinical presentation of patients with inflammatory heart disease
1. **Acute coronary syndrome-like:**
a. Acute chest pain frequently presents after respiratory or gastrointestinal infection, associated with severe or recurrent symptoms in the absence of angiographic evidence of coronary artery disease (CAD)
b. ST/T wave changes: ST-segment elevation or depression or T-wave inversion
c. With or without normal global or regional LV and/or RV dysfunction on echocardiography or CMR
d. With or without increased TnT/TnI that may have a time course similar to acute myocardial infarction or a prolonged and sustained release over several weeks or months
2. **New onset or worsening heart failure in the absence of CAD and known causes of heart failure**
a. New onset or progressive heart failure over 2 weeks to 3 months
b. Impaired systolic LV and/or RV function, with or without dilated LV and/or RV on echocardiography or CMR
c. Symptoms possibly started after a respiratory or a gastrointestinal infection, or in the peripartum period
d. Nonspecific ECG signs, sometimes bundle branch block and/or ventricular arrhythmias and/or AV-block
3. **Chronic heart failure in the absence of CAD and known causes of heart failure (see Point 2 above)**
a. Heart failure symptoms (with recurrent exacerbations) of >3 months duration
b. Fatigue, palpitation, dyspnoea, atypical chest pain, and arrhythmia in ambulant patient
c. Impaired systolic LV and/or RV function on echocardiography or CMR suggestive of dilated cardiomyopathy or nonischemic cardiomyopathy
d. Nonspecific ECG signs, sometimes bundle branch block and/or ventricular arrhythmias and/or AV-block
4. **Life-threatening condition', in the absence of CAD and known causes of heart failure comprising:**
a. Life-threatening arrhythmias and aborted sudden death
b. Cardiogenic shock
c. Severely impaired LV function
Source: Based on Ref. [2].

Table 3. Clinical presentation of patients with IC.

4.10. Clinicopathological classification

Myocarditis is classified based on clinical presentation, function of left ventricle, Dallas, and immunohistochemical criteria on the following:

1. Fulminant myocarditis: a presentation with acute illness following a distinct viral syndrome. Histological study reveals multiple foci of active myocarditis. Clinical presentation consists of severe cardiovascular compromise and ventricular dysfunction. This subgroup typically either resolves spontaneously or results in death. Fulminant myocarditis in most of the cases is associated with giant cell or eosinophilic myocarditis.

2. Acute myocarditis: a presentation with insidious onset of illness and evidence of established ventricular dysfunction. This subgroup may progress to dilated cardiomyopathy.

3. Chronic active myocarditis: a presentation with insidious onset of illness with clinical and histological relapses with development of left ventricular dysfunction and associated chronic recurrent inflammatory changes.

4. Chronic persistent myocarditis: a presentation with insidious onset of illness characterized by a persistent histological infiltrate frequently with foci of myocyte necrosis. Clinically, no ventricular dysfunction is present despite other cardiovascular symptoms (such as palpitations or chest pain).

4.11. Diagnostics

4.11.1. Electrocardiography

Infectious cardiomyopathy is often accompanied by nonspecific ECG abnormalities (**Table 4**). The spectrum changes to include ST-segment elevation in multiple leads, generally concave, rarely of another shape. The occurrence of atrioventricular block with a mild enlargement of the left ventricle may suggest, e.g., IC in the course of Lyme disease, sarcoidosis, or multicellular myocarditis [2]. Infectious cardiomyopathy may also result in "idiopathic" atrial or ventricular arrhythmias and reduction of PQ-segment [36, 37]. The sensitivity of the ECG is determined at 47%, but the specificity remains unknown [38]. It is recommended to perform standard 12-lead ECG in patients with suspected IC [2].

4.11.2. Echocardiography

Abnormalities revealed by echocardiography are not specific for IC. However, the use of this method allows assessing both size of heart chambers and systolic and diastolic function of the heart in patients with IC. This modality can be also useful to exclude other causes of heart failure, such as valvular heart disease or other forms of cardiomyopathy (hypertrophic cardiomyopathy and restrictive cardiomyopathy). Performing echocardiography plays especially important role in the assessment of the heart before EMB—to exclude pericardial effusion and blood clots in the cavities of the heart, which are present in 25% of the patients [39]. Moreover, evaluation of echocardiographic parameters has a prognostic significance. Patients with fulminant IC often have normal heart chamber dimensions but increased intraventricular septum thickness due to myocardial edema, while in patients with acute IC dilatation of left ventricle and normal wall thickness can be observed [3, 40].

Diagnostic criteria	
1.	**ECG/Holter/stress test features**
	Newly abnormal 12 lead ECG and/or Holter and/or stress testing, any of the following: I to III degree atrioventricular block, or bundle branch block, ST/T wave change (ST or non-ST elevation, T-wave inversion), sinus arrest, ventricular tachycardia or fibrillation ora systole, atriafl fibrillation, reduced R-wave height, intraventricular conduction delay (widened QRS complex), abnormal Q-waves, low voltage, frequent premature beats, supraventricular tachycardia
2.	**Myocardiocytolysis markers**
	Elevated TnT/TnI
3.	**Functional and structural abnormalities on cardiac imaging (echo/angio/CMR)** new, otherwise unexplained LV and/or RV structure and function abnormality (including incidental finding in apparently asymptomatic subjects): regional wall motion nor global systolic or diastolic function abnormality, with or without ventricular dilatation, with or without increased wall thickness, with or without pericardial effusion, with or without endocavitary thrombi
4.	**Tissue characterization by CMR**
	Edema and/or LGE of classical myocarditic pattern
Source: Based on Ref. [2].	

Table 4. Diagnostic criteria for clinically suspected IC.

4.11.3. Cardiac magnetic resonance

The use of CMR, with the assessment of early gadolinium enhancement (EGE) and late gadolinium enhancement (LGE), is helpful in making the diagnosis of IC. In T1-weighted imaging with the assessment of the EGE, hyperintense areas show myocardium with a good blood supply, whereas the assessment of the LGE in T1-weighted imaging allows to visualize the irreversible myocardial injury resulting from the replacement of myocardial cells by fibrous tissue. Scarring and fibrosis delineated with the use of LGE-imaging are hyperechoic in contrast to normal myocardial cells. Scarring that is present in IC is located intramuscularly (typically in chronic IC) or subepicardially (typically in acute IC) [41, 42]. Location of changes in CMR enables to distinguish postinfarction scars that occur subendocardially or include the entire myocardial wall from the scars arising in the course of IC. Moreover, T2-weighted imaging reveals swelling of the myocardium, which is visible as a hyperechogenic area. Swelling in IC can be both global and regional. It reflects the reversible myocardial damage and can be present even in the absence of LGE hyperintense regions [43–45]. Cardiac magnetic resonance should be performed before EMB in hemodynamically stable patients, however, in life-threatening conditions, in which urgent EMB is necessary, it is not recommended to perform CMR [2, 46, 47].

4.11.4. Endomyocardial biopsy

Endomyocardial biopsy plays an important role in the diagnosis of IC. Nevertheless, in many clinics, it is performed only in the minority of cases with a suspicion of IC or it is not performed at all because of the lack of technical possibilities and experience. However, it is important to perform EMB in every patient with suspected IC, as it is considered to be a gold standard in making the diagnosis of IC [2, 3]. In the absence of feasibility of performing EMB, patients should be transferred to a reference center [48]. According to Schultheiss, EMB should be performed in every case of suspected IC [18, 49]. This method indicates the etiology and shows type of inflammatory infiltration, which may have therapeutic implications. According to Dallas criteria, making the diagnosis of acute IC is possible based on the presence of both lymphocyte infiltration and necrosis of cardiomyocytes, while borderline IC is defined as the presence of lympocyte infiltration and lack of cardiomyocytes necrosis [48]. Together with molecular, histological, and immunohistochemical examinations, EMB allows to start antiviral treatment or immunosuppression safely. Performing EMB has the highest level of recommendation in life-threatening IC [46]. Endomyocardial biopsy should be performed early in the course of a disease and at least 8–10 specimens should be taken, each 1–2 mm in size. Samples should be examined histologically, by immunohistochemistry and for the presence of viral genome with the use of PCR (to exclude systemic infection, it is recommended to perform viral PCR in peripheral blood at the same time). If it is necessary, EMB should be repeated to monitor the effectiveness of therapy or when sampling error is suspected [2].

When ≥1 clinical presentation and ≥1 diagnostic criteria are fulfilled, coronary angiography and EMB are recommended [2].

Infectious cardiomyopathy is clinically suspected if ≥1 clinical presentation and ≥1 diagnostic criteria from different categories are fulfilled, in the absence of:

1. angiographically detectable coronary artery disease (coronary stenosis ≥50%);
2. known pre-existing cardiovascular disease or extra-cardiac causes that could explain the syndrome (e.g., valve disease, congenital heart disease, and hyperthyroidism). Suspicion is higher with higher number of fulfilled criteria. If the patient is asymptomatic, ≥2 diagnostic criteria should be met [2].

4.12. Treatment

In the course of IC, cardiomyocytes can be damaged by direct action of the virus, antiviral immune response, or autoimmune response. As the cardiomyocytes are not able to regenerate, improvement of myocardial function mainly depends on the tissue not affected by inflammation. Response to treatment depends on the cause of IC, and the severity of irreversible changes presents at the moment of initiation of treatment [50].

Regardless of the cause, IC therapy is based on optimal treatment of heart failure, consisting of the use of angiotensin-converting enzyme inhibitors (ACE-I)/angiotensin receptor blockers and/or β-adrenergic receptors' blockers [50–52]. There are well-known studies that confirm the efficacy of captopril and candesartan in the treatment of IC [53, 54]. Moreover, it is recommended to reduce physical activity during the acute phase of IC and for at least 6 months after the onset of the disease [2].

4.12.1. *Antiviral treatment*

Elimination of viruses from cardiomyocytes results in decrease in the symptoms reported by patients. It also affects the heart chambers' size, improvement of left ventricle EF, and reduction of long-term mortality [55]. Targeted antiviral therapy can result in total elimination of the virus genome or, even if the total elimination is not possible, it can reduce the patient's complaints. Nevertheless, starting antiviral therapy is useful only early in the course of a disease, when irreversible changes in the myocardium are not present yet [18]. In IC caused by HHV6, valacyclovir, and ganciclovir can be used [2, 17]. The use of interferon β (IFN-β) enables to eliminate adenoviruses and enteroviruses from cardiomyocytes, improving also heart efficiency. After treatment with IFN-β, increase in EF, decrease in left ventricle, reduction in heart failure symptoms, and smaller inflammatory infiltration were observed [55]. Interferon β can also be used in IC caused by PVB19—it can reduce the symptoms and endothelium dysfunction, but it has only little effect on the elimination of the virus [18]. Mechanism of beneficial clinical effects of IFN-β is not known, but IFN-β inhibits reactivation of PVB19 and improves the viability of endothelial cells [56]. Similarly, in IC caused by HHV6, treatment with IFN-β or ganciclovir does not eliminate virus from the myocardial tissue, probably because of viral genome integration with host genome. However, in patients with HHV6, IC ganciclovir reduces clinical symptoms [57].

4.12.2. *Immunosuppression*

Immunosuppression with the use of steroids, combination of steroids and azathioprine or azathioprine, cyclosporine A, and steroids is safe and efficient in IC. So far there is no data about the use of other Immunosuppresive drugs in IC treatment [2]. It is important to perform EMB before initiation of immunosuppression to exclude viral etiology of IC [50] because only patients with autoimmune IC benefit from immunosuppression [58–60]. Therefore, immunosuppression should be considered in patients with autoimmune IC, including giant-cell IC, sarcoidosis, IC in the course of "noncardiac" autoimmune diseases, who do not have contraindications for immunosuppressive therapy. The use of steroids is indicated in sarcoidosis with ventricle dysfunction and/or arrhythmia and in some cases of noninfectious eozynophilic IC or toxic IC with concomitant heart failure and/or arrhythmia. When there are no contraindications, immunosuppression can be also considered in noninfectious lymphocytic IC resistant to standard therapy [2].

4.12.3. *High-dose intravenous immunoglobulin*

No consensus exists on the benefits of high-dose intravenous immunoglobulin (IVIG) in the treatment of IC. Although there are reports confirming the improvement of left ventricular function and increase in one-year survival after application of IVIG [61], finally, it appears that this therapy has no positive effect on progression of IC [62, 63].

4.12.4. Immunoabsorption

The aim of immunoabsorption (IA) is elimination of antibodies against cardiac proteins [64]. There are some studies that confirm the efficacy of IA in dilated cardiomyopathy [65, 66]. However, multicenter, randomized studies are needed to recommend the use of IA in a standard IC therapy.

5. Other heart infections

5.1. Bacterial infections

Bacterial myocarditis with no coexisting endocarditis occurs extremely rarely. Usually, it results from massive bacteremia. *Staphylococcus aureus* is a main etiological factor of bacterial myocarditis. Nevertheless, cardiac involvement in the course of streptococcal (*Streptococcus pyogenes, Streptococcus viridans,* and *Streptococcus pneumoniae*) infection has also been reported [67]. Moreover, myocarditis can be the result of meningococcal disease or can be associated with *Salmonella, Listeria monocytogens,* or *Corynebacterium diphtheria* infection [68–71]. Bacteremia, neutropenia, myocardial infarction, osteomyelitis, and recent surgical procedures are considered to be main risk factors of bacterial myocarditis. Clinical manifestation is dominated by sepsis and heart failure symptoms. To confirm the diagnosis, EMB should be performed, revealing active myocarditis with evidence of bacterial invasion or positive tissue cultures [71]. Standard treatment consists of aggressive targeted antibiotic or antitoxin therapy and appropriate hemodynamic support, in conjunction with the treatment of arrhythmias or mechanical complications [67, 71].

5.1.1. Mycobacterium tuberculosis

Myocarditis is a very rare manifestation of Mycobacterium tuberculosis infection. There are three types of myocardial tuberculosis: nodular tubercles of the myocardium, miliary tubercles of the myocardium, and diffuse infiltrative type associated with tuberculous pericarditis. Cardiac tissue can be infected by hematogenous spread, by retrograde lymphatic spread from mediastinal lymph nodes, or directly from the pericardium. In patients with strong suspicion of cardiac tuberculosis, EMB should be performed to confirm the diagnosis. Clinical presentation is nonspecific and varies from ventricular fibrillation, long QT syndrome, congestive heart failure, and DCM to sudden cardiac arrest. However, a large number of patients are completely asymptomatic. Anti-tuberculosis therapy is usually effective; nevertheless, it does not reduce the risk of sudden cardiac death [72].

5.1.2. Tropheryma whipplei

Whipple's disease is a rare bacterial infection, which usually affects the intestinal tract, but it can also involve other organs. Cardiac manifestation of Whipple's disease occurs in 35–60% of affected patients. Infectious endocarditis with negative blood cultures develops most commonly. Whipple's disease may also present as adhesive pericarditis and myocardial fibrosis.

Lymphocytic myocarditis is unusual [73]. Cardiac involvement can clinically present as congestive heart failure, conduction disturbances, arrhythmias, or even sudden cardiac death. It is suggested that chronic damage of heart tissue is the cause of death in most patients with end-stage disease [74]. It is difficult to confirm the diagnosis due to lack of culture and serodiagnostic methods. Currently, detection of *T. whipplei* by PCR is a method of choice to establish the diagnosis. Treatment of Whipple's disease remains empirical; it is suggested to use trimethoprim-sulfamethoxazole for at least 1 year, or, alternatively, an initial parenteral therapy with penicillin and streptomycin for 2 weeks followed by trimethoprim-sulfamethoxazole [73].

5.2. Spirochetes infection

5.2.1. *Borrelia burgdorferi*

Lyme disease (LD) that is caused by *B. burgdorferi* mostly affects skin, heart, nervous system, and joints [75]. The most common cardiac manifestation of LD is conduction and rhythm disturbances, most frequent of which is atrioventricular (AV) block [76]. However, LD can also result in myocarditis and new-onset of DCM, especially in the highly endemic area for LD [75, 77]. Serological diagnosis in patients with cardiac LD may be difficult, as IgM and IgG antibodies against *B. burgdorferi* are frequently negative at first; a measurable level of antibodies develops in the course of illness [75, 78]. Therefore, EMB can be extremely useful in making the diagnosis of DCM caused by *B. burgdorferi* [79]. Early treatment with antibiotic therapy (intravenous infusion of ceftriaxone) is effective and leads to significant improvement of left ventricle ejection fraction and reduction of heart failure symptoms [75, 79].

5.3. Fungal infection

Fungal myocarditis mostly develops in immunodeficient patients. Therefore, it can be often clinically latent or masked by neurological or respiratory symptoms [80].

5.3.1. *Aspergillus*

Cardiac aspergillosis occurs mostly in patients with immunodeficiency or immunosuppression such as cancer, hematological conditions, or organ transplantation. Cardiac involvement occurs as a result of disseminated *Aspergillus* infection. It is associated with high mortality rate because of late diagnosis and lack of effective therapy [81].

5.3.2. *Blastomycosis*

Cardiac blastomycosis can develop by an extension from pericardial blastomycosis, by a direct involvement of heart tissue, or by a lymphatic spread from mediastinal lymph nodes. It often leads to congestive heart failure, with heart chambers dilatation and little hypertrophy. The course of cardiac blastomycosis has many common features with cardiac tuberculosis [82].

5.3.3. *Candida*

Candida is not pathogenic among immunocompetent hosts, but it can cause severe mucosal or systemic infections in immunocompromised patients [83]. *Candida* invasion of the heart significantly complicates the clinical course of candidiasis and aggravates the patients' condition and should be suspected when arrhythmia, conduction disturbance, or other QRS changes occur in patients with systemic candidiasis [84].

5.4. Protozoan infections

5.4.1. *Trypanosoma cruzi*

Chagas disease is caused by infection with *Trypanosoma cruzi* (*T. cruzi*), which is transmitted by blood-sucking insects and small mammals. The disease is common in the southwestern part of United States, Mexico, Central, and South America [85]. Contact of skin lesions, mucosal surfaces, or the conjunctiva with parasites present in the feces of the insect leads to infection with *T. cruzi*. In nonendemic countries, transmission is also possible with blood transfusion, organ transplantation, and vertical way [86].

In the course of Chagas disease, two phases are described: an acute and a chronic phase [86]. Patients with acute Chagas disease may present nonspecific symptoms or may be completely asymptomatic. Moreover, acute myocarditis, pericardial effusion, and/or meningoencephalitis can develop in the course of acute infection [85]. In a majority of patients, the acute phase subsides spontaneously after 6–8 weeks [86]. In some of the infected patients, chronic Chagas disease develops with the symptoms from various organs [86]. Patients with chronic Chagas cardiomyopathy can present symptoms of heart failure, arrhythmias, thromboembolism (systemic or pulmonary), and chest pain [85]. Echocardiography may be useful in making the diagnosis of Chagas cardiomyopathy. It can reveal a specific pattern of segmental myocardial contractility disturbance, mainly localized in left ventricular apex and inferior-posterior wall [86]. Moreover, in chronic Chagas cardiomyopathy, echocardiography can show severe dilation of the heart chambers characteristic aneurysm localized in left ventricle's apex [85]. Because of high risk of thromboembolism, transesophageal echocardiography can be helpful to identify cardiac sources of emboli and make decision about anticoagulant treatment [85]. Histopathologically myocytolysis, reparative fibrosis, and lymphocytic infiltrates are seen in Chagas heart disease. Treatment of Chagas cardiac disease consists of targeted antiparasitic therapy and treatment of heart failure, arrhythmias, and thromboembolism [86]. Benznidazole is used to eliminate *T.cruzi*, and it is effective in acute phase [87]. Its efficacy in chronic Chagas cardiomyopathy is still discussed [86]. Angiotensin-converting enzyme (ACE) inhibitors and β-blockers can be useful in heart failure therapy. Because of high risk of thromboembolism in Chagas disease, oral anticoagulation should be considered with cardioembolic risk score for Chagas disease patients [86]. Moreover, pacemaker or ICD implantation may contribute to a better survival in some patients with Chagas disease [87].

5.5. Parasitic infection

5.5.1. Echinococcus

Echinococcal infection develops after consumption of *Echinococcus* eggs from the feces of infected dogs or other canids. In the majority of cases, the disease involves liver or lungs. Heart is a very rare localization of parasites' cysts. Cardiac echinococcosis can manifest as arrhythmias, myocardial infarction, cardiac tamponade, pulmonary hypertension syncope, purulent pericarditis, and sudden cardiac death. The basis of making the diagnosis is serology and echocardiography, which can visualize myocardial or pericardial hydatid cysts. Moreover, with the use of CMR or computed tomography calcification of the cysts' walls can be shown. Albendazole or mebendazole should be used in the treatment of cardiac echonococcosis [88].

6. Autoimmune heart inflammation

6.1. Sarcoidosis

Sarcoidosis is a systemic granulomatous disease of unknown etiology. Clinical presentation varies among patients. Sarcoidosis mostly affects skin, lymph nodes, lungs, eyes, and the central nervous system. Cardiac involvement will occur in approximately 5% of the patients with sarcoidosis [89] and varies in the different geographical regions, but it is considered to be very important prognostic factor in this disease [90]. Cardiac sarcoidosis may present as acute heart failure, ventricular arrhythmia, conduction disturbances, and even sudden death. Diagnosing cardiac sarcoidosis may be difficult due to nonspecific ECG and echocardiographic findings; therefore, it is often misdiagnosed. To make the right diagnosis, the use of endomyocardial biopsy (EMB), cardiac magnetic resonance (CMR), and ^{18}F-fluorodeoxyglucose positron emission tomography may be helpful. Patients should be treated with corticosteroids, which help to control inflammatory process, prevent fibrosis, and protect from aggravation of the cardiac function [90].

6.2. Churg-Strauss syndrome (CSS)

Churg-Strauss syndrome is a rare systemic vasculitis, which affects small- and medium-sized blood vessels, characterized by eosinophil infiltration of various tissues [91]. It occurs in patients with an atopic condition, typically with a previous history of asthma or allergy disease. According to different sources, cardiac involvement is reported in 16–92% of patients with CCS [92, 93]. Cardiac changes are associated with a poor prognosis and high mortality, if not treated [94]. There are two types of cardiac involvement in CSS: vasculitis-related ischemia and eosinophilic infiltration of the myocardium. It can present as myocarditis with cardiomyopathy, pericarditis, pericardial effusion, heart failure, ventricular and supraventricular arrhythmias, and sudden cardiac death. Heart involvement is characterized by both fibrosis and an active inflammatory process. Changes visualized by CMR with LGE are mostly localized in the subendocardium [95, 96], but they can be also observed in the intramural and subepicardial myocardium [97]. Patients with cardiac involvement are mainly antineutrophil cytoplasmic antibody (ANCA)-negative. The management of myocarditis in the course of CCS includes standard therapy for heart failure and immunosuppressive treatment with steroids [98]. Initiation of treatment allows recovery of cardiac function and reduces symptoms of heart failure.

6.3. Systemic lupus erythematosus (SLE)

Systemic lupus erythematosus is an autoimmune disease, which usually occurs in young females. Cardiac involvement is one of the most frequent manifestations. All anatomical heart structures can be affected: pericardium, myocardium, valves, coronary arteries, and the conduction system [99]. Several autoantibodies, such as anti-phospholipid antibodies (aPL), anti-SSA/Ro antibodies, and anti-endothelial cells antibodies, can contribute to heart damage in SLE. Antibodies-SSA/Ro and anti-SSB/La antigens are responsible for the development of heart conduction disorders in the neonatal lupus syndrome.

Myocarditis is uncommon, but a serious presentation of SLE can lead to cardiac dysfunction or even sudden cardiac death [100]. Early diagnosis of lupus myocarditis is important because of the likely progression to arrhythmias, conduction disturbances, dilated cardiomyopathy, and heart failure [101]. Echocardiography is a sensitive and specific technique, and it can not only reveal global hypokinesis in patients with SLE myocarditis but also visualize other cardiac manifestations of SLE, such as pericarditis or valvular lesions [102]. In patients with lupus myocarditis, CMR shows LGE; however, it cannot differentiate these changes from myocarditis of other etiology [99]. Therefore, endomyocardial biopsy is the gold standard technique in making the diagnosis [103]. Histopathological examination shows immune complexes with mononuclear cell infiltrates, perivascular inflammation or arteriopathy, and necrosis of the cardiomyocytes [99]. Early treatment with high-dose steroids is the basis of lupus myocarditis therapy. In severe cases, intravenous pulse corticosteroid should be administered. Azathioprine, cyclophosphamide, or intravenous immunoglobulines (IVIG) may be useful [103].

7. Summary

Both the infectious agent and development of inflammatory response to infection can lead to irreversible myocardial injury, which affects the outcome of short- and long-term prognosis. In the case of the rapid elimination of the infectious agent and rapid withholding of inflammatory process, changes in myocardium are small. If the immune response does not lead to complete elimination of infectious agent or inflammation progresses after removing the virus, chronic myocardial damage may develop. Persistence of the virus in myocardium, postinfectious immune reaction, autoimmunity, and primary cardiac damage may result in the development of progressive ventricular dysfunction, development of cardiac arrhythmias, and exacerbation of symptoms [18]. Because of long-term consequences, it is important to diagnose IC quickly and start appropriate treatment. However, IC is still diagnostic challenge.

Infective cardiomyopathy is often underdiagnosed because of a wide spectrum of factors causing IC—infectious, toxic, immunologic, and various clinical manifestations [3]. The processes responsible for the development of IC take place at the cellular level, which is why it is important to make the diagnosis not only based on clinical symptoms and imaging but also to confirm it with the use of histological, immunohistochemical, and molecular studies [18]. Progress in the diagnosis and understanding of the pathomechanisms responsible for the development of IC contributed to the use of new therapeutic options. Immunosuppresive and immunomodulative treatment is still of limited use [2]. However, in some cases of viral IC, targeted antiviral treatment can be added to standard heart failure therapy resulting in improvement of the prognosis [18].

Acknowledgements

Funding provided by The National Science Center (Poland) grant No. 2014/13/B/NZ4/03832.

Author details

Agnieszka Pawlak[1,2*] and Robert Julian Gil[1,2]

*Address all correspondence to: a.pawlak1@wp.pl

1 Mossakowski Medical Research Centre, Polish Academy of Sciences, Warsaw, Poland

2 Central Clinical Hospital of the Ministry of Interior, Department of Invasive Cardiology, Warsaw, Poland

References

[1] Kearney, M.T., et al., Viral myocarditis and dilated cardiomyopathy: mechanisms, manifestations, and management. Postgrad Med J, 2001. 77(903): pp. 4–10.

[2] Caforio, A.L., et al., Current state of knowledge on aetiology, diagnosis, management, and therapy of myocarditis: a position statement of the European Society of Cardiology Working Group on Myocardial and Pericardial Diseases. Eur Heart J, 2013. 34(33): pp. 2636–48, 48a–d.

[3] Kindermann, I., et al., Update on myocarditis. J Am Coll Cardiol, 2012. 59(9): pp. 779–92.

[4] Richardson, P., et al., Report of the 1995 World Health Organization/International Society and Federation of Cardiology Task Force on the Definition and Classification of cardiomyopathies. Circulation, 1996. 93(5): pp. 841–2.

[5] Maisch, B. and S. Pankuweit, Standard and etiology-directed evidence-based therapies in myocarditis: state of the art and future perspectives. Heart Fail Rev, 2013. 18(6): pp. 761–95.

[6] Fabre, A. and M.N. Sheppard, Sudden adult death syndrome and other non-ischaemic causes of sudden cardiac death. Heart, 2006. 92(3): pp. 316–20.

[7] Doolan, A., N. Langlois, and C. Semsarian, Causes of sudden cardiac death in young Australians. Med J Aust, 2004. 180(3): pp. 110–2.

[8] Felker, G.M., et al., The spectrum of dilated cardiomyopathy. The Johns Hopkins experience with 1,278 patients. Medicine (Baltimore), 1999. 78(4): pp. 270–83.

[9] Andreoletti, L., et al., Viral causes of human myocarditis. Arch Cardiovasc Dis, 2009. 102(6–7): pp. 559–68.

[10] Kuhl, U., et al., High prevalence of viral genomes and multiple viral infections in the myocardium of adults with "idiopathic" left ventricular dysfunction. Circulation, 2005. 111(7): pp. 887–93.

[11] Kuhl, U., et al., Viral persistence in the myocardium is associated with progressive cardiac dysfunction. Circulation, 2005. 112(13): pp. 1965–70.

[12] Maisch, B., V. Ruppert, and S. Pankuweit, Management of fulminant myocarditis: a diagnosis in search of its etiology but with therapeutic options. Curr Heart Fail Rep, 2014. 11(2): pp. 166–77.

[13] Maisch, B. and S. Pankuweit, Current treatment options in (peri)myocarditis and inflammatory cardiomyopathy. Herz, 2012. 37(6): pp. 644–56.

[14] Klein, R.M., et al., Frequency and quantity of the parvovirus B19 genome in endomyocardial biopsies from patients with suspected myocarditis or idiopathic left ventricular dysfunction. Z Kardiol, 2004. 93(4): pp. 300–9.

[15] Mahrholdt, H., et al., Presentation, patterns of myocardial damage, and clinical course of viral myocarditis. Circulation, 2006. 114(15): pp. 1581–90.

[16] Pankuweit, S. and K. Klingel, Viral myocarditis: from experimental models to molecular diagnosis in patients. Heart Fail Rev, 2013. 18(6): pp. 683–702.

[17] Krueger, G.R. and D.V. Ablashi, Human herpesvirus-6: a short review of its biological behavior. Intervirology, 2003. 46(5): pp. 257–69.

[18] Kuhl, U. and H.P. Schultheiss, Viral myocarditis. Swiss Med Wkly, 2014. 144: p. w14010.

[19] Kandolf, R., et al., Molecular mechanisms and consequences of cardiac viral infections. Pathologe, 2008. 29(Suppl. 2): pp. 112–7.

[20] Bowles, N.E., et al., Detection of viruses in myocardial tissues by polymerase chain reaction. Evidence of adenovirus as a common cause of myocarditis in children and adults. J Am Coll Cardiol, 2003. 42(3): pp. 466–72.

[21] Kyto, V., et al., Cytomegalovirus infection of the heart is common in patients with fatal myocarditis. Clin Infect Dis, 2005. 40(5): pp. 683–8.

[22] Calabrese, F., et al., Overexpression of tumor necrosis factor (TNF)alpha and TNFalpha receptor I in human viral myocarditis: clinicopathologic correlations. Mod Pathol, 2004. 17(9): pp. 1108–18.

[23] Mamas, M.A., D. Fraser, and L. Neyses, Cardiovascular manifestations associated with influenza virus infection. Int J Cardiol, 2008. 130(3): pp. 304–9.

[24] Kuiken, T. and J.K. Taubenberger, Pathology of human influenza revisited. Vaccine, 2008. 26(Suppl. 4): pp. D59–66.

[25] Gdynia, G., et al., Sudden death of an immunocompetent young adult caused by novel (swine origin) influenza A/H1N1-associated myocarditis. Virchows Arch, 2011. 458(3): pp. 371–6.

[26] Sudano, I., et al., Cardiovascular disease in HIV infection. Am Heart J, 2006. 151(6): pp. 1147–55.

[27] Magnani, J.W. and G.W. Dec, Myocarditis: current trends in diagnosis and treatment. Circulation, 2006. 113(6): pp. 876–90.

[28] Barbaro, G., et al., Incidence of dilated cardiomyopathy and detection of HIV in myocardial cells of HIV-positive patients. Italian Group for the Study of Cardiology Patients Suffering from AIDS. N Engl J Med, 1998. 339(16): pp. 1093–9.

[29] Matsumori, A., et al., Myocarditis and heart failure associated with hepatitis C virus infection. J Card Fail, 2006. 12(4): pp. 293–8.

[30] Sanchez, M.J. and N.V. Bergasa, Hepatitis C associated cardiomyopathy: potential pathogenic mechanisms and clinical implications. Med Sci Monit, 2008. 14(5): pp. RA55–63.

[31] Matsumori, A., Role of hepatitis C virus in cardiomyopathies. Ernst Schering Res Found Workshop, 2006. 55: pp. 99–120.

[32] Maze, S.S. and R.J. Adolph, Myocarditis: unresolved issues in diagnosis and treatment. Clin Cardiol, 1990. 13(2): pp. 69–79.

[33] Hufnagel, G., et al., The European Study of Epidemiology and Treatment of Cardiac Inflammatory Diseases (ESETCID). First epidemiological results. Herz, 2000. 25(3): pp. 279–85.

[34] Dec, G.W., Jr., et al., Active myocarditis in the spectrum of acute dilated cardiomyopathies. Clinical features, histologic correlates, and clinical outcome. N Engl J Med, 1985. 312(14): pp. 885–90.

[35] Schultz, J.C., et al., Diagnosis and treatment of viral myocarditis. Mayo Clin Proc, 2009. 84(11): pp. 1001–9.

[36] Wang, K., R.W. Asinger, and H.J. Marriott, ST-segment elevation in conditions other than acute myocardial infarction. N Engl J Med, 2003. 349(22): pp. 2128–35.

[37] Dennert, R., H.J. Crijns, and S. Heymans, Acute viral myocarditis. Eur Heart J, 2008. 29(17): pp. 2073–82.

[38] Liu, P.P. and A.T. Yan, Cardiovascular magnetic resonance for the diagnosis of acute myocarditis: prospects for detecting myocardial inflammation. J Am Coll Cardiol, 2005. 45(11): pp. 1823–5.

[39] Blauwet, L.A. and L.T. Cooper, Myocarditis. Prog Cardiovasc Dis, 2010. 52(4): pp. 274–88.

[40] Felker, G.M., et al., Echocardiographic findings in fulminant and acute myocarditis. J Am Coll Cardiol, 2000. 36(1): pp. 227–32.

[41] Petryka, J., et al., Cardiovascular magnetic resonance in the diagnosis of myocarditis. Kardiol Pol, 2010. 68(7): pp. 824–9.

[42] Hunold, P., et al., Myocardial late enhancement in contrast-enhanced cardiac MRI: distinction between infarction scar and non-infarction-related disease. Am J Roentgenol, 2005. 184(5): pp. 1420–6.

[43] Friedrich, M.G., et al., Cardiovascular magnetic resonance in myocarditis: A JACC White Paper. J Am Coll Cardiol, 2009. 53(17): pp. 1475–87.

[44] Abdel-Aty, H., et al., Delayed enhancement and T2-weighted cardiovascular magnetic resonance imaging differentiate acute from chronic myocardial infarction. Circulation, 2004. 109(20): pp. 2411–6.

[45] Aletras, A.H., et al., Retrospective determination of the area at risk for reperfused acute myocardial infarction with T2-weighted cardiac magnetic resonance imaging: histopathological and displacement encoding with stimulated echoes (DENSE) functional validations. Circulation, 2006. 113(15): pp. 1865–70.

[46] Cooper, L.T., et al., The role of endomyocardial biopsy in the management of cardiovascular disease: a scientific statement from the American Heart Association, the American College of Cardiology, and the European Society of Cardiology. Endorsed by the Heart Failure Society of America and the Heart Failure Association of the European Society of Cardiology. J Am Coll Cardiol, 2007. 50(19): pp. 1914–31.

[47] Yilmaz, A., et al., Comparative evaluation of left and right ventricular endomyocardial biopsy: differences in complication rate and diagnostic performance. Circulation, 2010. 122(9): pp. 900–9.

[48] Aretz, H.T., Myocarditis: the Dallas criteria. Hum Pathol, 1987. 18(6): pp. 619–24.

[49] Kuhl, U., et al., Interferon-Beta improves survival in enterovirus-associated cardiomyopathy. J Am Coll Cardiol, 2012. 60(14): pp. 1295–6.

[50] Schultheiss, H.P., U. Kuhl, and L.T. Cooper, The management of myocarditis. Eur Heart J, 2011. 32(21): pp. 2616–25.

[51] Dickstein, K., et al., ESC Guidelines for the diagnosis and treatment of acute and chronic heart failure 2008: the Task Force for the Diagnosis and Treatment of Acute and Chronic Heart Failure 2008 of the European Society of Cardiology. Developed in collaboration with the Heart Failure Association of the ESC (HFA) and endorsed by the European Society of Intensive Care Medicine (ESICM). Eur Heart J, 2008. 29(19): pp. 2388–442.

[52] Hunt, S.A., et al., 2009 Focused update incorporated into the ACC/AHA 2005 Guidelines for the Diagnosis and Management of Heart Failure in Adults. A Report of the American College of Cardiology Foundation/American Heart Association Task Force on Practice Guidelines Developed in Collaboration With the International Society for Heart and Lung Transplantation. J Am Coll Cardiol, 2009. 53(15): pp. e1–e90.

[53] Rezkalla, S.H., S. Raikar, and R.A. Kloner, Treatment of viral myocarditis with focus on captopril. Am J Cardiol, 1996. 77(8): pp. 634–7.

[54] Saegusa, S., et al., Oral administration of candesartan improves the survival of mice with viral myocarditis through modification of cardiac adiponectin expression. Cardiovasc Drugs Ther, 2007. 21(3): pp. 155–60.

[55] Kuhl, U., et al., Interferon-beta treatment eliminates cardiotropic viruses and improves left ventricular function in patients with myocardial persistence of viral genomes and left ventricular dysfunction. Circulation, 2003. 107(22): pp. 2793–8.

[56] Schmidt-Lucke, C., et al., Interferon beta modulates endothelial damage in patients with cardiac persistence of human parvovirus b19 infection. J Infect Dis, 2010. 201(6): pp. 936–45.

[57] Kuhl, U., et al., Chromosomally integrated human herpesvirus 6 in heart failure: prevalence and treatment. Eur J Heart Fail, 2015. 17(1): pp. 9–19.

[58] Juhl, U., B.E. Strauer, and H.P. Schultheiss, Methylprednisolone in chronic myocarditis. Postgrad Med J, 1994. 70(Suppl. 1): pp. S35–42.

[59] Frustaci, A., et al., Immunosuppressive therapy for active lymphocytic myocarditis: virological and immunologic profile of responders versus nonresponders. Circulation, 2003. 107(6): pp. 857–63.

[60] Frustaci, A., M.A. Russo, and C. Chimenti, Randomized study on the efficacy of immunosuppressive therapy in patients with virus-negative inflammatory cardiomyopathy: the TIMIC study. Eur Heart J, 2009. 30(16): pp. 1995–2002.

[61] Drucker, N.A., et al., Gamma-globulin treatment of acute myocarditis in the pediatric population. Circulation, 1994. 89(1): pp. 252–7.

[62] McNamara, D.M., et al., Controlled trial of intravenous immune globulin in recent-onset dilated cardiomyopathy. Circulation, 2001. 103(18): pp. 2254–9.

[63] Klugman, D., et al., Pediatric patients hospitalized with myocarditis: a multi-institutional analysis. Pediatr Cardiol, 2010. 31(2): pp. 222–8.

[64] Felix, S.B., et al., Removal of cardiodepressant antibodies in dilated cardiomyopathy by immunoadsorption. J Am Coll Cardiol, 2002. 39(4): pp. 646–52.

[65] Felix, S.B., et al., Hemodynamic effects of immunoadsorption and subsequent immunoglobulin substitution in dilated cardiomyopathy: three-month results from a randomized study. J Am Coll Cardiol, 2000. 35(6): pp. 1590–8.

[66] Doesch, A.O., et al., Effects of protein A immunoadsorption in patients with advanced chronic dilated cardiomyopathy. J Clin Apher, 2009. 24(4): pp. 141–9.

[67] Wasi, F. and J. Shuter, Primary bacterial infection of the myocardium. Front Biosci, 2003. 8: pp. s228–31.

[68] Taldir, G., et al., Acute right-sided heart failure caused by *Neisseria meningitidis*. J Clin Microbiol, 2013. 51(1): pp. 363–5.

[69] Childs, L. and S. Cupta, *Salmonella enteritidis* induced myocarditis in a 16-year-old girl. BMJ Case Rep, 2012. Nov 27. doi: 10.1136/bcr-2012-007628.

[70] Sagar, S., P.P. Liu, and L.T. Cooper, Jr., Myocarditis. Lancet, 2012. 379(9817): pp. 738–47.

[71] Haddad, F., et al., Active bacterial myocarditis: a case report and review of the literature. J Heart Lung Transplant, 2007. 26(7): pp. 745–9.

[72] Michira, B.N., F.O. Alkizim, and D.M. Matheka, Patterns and clinical manifestations of tuberculous myocarditis: a systematic review of cases. Pan Afr Med J, 2015. 21: p. 118.

[73] Dutly, F. and M. Altwegg, Whipple's disease and *Tropheryma whippelii*. Clin Microbiol Rev, 2001. 14(3): pp. 561–83.

[74] de Takats, P.G., et al., Symptomatic cardiomyopathy as a presentation in Whipple's disease. Postgrad Med J, 1995. 71(834): pp. 236–9.

[75] Palecek, T., et al., Presence of *Borrelia burgdorferi* in endomyocardial biopsies in patients with new-onset unexplained dilated cardiomyopathy. Med Microbiol Immunol, 2010. 199(2): pp. 139–43.

[76] Lelovas, P., et al., Cardiac implications of Lyme disease, diagnosis and therapeutic approach. Int J Cardiol, 2008. 129(1): pp. 15–21.

[77] Cox, J. and M. Krajden, Cardiovascular manifestations of Lyme disease. Am Heart J, 1991. 122(5): pp. 1449–55.

[78] Bateman, H. and L. Sigal, Update on Lyme Carditis. Curr Infect Dis Rep, 2000. 2(4): pp. 299–301.

[79] Kuchynka, P., et al., Recent-onset dilated cardiomyopathy associated with *Borrelia burgdorferi* infection. Herz, 2015. 40(6): pp. 892–7.

[80] Hofman, P., et al., Fungal myocarditis in acquired immunodeficiency syndrome. Arch Mal Coeur Vaiss, 1992. 85(2): pp. 203–8.

[81] Xie, L., et al., Cardiac aspergillosis in patients with acquired immunodeficiency syndrome: a case report and review of the literature. Arch Pathol Lab Med, 2005. 129(4): pp. 511–5.

[82] Baker, R.D. and E.W. Brian, Blastomycosis of the heart: Report of two cases. Am J Pathol, 1937. 13(1): pp. 139–147.

[83] Smeekens, S.P., et al., Genetic susceptibility to Candida infections. EMBO Mol Med, 2013. 5(6): pp. 805–13.

[84] Franklin, W.G., A.B. Simon, and T.M. Sodeman, *Candida* myocarditis without valvulitis. Am J Cardiol, 1976. 38(7): pp. 924–8.

[85] Aiello, V.D. and F.P. de Campos, Chronic Chagas cardiomyopathy. Autops Case Rep, 2015. 5(3): pp. 7–9.

[86] Biolo, A., A.L. Ribeiro, and N. Clausell, Chagas cardiomyopathy—where do we stand after a hundred years? Prog Cardiovasc Dis, 2010. 52(4): pp. 300–16.

[87] Rassi, A., Jr., A. Rassi, and W.C. Little, Chagas heart disease. Clin Cardiol, 2000. 23(12): pp. 883–9.

[88] Hidron, A., et al., Cardiac involvement with parasitic infections. Clin Microbiol Rev, 2010. 23(2): pp. 324–49.

[89] Birnie, D.H., et al., Cardiac manifestations of sarcoidosis: diagnosis and management. Eur Heart J, 2016 Jul 28. pii: ehw328.

[90] Kusano, K.F. and K. Satomi, Diagnosis and treatment of cardiac sarcoidosis. Heart, 2016. 102(3): pp. 184–90.

[91] Correia, A.S., et al., Churg-Strauss syndrome presenting with eosinophilic myocarditis: a diagnostic challenge. Rev Port Cardiol, 2013. 32(9): pp. 707–11.

[92] Sinico, R.A., et al., Prevalence and clinical significance of antineutrophil cytoplasmic antibodies in Churg-Strauss syndrome. Arthritis Rheum, 2005. 52(9): pp. 2926–35.

[93] Guillevin, L., et al., Churg-Strauss syndrome. Clinical study and long-term follow-up of 96 patients. Medicine (Baltimore), 1999. 78(1): pp. 26–37.

[94] Knockaert, D.C., Cardiac involvement in systemic inflammatory diseases. Eur Heart J, 2007. 28(15): p. 1797–804.

[95] Wassmuth, R., et al., Cardiovascular magnetic resonance imaging detects cardiac involvement in Churg-Strauss syndrome. J Card Fail, 2008. 14(10): pp. 856–60.

[96] Neumann, T., et al., Cardiac involvement in Churg-Strauss syndrome: impact of endomyocarditis. Medicine (Baltimore), 2009. 88(4): pp. 236–43.

[97] Szczeklik, W., et al., Multimodality assessment of cardiac involvement in Churg-Strauss syndrome patients in clinical remission. Circ J, 2011. 75(3): pp. 649–55.

[98] Chen, M.X., et al., Eosinophilic myocarditis due to Churg-Strauss syndrome mimicking reversible dilated cardiomyopathy. Heart Lung, 2014. 43(1): pp. 45–7.

[99] Miner, J.J. and A.H. Kim, Cardiac manifestations of systemic lupus erythematosus. Rheum Dis Clin North Am, 2014. 40(1): pp. 51–60.

[100] Zhang, L., et al., Lupus Myocarditis: a case-control study from China. Chin Med J (Engl), 2015. 128(19): pp. 2588–94.

[101] Wijetunga, M. and S. Rockson, Myocarditis in systemic lupus erythematosus. Am J Med, 2002. 113(5): pp. 419–23.

[102] Doria, A., et al., Cardiac involvement in systemic lupus erythematosus. Lupus, 2005. 14(9): pp. 683–6.

[103] Tincani, A., et al., Heart involvement in systemic lupus erythematosus, anti-phospholipid syndrome and neonatal lupus. Rheumatology (Oxford), 2006. 45(Suppl. 4): pp. iv8–13.

Permissions

All chapters in this book were first published in CTT, by InTech Open; hereby published with permission under the Creative Commons Attribution License or equivalent. Every chapter published in this book has been scrutinized by our experts. Their significance has been extensively debated. The topics covered herein carry significant findings which will fuel the growth of the discipline. They may even be implemented as practical applications or may be referred to as a beginning point for another development.

The contributors of this book come from diverse backgrounds, making this book a truly international effort. This book will bring forth new frontiers with its revolutionizing research information and detailed analysis of the nascent developments around the world.

We would like to thank all the contributing authors for lending their expertise to make the book truly unique. They have played a crucial role in the development of this book. Without their invaluable contributions this book wouldn't have been possible. They have made vital efforts to compile up to date information on the varied aspects of this subject to make this book a valuable addition to the collection of many professionals and students.

This book was conceptualized with the vision of imparting up-to-date information and advanced data in this field. To ensure the same, a matchless editorial board was set up. Every individual on the board went through rigorous rounds of assessment to prove their worth. After which they invested a large part of their time researching and compiling the most relevant data for our readers.

The editorial board has been involved in producing this book since its inception. They have spent rigorous hours researching and exploring the diverse topics which have resulted in the successful publishing of this book. They have passed on their knowledge of decades through this book. To expedite this challenging task, the publisher supported the team at every step. A small team of assistant editors was also appointed to further simplify the editing procedure and attain best results for the readers.

Apart from the editorial board, the designing team has also invested a significant amount of their time in understanding the subject and creating the most relevant covers. They scrutinized every image to scout for the most suitable representation of the subject and create an appropriate cover for the book.

The publishing team has been an ardent support to the editorial, designing and production team. Their endless efforts to recruit the best for this project, has resulted in the accomplishment of this book. They are a veteran in the field of academics and their pool of knowledge is as vast as their experience in printing. Their expertise and guidance has proved useful at every step. Their uncompromising quality standards have made this book an exceptional effort. Their encouragement from time to time has been an inspiration for everyone.

The publisher and the editorial board hope that this book will prove to be a valuable piece of knowledge for researchers, students, practitioners and scholars across the globe.

List of Contributors

Gisèle Bonne and Antoine Muchir
Center of Research in Myology, Paris, France

Hakan Altay and Seckin Pehlivanoglu
Cardiology Department, Faculty of Medicine, Baskent University, Istanbul Hospital, Turkey

Tatsuya Ishikawa
Research Institute for Brain and Blood Vessels-AKITA, Akita, Japan

Tatsushi Mutoh
Research Institute for Brain and Blood Vessels-AKITA, Akita, Japan
Institute of Development, Aging and Cancer, Tohoku University, Sendai, Japan

Tomoko Mutoh and Yasuyuki Taki
Institute of Development, Aging and Cancer, Tohoku University, Sendai, Japan

Shuai Wang and Daoquan Peng
Department of Cardiovascular Medicine, The Second Xiangya Hospital of Central South University, Changsha, Hunan, China

Peter Magnusson
Cardiology Research Unit, Department of Medicine, Karolinska Institute, Karolinska University Hospital, Solna, Stockholm, Sweden
Centre for Research and Development, Uppsala University/Region Gävleborg, Gävle, Sweden

Christian R. Hamilton-Craig
Centre for Advanced Imaging, University of Queensland, Brisbane, Australia
Department of Radiology, University of Washington, Seattle, WA, USA

Graham J. Galloway
Centre for Advanced Imaging, University of Queensland, Brisbane, Australia
Translational Research Institute, Brisbane, Australia

Mark W. Strudwick
Medical Imaging and Radiation Science, Monash University, Australia

Özge Altaş Yerlikhan and Hakan Hançer
Department of Cardiac Transplantation and Ventricular Assist Device, Kartal Koşuyolu YIEA Hospital, Istanbul, Turkey

Kaan Kırali
Department of Cardiac Transplantation and Ventricular Assist Device, Kartal Koşuyolu YIEA Hospital, Istanbul, Turkey
Department of Cardiovascular Surgery, Faculty of Medicine, Sakarya University, Sakarya, Turkey

Coskun Celtik and Nelgin Gerenli
Pediatric Gastroenterology, Health Sciences University, Istanbul Umraniye Training and Research Hospital, Istanbul, Turkey

Halil Haldun Emiroglu
Pediatric Gastroenterology, Selcuk University, Faculty of Medicine, Konya, Turkey

Nimet Cındık
Pediatric Cardiology, Health Sciences University, Istanbul Umraniye Training and Research Hospital, Istanbul, Turkey

Agnieszka Pawlak and Robert Julian Gil
Mossakowski Medical Research Centre, Polish Academy of Sciences, Warsaw, Poland
Central Clinical Hospital of the Ministry of Interior, Department of Invasive Cardiology, Warsaw, Poland

Index